AF376244

The Decubitus Ulcer in Clinical Practice

Springer
Berlin
Heidelberg
New York
Barcelona
Budapest
Hong Kong
London
Milan
Paris
Santa Clara
Singapore
Tokyo

L.C. Parish   J.A. Witkowski
J.T. Crissey   (Eds.)

The Decubitus Ulcer
in Clinical Practice

With 76 Figures and 24 Tables

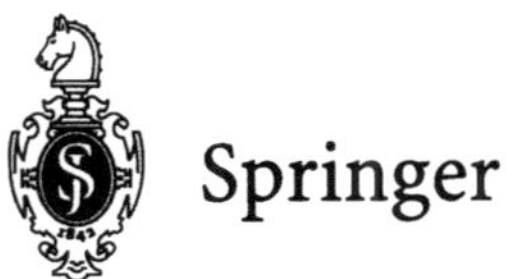

Springer

Lawrence Charles Parish, M.D.
1819 JF Kennedy Boulevard
Philadelphia, PA 19103, USA

Joseph A. Witkowski, M.D.
3501 Ryan Avenue
Philadelphia, PA 19136, USA

John Thorne Crissey, M.D.
608 Sierra Madre Boulevard
San Marino, CA 91108, USA

ISBN- 13: 978-3-642-64436-8   e-ISBN- 13: 978-3-642-60509-3
DOI: 10.1007/978-3-642-60509-3

Library of Congress Cataloging-in-Publication Data. The decubitus ulcer in clinical practice/ L.C. Parish, J.A. Witkowski, J.T. Crissey (eds.). p. cm. Includes bibliographical references and index. 1. Bedsores – Treatment. I. Parish, Lawrence Charles. II. Witkowski, Joseph A. III. Crissey, John Thorne, 1924- [DNLM: 1. Decubitus Ulcer. WR 598 D2981 1997] RL675.D43 1997 616.5′45–DC20 DNLM/DLC for Library of Congress 96-31691

Cover design: Design & Production GmbH, Heidelberg

Typesetting: Scientific Publishing Services (P) Ltd, Madras

SPIN: 10519700   23/3134/SPS – 5 4 3 2 1 0 – Printed on acid-free paper

Preface

The bedsore problem is ancient and has never been far removed from the daily concerns of those whose business it is to deal with chronic disease. It is only in the last 2 decades, however, that attention has been devoted to this entity that is more commensurate with its significance. The advent of contemporary decubitus thought can be traced to the clinical trials on the use of dextranomer isomer for wound healing in the 1970s [1] and the introduction of technologically advanced occlusive dressings in the 1980s [2].

In 1983 we summarized the knowledge of pressure sores as it existed at that time and presented it in a text entitled *The Decubitus Ulcer* [3]. In the ensuing years, new concepts have evolved and views on wound healing have radically changed [4]. Older ideas on etiology have been challenged [5], and once standard nomenclature has been opened to debate [6]. To deal with these changes the National Pressure Ulcer Advisory Panel (NPUAP) was organized, and one of us (JAW) has served as president.

Although much remains to be learned about decubitus ulcers, progress has been made. We can now describe the morphologic changes associated with this dermatologic problem with greater accuracy and in terms more standardized than ever before. Similarly, worldwide agreement on the staging parameters of this entity is within reach and will place statistical comparisons in matters of incidence and therapeutic approach on a firmer basis. Progress has also been made in understanding the pathogenesis of decubitus ulcers and wound healing in general. These observations, along with therapeutic innovations empirically derived but nonetheless valuable, have improved the success rate in dealing with this difficult problem. We feel, therefore, that the time has come to review the new and developing material and in combining it with the basics from our previous text make it readily available to health care providers on the firing line.

The team approach is essential to success in the management of decubitus ulcers. It is the duty of the nurse to assess and intervene and the physician to diagnose and treat. The assistance of laboratory personnel and other members of the health care team is also required, and of utmost importance is the development and maintenance of lines of communication with the patient and the patient's family. Only in this way can we avoid the unhappy scenario – family blaming nurse, nurse blaming physician – played out now on a regular basis in hospitals and nursing care facilities throughout the world.

We are most grateful to our contributors and to our publisher, Springer-Verlag, and particularly to Dr. Wolfram Wiegers.

Philadelphia and Los Angeles   Lawrence Charles Parish
October 1996   Joseph A. Witkowski
                                        John Thorne Crissey

1. Parish LC, Collins E (1979) Decubitus ulcers: a comparative study. Cutis 23:106–110
2. Eaglstein WH (1984) Effect of occlusive dressings on wound healing. Clin Dermatol 2(3):107–111
3. Parish LC, Witkowski JA, Crissey JT (1983) The decubitus ulcer. Masson, New York, pp 1–134
4. Witkowski JA, Parish LC (1993) Skin failure and the pressure ulcer. Decubitus 6(5):4
5. Yarkony GM (1994) Pressure ulcers: a review. Arch Phys Med Rehabil 75:908–917
6. Parish LC, Witkowski JA, Millikan LE (1988) Cutaneous torsion stress alias the decubitus ulcer: a felony. Int J Dermatol 27:375–376

Contents

Therapy – Specific

Additional Concepts

Contributors

Barbara M. Bates-Jensen
Assistant Professor of Clinical Nursing, University of Southern
California, Department of Nursing, 1540 East Alcazar Street,
Los Angeles, CA 90033, USA

Laura L. Bolton, Ph.D.
Adjunct Associate Professor of Surgery, University of Medicine
and Dentistry of New Jersey, Piscataway, New Jersey, and Worldwide
Director of Scientific Affairs, ConvaTec, Skillman, New Jersey.
P.O. Box 5254, Princeton, NJ 08453, USA

Edward C. Bradley, S.J., M.D.
Clinical Associate Professor of Medicine, Jefferson Medical College
of Thomas Jefferson University, Philadelphia, Pennsylvania.
1000 Walnut Street, #502, Philadelphia, PA 19107, USA

Louis P. Bucky, M.D.
Assistant Professor of Surgery, University of Pennsylvania School
of Medicine, Philadelphia, Pennsylvania. 3400 Spruce Street,
Philadelphia, PA 19104, USA

Ronni Chernoff, Ph.D., R.D.
Professor of Nutrition and Dietetics, College of Heralth Related
Professions, University of Arkansas for Medical Sciences,
Little Rock, Arkansas. GRECC(182), VA Medical Center, 4300 West
7th Street, Little Rock, AR 72205, USA

George W. Cherry, D.Phil.
Senior Clinical Scientist, Oxford Wound Healing Institute,
Department of Dermatology, Churchill Hospital, Headington,
Oxford, OX3 7LJ, England

Helen M. Cioschi, M.S.N., C.R.N.P.
Vice President/Clinical Operations, Magee Rehabilitation,
Philadelphia, Pennsylvania. Six Franklin Plaza, Philadelphia,
PA 19102, USA

Joan R. Coates, D.V.M., M.S.
Assistant Professor of Neurology and Neurosurgery, University
of Georgia College of Veterinary Medicine, Athens, GA 30602,
USA

John Thorne Crissey, M.D.
Clinical Professor of Medicine (Dermatology), University
of Southern California School of Medicine, Los Angeles, California.
608 Sierra Madre Boulevard, San Marino, CA 91108, USA

J Carl Craft, M.D.
Head, Macrolide Venture, Abbott Laboratories, Abbott Park,
Illinois. 100 Abbott Park Road, Abbott Park, IL 60064, USA

Nicholas Cullum, Ph.D., R.G.N.
Research Fellow, Centre for Health Economics, University of York,
York, Y01 5DD, England

Jannes J.E. van Everdingen, M.D., Ph.D.
Secretary, Medical Scientific Council, National Organization
for Quality Assurance in Hospitals, Utretcht, The Netherlands

Jeen R.E. Haalboom, M.D., Ph.D.
Associate Professor of Internal Medicine, University of Utrecht,
Utrecht, The Netherlands. Chairman, Dutch Pressure Sore
Prevention and Treatment Consensus Meeting. University Hospital
Utrecht, The Netherlands. Utrecht, The Netherlands

R. Reid Hanson Jr., D.V.M.
Professor of Large Animal Surgery, Auburn University College
of Veterinary Medicine, Auburn University, Alabama. Scott-Ritchey
Research Center, Auburn University, AL 36840, USA

Beth Jacobs, R.N.
Wound Care Specialist, Magee Rehabilitation, Philadelphia,
Pennsylvania. Six Franklin Plaza, Philadelphia, PA 19102,
USA

Donato LaRossa, M.D.
Professor of Surgery, University of Pennsylvania School of Medicine,
Philadelphia, Pennsylvania. 3400 Spruce Street, Philadelphia,
PA 19104, USA

Susan A. Larson, J.D.
Partner of Wright, Young & McGilvery, Blue Bell, Pennsylvania.
1400 Union Meeting Road, Blue Bell, PA 19422, USA

Charles Parish, Ph.D.
Professor of Linguistics (Emeritus), University of Southern Illionois
at Carbondale, Carbondale, Illinois. 600 West Oak Street,
Carbondale, IL 62901, USA

Lawrence Charles Parish, M.D.
Clinical Professor of Dermatology and Cutaneous Biology
and Director of the Jefferson Center for International Dermatology,
Jefferson Medical College of Thomas Jefferson University,
Philadelphia, Pennsylvania, Visiting Professor of Dermatology,
Yonsei University College of Medicine, Seoul, Korea, and Visiting
Professor of Dermatology and Venereology, Zagazig University,
Zagazig, Egypt. 1819 J.F. Kennedy Boulevard, #465, Philadelphia,
PA 19103, USA

Lia van Rijswijk, R.N., E.T.
Nurse Consultant, Newtown, Pennsylvania. P.O. Box 5254,
Princeton, NJ 08453, USA

Terence J. Ryan, D.M., F.R.C.P.
Professor of Dermatology, Oxford University, Oxford, England,
Visiting Professor of Dermatology and Cutaneous Biology, Jefferson
Medical College of Thomas Jefferson University, Philadelphia,
Pennsylvania. Churchill Hospital, Headington, Oxford, OX3 7LJ,
England

William E. Staas Jr., M.D.
Professor of Rehabilitation Medicine, Jefferson Medical College
of Thomas Jefferson University and President/Medical Director,
Magee Rehabilitation, Philadelphia, Pennsylvania. Six Franklin
Plaza, Philadelphia, PA 19102, USA

Thomas P. Stewart, Ph.D.
Adjunct Assistant Professor, State University of New York. Vice-
President – Clinical Affairs, Gaymar Industries, Inc., Orchard Park,
New York. 10 Centre Drive, Orchard Park, NY 14127, USA

Steven F. Swaim, D.V.M., M.S.
Professor of Small Animal Surgery, Auburn University College
of Veterinary Medicine, Auburn University, Alabama. Scott-Ritchey
Research Center, Auburn University, AL 36840, USA

Joseph A. Witkowski, M.D.
Clinical Professor of Dermatology, University of Pennsylvania
School of Medicine, and Professor of Dermatology, Pennsylvania
College of Podiatric Medicine, Philadelphia, Pennsylvania. 3501
Ryan Avenue, Philadelphia, PA 19136, USA

George L. Young, J.D.
Partner of Wright, Young & McGilvery, Blue Bell, Pennsylvania.
1400 Union Meeting Road, Blue Bell, PA 19422, USA

Background

1 Bedsores over the Centuries

Decubitus ulcers, pressure sores, or bedsores (take your choice) have been recognized since antiquity. From the sixteenth through the eighteenth century they were considered occasionally and usually indirectly in treatises on gangrene [1]. The subject, however, was evidently so much a matter of common knowledge in possession of everyone concerned at the time with patient care that discussions in print were seldom considered necessary, and certainly no great literature devoted to it existed prior to 1800.

Early Advances

Effective steps in the prevention and treatment of the lesions were already being taken in the 1st decade of the nineteenth century. As early as 1806, for example, J.C. Aronssen of Berlin took the trouble to point out the importance of the bed itself in patient care and in his report furnished plans for the construction of a new and improved invalid chair of his own invention [2]. In 1815, William Heberden Jr. – another physician's son of genuine talent who suffered from having a too-famous father – published the description of a bed frame (Fig. 1), designed to reduce both pressure ischemia and the soiling of sheets and skin from incontinence [3]. His introductory paragraph demonstrates that these two key factors in the production of decubitus ulcers were well appreciated even at this early date:

As the ultimate object of the medical art is the removal or alleviation of those evils to which the human body is exposed, I make no scruple of laying before the College of Physicians some account of a contrivance from which I have lately experienced great benefit; though strictly speaking the calamity be no disease and the remedy no medicine. There is no one in the habit of attending the sick but must have had reason to deplore the wretched condition of those who, being bedridden through accident or infirmity, have contracted sores of a very painful and dangerous kind by long pressure, especially if the patient lie in the wet and filth of his own body which he is unable to restrain.

Heberden described the use of the frame in the treatment of severe decubitus ulcers that had developed in an 80-year-old woman who suffered from hemiplegia, and he reported these satisfying results:

The mischief seemed to be rapidly increasing under the unfavorable circumstances of a helpless old age when the contrivance I am going to described was adopted; by which the sick chamber was immediately rendered sweet and wholesome, the ulceration ceased, and in less

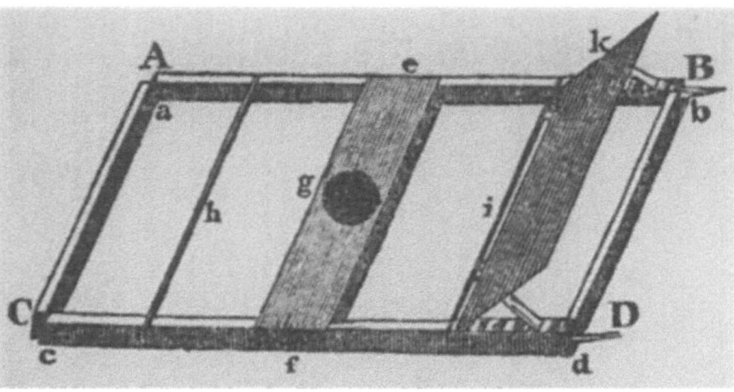

Fig. 1. Bedframe recommended in 1815 by William Heberden Jr. for the treatment and prevention of pressure sores. The mattress that covered it contained a large waterproofed opening designed to take pressure off the sacrum and permit passage of urine and feces into the hole (*g*); *e–f* is a drawer containing a bedpan and made to pull out from either side; *k* is a "sort of desk for the convenience of raising the patient's head"

than six weeks the sore places were perfectly healed and covered again with a sound skin, though the disabilities of all kinds which had originally occasioned the malady continued without any abatement for more than three months, for so long was the life protracted.

Other devices followed, slings and the like [4], and in 1873 the water bed made its appearance in the medical literature in these remarks on decubitus management by Sir James Paget [5]:

First of all look to the bed. Good bed-making is an indispensable thing in the prevention of bed sores. Several beds have been made especially for this purpose, of which the best is Dr. Arnott's. It consists of a chest full of water; on top of this is a waterproof sheet and over this an ordinary sheet on which the patient is laid. Here the patient is absolutely floating on water. The waterproof sheet is not drawn tight but adapts itself to every part of the patient. A patient might lie on this for years and never have a bedsore.

Specialty beds proliferated, and a review of the shapes and forms they assumed as shown in the medical trade catalogues of the nineteenth and early twentieth centuries confirms once again the ingenuity of which the human mind is capable when financial rewards are anticipated [6].

Pioneer Investigations

The clinical conclusions on the importance of pressure and soiling received experimental confirmation in 1852 with the publication of a remarkable set of observations carried out by the Franco-American genius, Charles Edward Brown-Sequard [7]. Consider this impressive extract from his communication on the subject (and ignore the peculiar syntax):

My opinion is well proved by the following experiments:
1st. I have put, three or four times a day for many days, a certain quantity of urine on the posterior part of the neck, in the neighborhood of the scapula, upon guinea-pigs. Before a week elapsed, the skin at the place acted on by the urine had lost its hair and epidermis. After a week more there was an ulceration of the skin, and 10 or 12 days later the skin was

destroyed, and there was an ulcer with a very bad aspect. This fact proves how powerful is the action of urine on the skin.

2nd. On guinea-pigs upon which the spinal cord was cut in the dorsal region, and on pigeons upon which the spinal cord was destroyed from the fifth costal vertebra to its termination, I found that no ulceration appeared when I took care to prevent any part of their bodies from being in a continued state of compression, and of washing them many times a day to remove the urine and faeces.

3rd. In cases where an ulceration had been produced, I have succeeded in curing it by washing and preventing compression.

4th. I have found that in animals having the spinal cord cut across, every kind of wounds and burns were cured as quickly as in healthy animals.

Therefore the ulcerations which occur in cases of paraplegia do not exist directly in consequence of the palsy; they can be avoided, and in many cases they can be cured.

The orderly march of progress, both clinical and experimental, evident in the foregoing observations came to an abrupt halt, however, with the misinterpretation of clinical facts on the part of the celebrated French neurologist, Jean Martin Charcot. In 1868, the Maître of the Salpêtrière published a persuasive and much-admired report [8] on the appearance of decubitus ulcers immediately after cord injuries in which he sponsored the proposition that the development of such lesions is tied directly to trophic disturbances, to impairments in tissue nutrition that result from interruption of the nerve supply, and is therefore inevitable. *"Troubles de la nutrition fort graves,"* Charcot called them and added:

In such cases, ulcerations and even areas of deep necrosis develop in the sacral region, the heels, and elsewhere, no more than a few days after the accident, so that the mechanical influence of pressure can be considered in these instances no more than a contributing factor.

The result of this unfortunate trophic talk was an era of therapeutic nihilism – unconscionable neglect might be a better term – in which the occurrence of decubitus ulcers was accepted in many quarters as a neurologic fact of life. The hopelessness and inevitability of decubitus and the suffering associated with it even became at times evidence in support of the euthanasia movements that have waxed and waned over the past 120 years [9]. A number of the leading medical contemporaries of Charcot, Sir James Paget for example, knew better and objected [10], but trophic fatalism prevailed until the 1914 explosion in Europe. In a landmark paper [11] delivered before the Academy of Medicine in Paris on May 18, 1915 (with the German forces scarcely 50 miles away and Foch at that very moment launching another futile attack before Arras and Vimy that would cost the French army an additional 100 00 casualties), Pierre Marie and Gustav Roussy urgently pressed the case for something better. Despite the sober and carefully chosen language in which their report was written, the text succeeds even now in summoning the horrors of the trench warfare that characterized that bloody conflict and generated cord injuries in unprecedented numbers.

The alleviation of pressure and the prevention of infection were the principle features in the Marie and Roussy program. The benefits to be expected in cord cases using the new approach were spelled out carefully in the report, and over the next 4 years the physicians, and above all the dedicated cadres of skilled nurses who toiled on behalf of the military, confirmed the judgement of the two men and provided convincing evidence that the dogmatic nihilism of the Charcot school was unwarranted. But the trophic concept died hard. As late as 1964, experiments were still being designed and carried out to settle the question once and for all [12].

In the nineteenth and early twentieth centuries, the importance of supportive therapy in the management of decubitus was stressed to a greater or lesser extent in most publications dealing with the subject. This excerpt from the 1882 *System of Surgery* of Samuel Gross [13] is typical of the attitudes of the period:

The constitutional treatment of bedsores must be conducted according to the general rules followed in typhoid states of the system, from whatever cause proceeding. Nutritious food, wine, brandy, milk punch, quinine, iron, and anodynes, are the means chiefly to be relied upon for upholding the flagging powers of nature. This treatment can hardly be commenced too soon whenever there is any tendency to the formation of bedsores, for the very fact that such a disposition exists is sufficient reason for redoubling our efforts to support the patient's system.

The discovery of the vitamins was followed inevitably by their recommendation as adjuncts to standard bedsore management [14], but the first attempt to test the benefits of improved nutrition in decubitus patients on a more scientific basis appears to be the 1943 study of John H. Mulholland and his coworkers in New York [15]. Their work on dietary protein supplements furnished convincing evidence that a shift from negative to positive nitrogen balance accelerated the healing process.

Surgical Approaches

Considering the way things actually developed in the future, surgical approaches received surprisingly little attention in the nineteenth century and in the earlier decades of the twentieth. As late as 1939, for example, the noted surgeon Zachary Cope [16] saw nothing wrong with ending a dissertation on the management of decubitus ulcers with this remark: "When there is a large slough it may be advisable to cut it away, but that is about as much surgical intervention as is ever required". Signs of things to come had already appeared a year before those words were written, in the pioneering work of John Staige Davis of Baltimore [17], who demonstrated in 1938 the feasibility of revising scars and shifting skin and fat around in decubitus patients.

But again it was war that provided the major stimulus for change. The combination of large numbers of cord cases among the casualties of World War II and the added dimension of safety provided by the availability of penicillin and the other antibiotics encouraged surgical experiment. Throughout the 1940s, a variety of operative approaches were put forward, ranging from simple excision and suture of the ulcers to Z-plasty and rotation flaps, alone or in association with grafts of various types. In the decades that followed, the turning of larger flaps that included muscle, and the excision of bony prominences at pressure points came into their own as acceptable procedures [17].

Also belonging to this era was the introduction in 1958 of the concept of shearing force as a factor in the production of pressure sores [18]. The originator of the idea, Samuel Reichel (then of Baltimore), was concerned in his initial report solely with the effect of bed elevation on tissue overlying the sacrum, but the concept has been broadened profitably to include all those situations in which detrimental forces act parallel to the surface of the skin. Those developments that have taken place since belong to the arena of the present and are, of course, considered in the chapters that follow.

The Future

We harbor no illusions concerning the discovery of wholly satisfactory means of dealing with decubitus ulcers until answers can be found to the neurologic, orthopedic, and vascular problems that commonly precede them. Nevertheless, the medical, surgical, and mechanical approaches that have emerged from the historical dialectics described above have provided relief and hope for many sufferers even when the disasters that put them in jeopardy in the first place have continued unabated. "The freedom from pain and misery of an extensive sore and mortification are at least blessings of no trifling value," our earlier witness Dr. Heberden observed in his 1815 article on the bedframe, and who would deny the truth of that?

References

1. Quesnay M (1749) Traité de la gangrene, 1st edn. D'Houry, Paris
2. Aronssen JE (1806) Ueber die Wichtigkeit der Berücksichtigung des Krankenlagers bei der Heilung der Krankheiten, nebst Beschreibung und Abbildung eines neuen Krankenstuhls. J Pract Arznk Wundarznk 33:94–97
3. Heberden W (1815) Some account of a contrivance which was found of singular benefit in stopping the excoriation and ulceration consequent upon continued pressure in bed. Med Trans Coll phys Lond 5:39–40
4. Porter NI (1869) On a sling for treatment of bed-sores on sacrum or nates when the patient is obliged to rest in the recumbent position. Med Press Circ 8:453
5. Paget J (1873) Clinical lecture on bed-sores. Students J Hosp Gaz 1:144–147
6. Levine JM (1994) A historical perspective on specialty beds and other apparatus for the treatment of invalids. Adv Wound Care 7(5):51–52,54
7. Brown-Sequard CE (1852) Original communications. Med Exam 8:495–498
8. Charcot JM (1868) Sur quelques arthropathies qui paraissent dépendre d'une lésion du cerveau ou de la moelle épinière. Arch Phys 1:161–178, 308–314
9. Van der Sluis I (1979) The movement for euthanasia. Janus 66:131–172
10. Bliss MR (1995) Acute pressure area care: Sir James Paget's legacy. Lancet 339:221–223
11. Marie P, Roussy G (1915) Sur la possibilité de prévenir la formation des escarres dans les traumatismes de la moelle épinière par blessures de guerre. Bull Acad Med Paris 73:602–609
12. Wagner KJ (1964) Epithelial regeneration in anesthetic areas after spinal cord injuries. Plast Reconst Surg 34:268–274
13. Gross SD (1882) System of surgery, vol 1. Henry C. Lea, Philadelphia, pp 581–583

14. McCormick WJ (1941) Nutritional aspect of bedsores. Med Record 154:389–391
15. Mulholland JH, Tui C, Wright AM, Vinci V, Shafiroff B (1943) Protein metabolism and bedsores. Ann Surg 118:1015–1023
16. Cope VZ (1939) Prevention and treatment of bed-sores. Br Med J 1:737–738
17. Davis JS (1938) The operative treatment of scars following bedsores. Surgery 3:1
18. Vasconez LO, Schneider WJ, Jurkiewicz MJ (1977) Pressure sores. Curr probl Surg 14:1–62
19. Reichel SM (1958) Shearing force as a factor in decubitus ulcers in paraplegics. JAMA 166:762–763

2 Decubitus: The Word[*]

C. Parish

History and Early Use

Both the noun *decubitus* and the adjective *decubital* have been in use for more than 100 years, and both have been linked with "bedsore". In Power and Sedgwick [1], cited in the *Oxford English Dictionary* (OED; 1933) [2], "decubitus" is mentioned specifically as "a synonym for bedsore". In an unlisted reference under the entry "decubital", a certain Braithwaite (1876), in *Retrospect. Med.* LXXIII 4, cites "Dr. Handfield Jones on decubital inflammation" – a reasonably clear reference to bedsores.

In its origin, the word decubitus referred only to position: it means "lying down", "reclining". The etymology given in the OED repeats the Latin form: "decubitus: from decumbere, to lie down, to recline".

Early Twentieth-Century Usage

Although decubitus was obviously an "available" word, apparently it was not a favorite word. The pressure sores caused by lying in bed were called "bedsores" by Florence Nightingale in 1866 ("Where there is any danger of bedsores a blanket should never be placed under the patient". Cited under "bedsore" in OED.) Early twentieth-century preference also seems to be on the side of "bedsore": in 1915 Jay Frank Schamberg in his text, *Diseases of the Skin and Eruptive Fevers*, spoke of "bed-sores" in smallpox and typhoid fever. James H. Sequeira, in his text *Diseases of the Skin*, used only the term "bedsore" [3]. Such lesions, however, were evidently not then considered the province of the dermatologist, for there is no discussion at all of their prevention or management. Even in the first edition of George C. Andrews' *Diseases of the Skin* (1930) [4], the only mention of "bedsores" (or "bed-sores") is in connection with ultraviolet irradiation, said to be useful in their management. The word "decubitus" does not appear.

---

[*]Based upon the conepts of the late Harry L. Arnold Jr.

Later Twentieth-Century Usage

In the second edition of Andrews' *Diseases of the Skin* (1938) [4], however, what seems to be a sudden emergence of the word "decubitus" is found; a paragraph entitled "Acute Decubitus" deals with the management of "bed-sores" (two words – "bed sores" – in the index). "Decubitus" then appears in all subsequent editions as "Acute decubitus" in the entry heading, and "bed-sore" in the text. Andrews seems to be taking the older option of calling "bedsore" "decubitus". In the sixth edition of Andrews (1972), Domonkos changed the term to "decubitus ulcer" or "bedsore", and in the seventh edition the same terms are used. Sutton Jr. in his 11th edition (1956) [5], chose the adjectival form of the phrase, writing only "decubital ulcer".

Thus, following textual tradition, we can choose to say "decubitus ulcer", i.e., an ulcer from prolonged reclining, or we can say "decubital ulcer", i.e., an ulcer related to prolonged reclining, or we can simply say "decubitus", since medical professionals have been using the word with the same meaning as "bedsore".

Dictionary Summaries

Recent dictionaries summarize the situation well:

1. Webster II (*Webster's New International Dictionary*) (1935) [6] defines "decubitus" in this way: "In full, decubitus ulcer. A bedsore". If they gave a plural (they don't!) it would probably be "decubitus ulcers".
2. Webster III (1966) [7], more inclusive, gives the whole story of etymology, original meaning, and usage, and medical usage (selections follow): "1: a position assumed in lying down .... " (i.e., the Latin meaning), "2a: ULCER b: or decubitus ulcer; BEDSORE" (i.e., the medical application, plus syno-nyms), and also "3: prolonged lying down (as in bed)" (i.e., a sort of old-fashioned definition, not medical).

Plural Forms

Inevitably, a plural form has grown up with the use of the word "decubitus", even though there is no Latin linguistic justification for it: "decubiti". *Dor-land's Illustrated Medical Dictionary*, in its rewritten 25th edition (1974) [8] followed Blakiston's third edition (1972) [9] giving the plural of "decubitus" as "decubiti". They may have followed Beninson, who had written of "decubiti" in 1972 in the Demis, Dobson, and McGuire text [10]. This plural form is seen quite often, although it is more linguistically appropriate to call two occur-rences of "decubitus" "decubituses".

Conclusions and Recommendations

Classical – Latin and Greek – forms are usually more attractive to physicians, especially younger ones, so "decubitus" may win out over the pedestrian "bedsore" or "pressure sore". But in keeping with that choice, an anglicized plural like "decubituses" is technically preferable to a non-existent Latin plural "decubiti". (It may help to know that the British prefer "syllabuses", even though Americans prefer "syllabi!"). And there are the two other good alternatives as well: two pressure sores are two "decubital ulcers", or they are two "decubitus ulcers". Either one is more communicative to the rest of the world than decubituses perhaps. And as for "decubiti", all one can say is that since the average medical professional is unlikely to be also a student (and judge) of Latin grammar, it will certainly continue to be heard, even though it may arouse a *tsk-tsk* among the older members of the profession. In summary, the editors of this book recommend any of these forms: "decubitus ulcers", "decubital ulcers", "decubituses". They consider less desirable these forms: "decubitii" and "decubiti". And for the reason that it seems to treat the subject too informally – even cozily – they consider undesirable this form: "decubs" based upon the concepts of the late Harry L. Arnold Jr.

References

1. Power H, Sedgwick LW (1879–1899) Lexicon of medicine and allied sciences. Publications of the New Sydenham Society
2. Oxford English Dictionary (1933) Oxford University Press, London. (Compact edn. 1971)
3. Sequeira JH (1919) Diseases of the skin, 3rd edn. Blakiston, Philadelphia, p 409
4. Andrews GC (1930) Diseases of the skin, 1st edn. Saunders, Philadelphia, p 235 (2nd edn, 1938; p 199, 6th edn, 1973; p 55)
5. Sutton RL Jr (1956) Diseases of the skin, 11th edn. Mosby, St Louis, p 764
6. Webster's New International Dictionary of the English Language (1935) 2nd edn. Merriam, Springfield
7. Webster's Third New International Dictionary of the English Language (1966) Merriam, Springfield
8. Dorland's Illustrated Medical Dictionary (1948) 25th edn. Saunders, Philadelphia
9. Blakiston's Gould Medical Dictionary (1972) 3rd edn. McGraw-Hill, New York, p 410
10. Beninson J (1972) Leg ulcers. In: Demis D, Crounce RG, Dobson RL, McGuire J (eds) Clinical dermatology, Section II, Chap 45. Harper and Row, Hagerstown, pp 1–6
11. Arnold HL, Decubitus: the word. In: Parish LC, Witkowski JA, Crissey JT (1983) The decubitus ulcer. Masson, New York, pp 1–3

3 Incidence, Prevalence, and Classification

J.R.E. Haalboom, J.J.E. van Everdingen, and N. Cullum

Decubitus ulcers occur mainly, but not exclusively, in the elderly, bedridden, and severely ill. Increased longevity and associated morbidity are likely to lead to an increase in the prevalence and incidence of decubitus ulcers unless preventive steps are taken.

Recent advances in medical and nursing care have improved the prognosis of patients for whom treatment or cure was previously unlikely. At the same time, health care professionals now see complications that were previously seldom seen. The development of decubitus ulcers in hospital and community settings is quite common, for example, new decubitus ulcers occurred in 0.35%–11% of patients admitted to a district general hospital in the United Kingdom depending on the case mix [1]. Decubitus ulcers represent a major burden of sickness and reduced quality of life for patients and their carers. They are also costly in financial terms. In the United Kingdom, the cost of preventing and treating decubitus ulcers in a 600-bed large general hospital has been roughly estimated at between £600 000 and £3 million per year [2]. Because decubitus ulcers are viewed as largely preventable, occurrences increasingly lead to costly litigation [3]. Thus, for reasons of cost containment government departments and hospital managers are increasingly giving their attention to decubitus ulcers. In the United Kingdom and the Netherlands, for example, the government's Departments of Health have placed the measurement and reduction of decubitus ulcers prevalence high on the agenda [3, 4].

Decubitus ulcers have long been considered the domain of the nurse. In fact, poor nursing care has often been blamed as the cause [5–7]. Despite the fact that the existence of decubitus ulcers has been documented back to Egyptian times, research remains a backwater, with very few good-quality data available for effective prevention [8]. The persistence of a decubitus ulcer problem does not fit the image of contemporary medicine.

Decubitus ulcers are associated with pain, discomfort, and social isolation for the patient, with a high cost to the health care institution. The budgets of health care institutions are usually based on figures derived from admissions over the preceding years. In the Netherlands, for example, the mean duration of hospitalization was 10.8 days in 1994. Every new patient admitted increases the budget for the following year. Patients with a longer duration of stay are less attractive for a hospital because shorter stays pay proportionately more than longer stays. Patients with decubitus ulcers usually stay in hospital much longer, stays over 35 days are no exception [9]. Patients who develop decubitus ulcers not only require more nursing care, they also need special, and invariably more costly, mattresses and or bed systems. In the United Kingdom and elsewhere, the prevalence and incidence of decubitus ulcers have come to be regarded as indicators of the quality of care [3]; written guidelines and protocols for decubitus ulcer prevention and treatment are used in most institutions [10, 11].

Classification

If decubitus ulcer incidence and prevalence rates are to be used as indicators of the quality of care, we need to be able to measure the rates accurately, and accurately and reliably grade the severity of any ulcers which occur. The accurate classification of decubitus ulcer severity is also important in research. It is essential that everybody dealing with decubitus ulcers uses the same definitions. Unfortunately, unlike diseases such as cancer, there is no single, universally accepted classification system. This is understandable because there is not even a universally accepted explanation of the pathogenesis of decubitus ulcers (explanations range from friction and moisture on the skin [12] to occlusion–reperfusion damage [13]). This lack of consistency in decubitus ulcer grading makes it difficult to compare the different epidemiology studies. A decubitus ulcer incidence of 6% in country A and 12% in country B implies that country B has double the incidence; however, if in country A only patients with broken skin are regarded as having decubitus ulcers, while in country B patients with persistent erythema are included, then the figures cannot be compared. This problem is illustrated by a publication dealing with prevalence studies in four Western European countries, known to have comparable levels of hospital care: in Germany and Italy, the prevalence of decubitus ulcers was estimated to be 6%, in the Netherlands and the United Kingdom more than 12% [14]!

Therefore, an agreed system of classifying decubitus ulcers is essential. Such a system should be accompanied by clear guidelines on its use in order to maximize inter-rater reliability. Such a classification should have the following features: (a) it must be useful at the bedside; (b) it be useable by different members of the health care team; (c) it should have high inter-rater reliability; (d) the staging should be clearly linked to severity and prognosis (i.e., stage 2 should be worse than stage 1); and (e) its use should provoke the use of the appropriate interventions.

Various authors use definitions of both the appearance and staging of decubitus ulcers. Differences exist not only between countries with different cultures, but even within single countries. A summary of the classification systems used in the United Kingdom lists 13 classifications [15], 11 of which are traceable in the literature [16–25] (Table 1)! Most classifications are based on the work of Shea [16], who identified five distinctive stages of severity. Experience of patients with decubitus ulcers reveals, however, that some adaptation of the Shea classification system is necessary. Shea did not regard red skin (or erythema) as a decubitus ulcer; however, red unbroken skin seems

Table 1. Summary of the classifications of pressure sore severity commonly used in the United Kingdom (adapted from [15])

Stage	Reference				
	[16]	[17]	[18]	[19]	[20]
0	–	–	–	–	–
1	Limited to epidermis	Discoloration of the skin	Blanching hyperemia	(a) Skin is likely to break (b) Healed areas covered by a scab	Erythema of intact skin
2	Full thickness of dermis to junction of subcutaneous fat	Superficial ulcer	Non-blanching hyperemia	Superficial break in the skin	Partial thickness epidermal tissue
3	Fat obliterated, limited by deep fascia, undermining of the skin	Destruction of skin – no cavity	Ulceration progresses through the dermis only	Destruction of the skin without cavity	Full-thickness ulceration through to the junction with subcutaneous tissue
4	Bone at the base of the ulceration	Destruction of skin – cavity	Lesion extends into subcutaneous fat	Destruction of skin with cavity	Lesion extends into subcutaneous fat with lateral extension of the sore over the deep fascia
5	Closed large cavity through small sinus	–	Infective necrosis penetrates the deep fascia	–	Wound extends through deep fascia with destruction of muscle tissue; bone or tendon may be exposed
6	–	–	–	–	–

[21]	[22]	[23]	[24]	[25]
Inflammation with local heat, erythema, edema, and possible induration – more than 15 mm in diameter	–	–	–	–
Blood under skin or in a blister, or black discoloration under the skin – more than 5 mm in diameter, or clear blister/bullus more than 15 mm in diameter	Discoloration of skin, with persistent erythema after pressure is released; a blister may be forming	Red area (a) present longer than 30 min but less than 24 h (b) present longer than 24 h	Reddened pressure area (blanching hyperemia)	Non-blanchable erythema of intact skin
A break in the skin (epidermis) which may include damage to dermis but without black discoloration – more than 5 mm in diameter	Oedema, blistering epidermal skin loss, with exposure of thedermis; pain	Epidermis and/or dermis ulcerated with no subcutaneous fat observed	Bruising/blister (non-blanching hyperemia)	Partial-thickness skin loss involving epidermis and/or dermis
Destruction of the skin (epidermis and dermis) without an obvious cavity but possibly with black discoloration (possibly a slough) more than 5 mm in diameter	Loss of tissue through dermis, the edge distinct and surrounded by erythema and induration	Subcutaneous fat observed; no muscle involved	Shallow pressure sore (ulceration to dermis)	Full-thickness skin loss involving damage or necrosis of subcutaneous tissue that may extend down to, but not through, underlying fascia
Penetration of skin (epidermis and dermis) with a clearly visible cavity (with or without necrotic tissue) – more than 5 mm in diameter at the surface	Lesion extending into subcutaneous tissue and may penetrate deeper into the deep fascia and muscle	Muscle/fascia observed, but no bone observed	Deep ulceration to subcutaneous fat	Full-thickness skin loss with extensive destruction, tissue necrosis or damage to muscle, bone, or supporting structures
Necrotic, possibly infected and possibly suppurating sore – more than 40 mm in diameter overall, but with either no skin opening or one less than 15 mm in diameter	–	Bone observed, but no involvement of joint space	–	Very deep pressure sore (infective necrosis)
–	–	Involvement of joint space	–	–

to be of great importance in the sequence of decubitus ulcer development. Persistent erythema is an ominous sign, and further development of a decubitus ulcer may still be preventable in most cases. Thus, we would regard the identification of persistent erythema as an essential part of decubitus ulcer prevention. In fact, persistent erythema is a component of eight out of 13 classification systems used in the United Kingdom. Other differences between classification systems concern the involvement of different layers of the skin and underlying tissues. In clinical practice, the involvement of deeper structures such as tendon and bone is associated with protracted healing times and more complications; therefore, a classification system should contain a prognostic aspect which recognizes this.

In the United States, the National Pressure Ulcer Advisory Panel [26] developed a consensus-based classification system which was modified and utilized by the United States Department of Health and Human Services for their decubitus ulcer guidelines [27]. In the United Kingdom, a small consensus group also drew up a classification system. When used in its simplest form this was similar to that developed in the United States but had the capability of being used as a more complex, four-digit classification system to include a description of the wound bed and presence of infection [15] (Table 2).

It is striking that around the same time there were very similar developments in the Netherlands. In 1985, a consensus meeting agreed upon a classification system with four stages and subdivisions in every stage. In 1992, this early classification was modified in the light of additional clinical experience to leave a four-stage system comparable to those developed in the United Kingdom and the United States [28] (Figs. 1–4). The use of a classification of six to eight stages simply did not work in clinical practice; the greater the number of stages, the lower the inter-rater reliability; and the fewer stages there are, the higher the level of agreement. Surprisingly, only one study explored the issue of inter-rater reliability and reported that inter-rater agreement was achieved in only 68% of cases when using the Shea score! Such poor agreement is clearly unsatisfactory; however, an important plus of the Shea classification is its basis in pathology.

The absence of a reliable and accepted classification system has also led to the development of very simple systems, such as one in which an ulcer is graded according to its color (red, yellow, or black) [29]. In clinical practice, this simple approach may appear to confer some advantages, but in reality

Table 2. United Kingdom consensus classification of decubitus ulcers (adapted from [15])

Stage 0	No clinical evidence of a pressure sore
Stage 1	Discoloration of intact skin – light finger pressure applied to the site does not alter the discoloration
Stage 2	Partial-thickness skin loss or damage involving epidermis and/or dermis, and/or blister, abrasion, and shallow ulcer without undermining of adjacent tissue
Stage 3	Full-thickness skin loss involving damage or necrosis of subcutaneous tissue but not extending to underlying bone, tendon, or joint capsule
Stage 4	Full-thickness skin loss with extensive destruction and tissue necrosis extending to underlying bone, tendon or capsule; "deep decubitus"

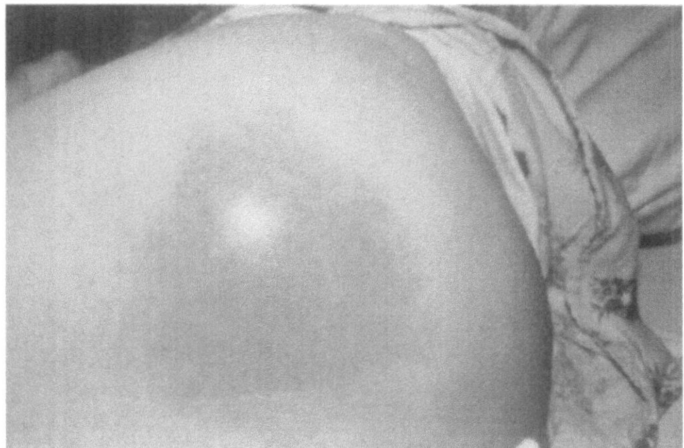

Fig. 1. Stage I decubitus (nonblanching erythema)

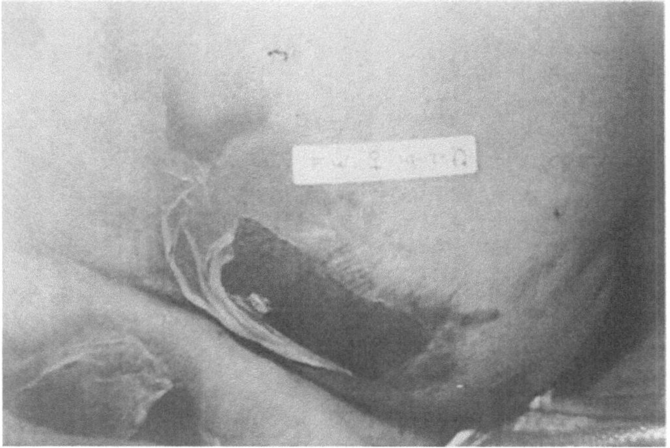

Fig. 2. Stage II decubitus (partial thickness skin loss)

such a system is potentially dangerous because it does not consider either the extent and depth of the lesion or its pathology [30]. These kinds of classification lead to an underestimation of the severity of decubitus ulcers and to undertreatment, and thus cannot be recommended.

In conclusion, decubitus ulcer classification or grading systems should have the following properties:

- They must be suitable for bedside use by all personnel
- They must have a prognostic quality
- They must have high inter-rater reliability
- They should invoke specific interventions

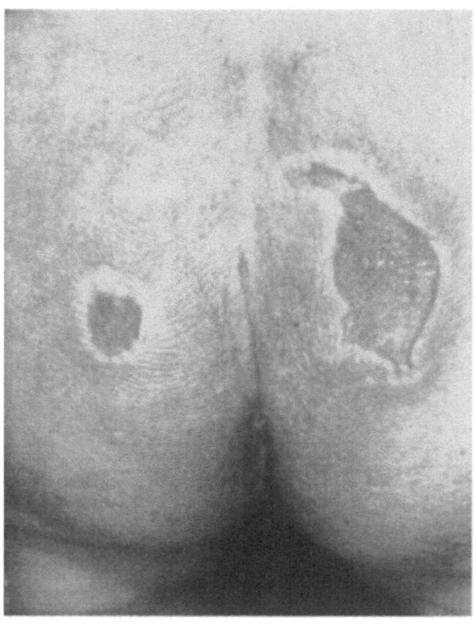

Fig. 3. Stage III decubitus (full-thickness skin loss not extending to underlying bone, tendon or capsule)

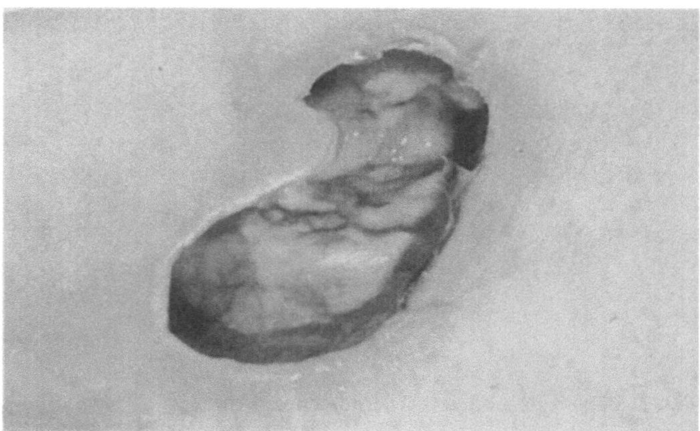

Fig. 4. Stage IV decubitus (full-thickness skin loss extending to underlying bone, tendon or capsule)

In the United States, the United Kingdom, and the Netherlands, consensus has been reached on the use of a four-stage classification (Table 2). All decubitus ulcer research should use this four-stage classification in order to allow the reliable comparison of prevalence and incidence figures, and the accurate interpretation of studies which evaluate the effectiveness of different prevention and treatment regimes. More detailed fundamental research into the pathophysiology of decubitus ulcer formation may ultimately bring about revision of the four-state system [13], but it is more likely that they will enforce the rationale of an international decubitus ulcer rating.

Incidence and Prevalence

The lack of a standard decubitus ulcer classification system further complicates the interpretation of prevalence and incidence data. Decubitus ulcer incidence is the rate of *new* ulcers developing. It is measured prospectively over a specific time period; while prevalence is the proportion of the population with decubitus ulcers at a given time in a particular institution or care setting. It will include both new and old cases plus ulcers which have been imported from elsewhere, as well as those developed in that institution. For example, in January 1995, the dykes in the Netherlands almost collapsed due to very high water levels, and in one night a hospital of 200 beds was evacuated. The patients were transferred to the disaster hospital associated with the Utrecht University Hospital, where the prevalence of decubitus ulcers was 6% on the day before the event and more than 9% the day after. The increase in prevalence was obviously not a result of a sudden decline in the quality of care, but rather due to a relatively large number of patients with existing decubitus ulcers who were imported to the institution.

Incidence is therefore the most useful measure because it best describes what is actually happening in an institution over time; prevalence is only a snapshot view and its value is very limited. However, incidence figures are much more difficult and costly to obtain. They require, at the very least, the accurate registration of all patients with decubitus ulcers in an institution. This is difficult to achieve in a hospital setting and even more troublesome to collect where patients are cared for in the community.

While decubitus ulcer prevalence and incidence are often viewed as indicators of the quality of care, it is important to remember that neither measure can be used as a measure of quality to be compared either between institutions or within an institution over time without a good measure of baseline risk or case mix. Keeping this in mind, examination of the literature reveals that, with minor exceptions, studies of the epidemiology of decubitus ulcers throughout Europe have produced remarkably similar figures. In general hospitals, *prevalence* figures between 5% and 15% [14, 24, 27, 30–34] have been reported; in tertiary care hospitals (intensive care facilities, university hospitals), decubitus ulcer prevalence is higher among patients in intensive care (up to 40%); and in nursing homes, the reported prevalence varies between 3.5% to more than 20% [24, 30, 34]. In spinal units, prevalence figures range between 5.8% and 50% [28, 32]. Recorded figures of decubitus ulcer *incidence* range from 1% to 11% [1, 12, 13, 33–35]. The importance of the difference between prevalence and incidence is illustrated here: while the prevalence of decubitus ulcers in spinal units is high, the incidence may be low: decubitus ulcers occur in spinally injured patients during the acute phase of their trauma, often in the non-specialist unit to which they were first admitted, and once they have occurred these ulcers heal very slowly. The incidence of ulcers in specialist spinal units tends to be fairly low as staff and patients are extensively trained in their prevention, but these units often admit patients who have developed their ulcers elsewhere.

There are no extensive investigations of decubitus ulcers in the home care, or community, situation. In the Glasgow region of Scotland [36] as well as in Aarhus in Denmark [37], reported prevalence figures comprise both hospital and home care. An unpublished study in the Nijmegen region (Continuous Survey of General Health Care, University of Nijmegen, the Netherlands, 1992) revealed that every Dutch general practitioner treats two to four patients with decubitus ulcers per standard practice of 2000 patients, representing a prevalence of 0.1%–0.2% of the total population.

Overall, some new admissions to hospitals have decubitus ulcers (< 2%) [1], but many more patients (25%–35%) have decubitus ulcers following admission to orthopedic or geriatric units and nursing homes. Most decubitus ulcers occur during the institutional stay – long periods in emergency rooms, X-rays, operating theaters, and on poor-quality mattresses and chairs [34]. It is also striking that decubitus ulcers often occur in patients of nursing homes who are temporarily transferred to a hospital [35]. Again highlighting the difference between prevalence and incidence measures.

Decubitus ulcers occur mainly in elderly patients, as is shown in Table 3 and Fig. 5 which illustrate the age distribution of patients in a prevalence study in Utrecht University Hospital in 1984 [33]. Table 3 distinguishes between surgical and non-surgical patients. It is in the non-surgical patients that the increasing prevalence with age is most obvious. In the surgical patients, those younger than 40 years were all treated in the intensive care unit after extensive trauma. Table 4 and Fig. 6 (which relate to the same study) list the typical locations of pressure sores and show that the back of the head, shoulders,

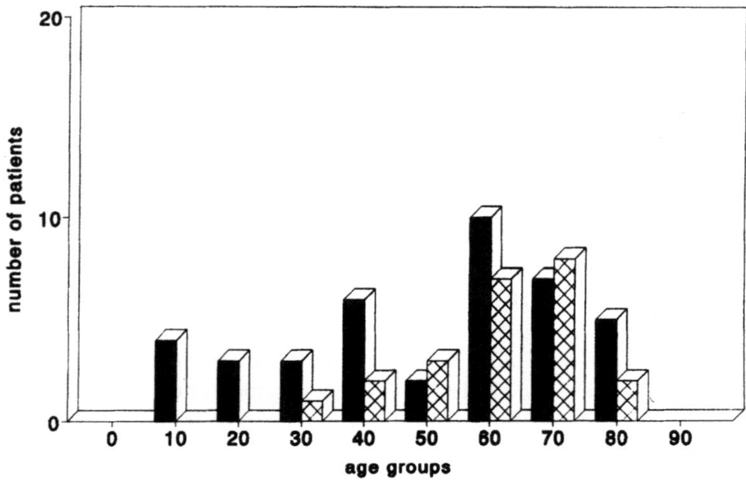

Fig. 5. Age distribution of decubitus ulcers (*solid columns,* surgical; *hatched columns,* nonsurgical)

Table 3. Age distribution of patients with decubitus ulcers. The figures are from a prevalence study in Utrecht University Hospital [33]

Patients	Age (years)								
	0–10	11–20	21–30	31–40	41–50	51–60	61–70	71–80	80+	Total (*n*)
Surgical (*n*)	0	4	3	3	6	2	10	7	5	40
Non-surgical (*n*)	0	0	0	1	2	3	7	8	2	23

Table 4. Distribution of location of decubitus ulcers in 63 patients. The figures are from a prevalence study in Utrecht University Hospital [33]

Location	Head (%)	Shoulders (%)	Elbows (%)	Hips (%)	Buttocks (%)	Heels (%)
	1	2	5	8	55	29

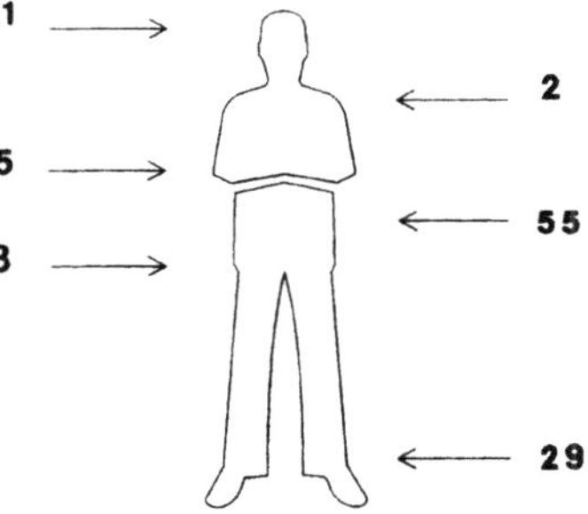

Fig. 6. Location of pressure sores (*n*=63)

elbows, hips, buttocks, and heels are the most commonly affected sites. These sites have in common a bone prominence thinly covered with tissue. As patients are usually treated lying on their back, the frontal risk points (knees, superior anterior pelvic spines, sternum, and shoulders) are not usually affected. However, that these are also areas at risk is illustrated by a recent pilot study in Utrecht University Hospital. All 396 surgical patients consecutively admitted over a 2-week period were investigated immediately after their arrival into the recovery room following surgery. Of these patients, 350 were operated on lying on their back, the remaining 46 were operated on while lying prone. From the first group, 27 patients (8%) showed symptoms of pressure damage (limited to stages 1 and 2 decubitus ulcers) in the typical locations, while 14 patients (30%) who had been prone showed such lesions. The fact that frontal decubitus ulcers usually do not further deteriorate in such patients can be explained by the fact that after surgery they are usually nursed lying on their backs.

Conclusions

The reported prevalence of decubitus ulcers varies between 5% and 15% in general hospitals, between 3.5% and more than 20% in nursing homes, and between 5.8% and 50% in spinal units. Reported incidence ranges between 1% and 11%. Prevalence in the home care setting is estimated to be 0.1%–0.2%. These figures suggest that, in a hospital of 600 beds, there are typically 30–90 patients with a decubitus ulcer at any point in time. In nursing homes, one in every five patients may be affected. Patients who experience a sore suffer pain and discomfort and protracted rehabilitation, they stay longer in hospital and consume considerably more resources than patients who do not develop pressure sores. Decubitus ulcers are therefore important for all these reasons.

References

1. Clark M, Watts S (1994) The incidence of pressure sores within a National Health Service trust hospital during 1991. J Adv Nurs 20:33–36
2. Touche Ross et al. (1993) The costs of pressure sores. Report to the Department of Health
3. Department of Health (1993) Pressure sores: a key quality indicator. Department of Health, London
4. NHS Executive (1994) Pressure sores – a preventable problem. VFM update no 12
5. Sutton JC, Wallace WA (1990) Pressure sores: the views and practices of senior hospital doctors. Clin Rehabil 4:137–143
6. Kulkarni J, Philbin M (1993) Pressure sore awareness survey in a university teaching hospital. J Tissue Viabil 3:77–79
7. Bennett G (1992) Medical undergraduate teaching in chronic wound care (a survey). Tissue viabil 2:50–51
8. Cullum N, Deeks J, Fletcher A, Sheldon T, Song F (in press) The prevention and treatment of pressure sores. Qual Health Care
9. Haalboom JRE (1991) The costs of pressure sores. Ned Tijdschr Geneeskd 135:606–610 (with a summary in English)
10. Abruzzese R (1991) Quality care and staging of ulcers. Decubitus 4:6–7
11. Klazinga N (1994) Improving pressure sore prevention rates through quality assurance. Wound Care 3:141–144
12. Allman RM (1989) Pressure ulcers among the elderly. N Engl J Med 320: 850–853
13. Houwing R, Jonasse Y, van Asbeck S, Haalboom JRE (1991) Pressure sores are caused by oxygen free radicals. Eur J Clin Invest 21:58
14. O'Dea K (1995) The prevalence of pressure sores in four European countries. J Wound Care 4:192–195
15. Reid J, Morison M (1994) Classification of pressure sore severity. Nurs Times 90:46–50
16. Shea JD (1975) Pressure sores. Clin Orthop Relat Res 112:89–100
17. Jordan MM, Clark MO (1977) Report on incidence of pressure sores in the patient community of the Greater Glasgow Health Board Area on 21 Jan 1976. University of Strathclyde, Glasgow
18. Torrance C (1983) Pressure sores: aetiology, treatment and prevention. Croom Helm, Beckenham
19. David JA, Chapman RG, Chapman EJ (1983) An investigation of the current methods used in nursing for the care of patients with established pressure sores. Nurs Practi Research Unit, Harrow
20. Johnson A (1985) A blueprint for the prevention and management of pressure sores. CARE Sci Pract 1:2, 8–13
21. Lowthian P (1987) The classification and grading of pressure sores. CARE Sci Pract 5:5–9

22. International Association for Enterostomal Therapy (1988) Dermal wounds: pressure sores. J Enterost Ther 15:4–17
23. Hibbs PJ (1988) Pressure area care for the City and Hackney Health Authority. City and Health Authority, London
24. Yarkony GM, Kirk PM, Carlson C, Roth EJ, Lovell L, Heinemann A, King R, Lee MY, Betts HB (1990) Classification of pressure ulcers. Arch Dermatol 126:1218–1219
25. Robertson W (1992) Policy for the prevention and treatment of pressure sores. Inverclyde, Cowal and Bute Unit, Aryll and Clyde Health Board, Greenock
26. National Pressure Ulcer Advisory Panel (1989) Pressure ulcers: incidence, economics and risk assessment. CARE Sci Pract 7:96–99
27. Agency for Health Care Policy and Research (1992) Pressure ulcers in adults: prediction and prevention. Clin Pract Guidelines 3:1–63
28. Haalboom JRE, Bakker H (1992) Herziening consensus preventie en behandeling decubitus. Ned Tijdsch Geneeskd 136:1306–1308 (with a summary in English)
29. Ziegler Cuzzell J (1988) The new RYB color code. Am J Nurs 88:1342–1346
30. Yarkony GM (1994) Pressure ulcers: a review. Arch Phys Med Rehabil 75:908–917
31. Allman RM, Laprade CA, Noel LB (1986) Pressure sores among hospitalized patients. Ann Intern Med 105:337–342
32. Knutsdottir S (1993) Spinal cord injuries in Iceland 1973–1989: a follow up study. Paraplegia 31:68–72
33. Haalboom JRE (1984) Decubitus in het ziekenhuis. Ned Tijdschr Geneeskd 128:1957–1958 (with a summary in English)
34. Leigh IH, Bennett G (1994) Pressure ulcers: prevalence, etiology, and treatment modalities. Am J Surg 167 [1A; Suppl]: 25–30
35. Rudman D, Slater EJ, Richardson TJ, Mattson DE (1993) The occurrence of pressure ulcers in three nursing homes. J Gen Intern Med 8:653–658
36. Barbanel JC, Nicol SM, Jordan MM (1977) Incidence of pressure spores in the Greater Glasgow Health Board Area. Lancet II:548–550
37. Petersen NC, Bittmann S (1971) The epidemiology of pressure sores. Scand J Plast Reconstr Surg 5:62–66

4 Assessment and Grading

Because of our aging population and advances in medical and surgical therapy permitting survival from catastrophic illness and injury, the incidence of decubitus ulcers is likely to increase unless greater attention is paid to prophylaxis. At present, there is more interest in treating and curing than in avoiding injury and illness. We must become more prevention oriented; with cost restraints limiting resources, not everyone can be offered perfect decubitus ulcer prevention. The patient at greatest risk must be identified before the problem begins. Our limited equipment and personnel have to be concentrated on those patients at highest risk.

Nurses have been identified as the patient's first line of defense in the prevention of decubitus ulcers [1]. Because they are involved in total care of the patient, nurses have assumed the responsibility for care of the patient's skin [2, 3]. As a result, nurses have become the primary care givers for the prevention and treatment of decubitus ulcers [4]. They are responsible for identifying the patients at greatest risk.

Assessment Scales

While many nurses can identify patients at risk and are able to prevent a problem before it occurs [5], some, because of lack of experience, knowledge, or interest, are not able to do so. To help these care givers identify high-risk patients, a number of risk assessment scales have been developed. Risk assessment scales are based on the fact that, while no one is immune to decubitus ulcer formation beyond some critical point, certain factors place patients at a particularly high risk of pressure damage. These factors are easily recognized. Several schemes for the identification of these factors have been developed. In the Norton scale (Table 1) risk factors considered are physical condition, mental state, activity, mobility, and incontinence [6]. The Braden scale (Table 2) identifies three determinants of pressure, i.e., sensory perception, activity, and mobility; and three factors influencing tolerance of the skin to pressure, i.e., moisture, nutrition, and friction and shear [7]. Numerical values ranging from 1 to 3 or 4 are assigned to each factor. A score of 1 is least

Table 1. The Norton scale (adapted from [6])

		Physical condition		Mental condition		Activity		Mobility		Incontinent		Total score
		Good	4	Alert	4	Ambulant	4	Full	4	Not	4	
		Fair	3	Apathetic	3	Walk/help	3	Slightly limited	3	Occasional	3	
		Poor	2	Confused	2	Chairbound	2	Very limited	2	Usually/Urine	2	
		Very bad	1	Stupor	1	Stupor	1	Immobile	1	Doubly	1	
Name	Date											

favorable while a score of 3 or 4 is most favorable. The scores for each factor are then tabulated. Low total scores indicate high risk and high scores low risk. The cut-off score indicating high risk for the Norton scale is 14 [8] while on the Braden scale it is 12. Both the cut-off score and the risk factors may vary with the patient setting [9, 10]. These total scores should influence the nurse's decision with respect to the appropriate interventions for the patient.

Assessment scales also serve other useful purposes. In addition to determining risk, they indicate the probability of healing of existing decubitus ulcers. They also serve as reminders of the factors that place patients at risk, permit easy communication among health care personnel of the patient's risk, and ensure systematic evaluation of risk factors.

Because decubitus ulcers usually occur within the first 10 days of admission to an acute care institution, assessment should be performed on admission. Any acute deterioration of the patient's clinical status requires immediate reassessment.

Skin and Ulcer Assessment

In addition to assessing risk, health care givers should inspect the patient's skin for early changes of pressure damage. Skin assessment should be performed routinely and systematically. It should be done daily, usually at the time of the patient's bath [11]. The characteristic erythema over bony prominences, particularly when accompanied by increased local temperature and tenderness (if sensory nerves are intact) should serve as a warning sign. In the skin of black patients, darkening may obscure underlying erythema. Increased temperature can be detected with the back of the hand [12]. Health care personnel unaware of these early changes in the skin can condemn the patient to an ulcer and prolonged healing time, and contribute to increasing hospital costs and an increased burden on nursing facilities.

Table 2. The Braden scale for predicting decubitus ulcer risk (adapted from [7])

Patient's Name_____________ Evaluator's Name_________________________

Sensory perception Ability to respond meaningfully to pressure-related discomfort	1. Completely limited: Unresponsive (does not moan, flinch, or grasp) to painful stimuli, due to diminished level of consciousness or sedation, OR limited ability to feel pain over most of body surface	2. Very limited: Responds only to painful stimuli; cannot communicate discomfort except by moaning or restlessness, OR has a sensory impairment which limits the ability to feel pain or discomfort over 1/2 of body
Moisture Degree to which skin is exposed to moisture	1. Constantly moist: Skin is kept moist almost constantly by perspiration, urine, etc.; dampness is detected every time patient is moved or turned	2. Moist: Skin is often but not always moist; linen must be changed at least once a shift
Activity Degree of physical activity	1. Bedfast: Confined to bed	2. Chairfast: Ability to walk severely limited or nonexistent; cannot bear own weight and/or must be assisted into chair or wheelchair
Mobility Ability to change and control body position	1. Completely immobile: Does not make even slight changes in body or extremity position without assistance	2. Very limited: Makes occasional slight changes in body or extremity position but unable to make frequent or significant changes independently
Nutrition Usual food intake pattern	1. Very poor: Never eats a complete meal; rarely eats more than 1/3 of any food offered; eats two servings or less of protein (meat or dairy products) per day; takes fluids poorly; does not take a liquid dietary supplement, OR is NPO and/or maintained on clear liquids or IV for more than 5 days	2. Probably inadequate: Rarely eats a complete meal and generally eats only about 1/2 of any food offered; protein intake includes only three servings of meat or dairy products per day; occasionally will take a dietary supplement, OR receives less than optimum amount of liquid diet or tube feeding
Friction and shear	1. Problem: Requires moderate to maximum assistance in moving; complete lifting without sliding against sheets is impossible; frequently slides down in bed or chair requiring frequent repositioning with maximum assistance; spasticity, contractures, or agitation leads to almost constant friction	2. Potential problem: Moves feebly or requires minimum assistance; during a move skin probably slides to some extent against sheets, chair, restraints, or other devices; maintains relatively good position in chair or bed most of the time but occasionally slides down

NPO, nothing by mouth; IV, intravenously; TPN, total parenteral nutrition.

	Date of Assessment				
3. Slightly limited: Responds to verbal commands but cannot always communicate discomfort or need to be turned, OR has some sensory impairment which limits ability to feel pain or discomfort in one or two extremities	4. No impairment: Responds to verbal commands; has no sensory deficit which would limit ability to feel or voice pain or discomfort				
3. Occasionally moist: Skin is occasionally moist, re quiring an extra linen change approximately once a day	4. Rarely moist: Skin is usually dry; linen requires changing only at routine intervals				
3. Walks occasionally: Walks occasionally during day but for very short distances, with or without assistance; spends majority of each shift in bed or chair	4. Walks frequently: Walks outside the room at least twice a day and inside room at least once every 2 h during waking hours				
3. Slightly limited: Makes frequent though slight changes in body or extremity position independently	4. No limitations: Makes major and frequent changes in position without assistance				
3. Adequate: Eats over half of most meals. Eats a total of four servings of protein (meat, dairy products) each day; occasionally will refuse a meal, but will usually take a supplement if offered, OR is on a tube feeding or TPN regimen, which probably meets most of nutritional needs	4. Excellent: Eats most of every meal. Never refuses a meal; usually eats a total of four or more servings of meat and dairy products; occasionally eats between meals; does not require supplementa-tion				
3. No apparent problem: Moves in bed and in chair independently and has sufficient muscle strength to lift up completely during move; maintains good position in bed or chair at all times					
Total score					

If more advanced pressure changes are present, the depth of the tissue destruction should be graded using the National Pressure Ulcer Advisory Panel (NPUAP) classification of pressure ulcers [13]:

Stage I Nonblanchable erythema of intact skin – this should not be confused with erythema which blanches on pressure (reactive hyperemia)
Stage II Full-thickness loss of skin involving epidermis and/or dermis – the ulcer is superficial and presents clinically as a blister, abrasion, or shallow crater
Stage III Full-thickness loss of skin including the subcutaneous tissue that may extend down to, but not through the underlying fascia – the ulcer presents clinically as a deep crater, with or without undermining of the adjacent skin
Stage IV Full-thickness loss of skin including the subcutaneous tissue, muscle, bone, or supporting structures such as tendon or joint capsule – the ulcer presents clinically as a deep crater with or without undermining and sinus tract formation

A stage I decubitus ulcer in the black patient may be identified by local pain and tenderness and darkening of the skin. The area is often cool to the touch. The skin may be soft, edematous, or slightly indurated. When an eschar is present, accurate staging is not possible until the eschar is removed. The findings of the assessment should be placed on a diagram identifying pressure points.

Because the NPUAP staging system lacks sensitivity and specificity to change, the Pressure Sore Staging System (PSSS; Appendix 1) is used to evaluate ulcers [14]. The PSSS assessment method includes a composite of wound characteristics providing a better indication of overall ulcer status. It encompasses 13 subscale items including size, depth, edges, undermining, necrotic tissue type and amount, exudate type and amount, skin color surrounding the ulcer, peri-ulcer edema and induration, granulation tissue and epithelialization. These are rated 1 to 5, with 5 being the worst for that characteristic. These subscale items can be added together for a total score ranging from 13 (least severe) to 65 (most severe). The total score can be used as an overall indicator of ulcer status and permits documentation of clinical progress [15].

Conclusions

Reducing the incidence of decubitus ulcers requires vigilance and interest on the part of everyone concerned. Assessment scales and methods are a means to this end.

References

1. Krainski MM (1992) Pressure ulcers and the elderly: a review of the literature 1980–1990. Ostomy/Wound Management 38:22–37
2. Towey AP, Erland SM (1988) Validity and reliability of an assessment tool for pressure ulcer risk. Decubitus 1:40–48
3. Pieper B, Mott M (1995) Nurses knowledge of pressure ulcer prevention, staging, and description. Adv Wound Care 8:34–48
4. Pieper B, Mikals C, Mance B, Adams W (1990) Nurses documentation about pressure ulcers. Decubitus 3:32–34
5. Maklebust J, Sieggren M (1991) Pressure ulcers: guidelines for prevention and nursing management. S–N Publ, West Dundee, p 59
6. Norton D, McLaren R, Exton-Smith AN (1962) An investigation of geriatric nursing problems in hospital. National Corporation for Care of Old People, London
7. Braden BJ, Bergstrom N (1989) Clinical utility of the Braden scale for predicting pressure ulcer risk. Decubitus 2:44–51
8. Norton D (1989) Calculating the risk: reflections on the Norton scale. Decubitus 2:24–31
9. Smith DM (1995) Pressure ulcers in the nursing home. Ann Intern Med 123:433–442
10. National Pressure Ulcer Advisory Panel (1996) Etiology, assessment, and early intervention. Dermatol Nurs 8:41–47
11. Ayella E (1992) Teaching the assessment of patients with pressure ulcers. Decubitus 5:53–54
12. Parish LC, Witkowski JA, Crissey JT (1983) The decubitus ulcer. Masson, New York, p 120
13. National Pressure Ulcer Advisory Panel (1989) Pressure ulcers: incidence, economics, risk assessment. Consensus development conference statement. Decubitus 2:24–28
14. Bates-Jensen B (1990) A new pressure ulcer status tool. Decubitus 3:14–15
15. Bates-Jensen B, McNees P (1995) Toward an intelligent wound assessment system. Ostomy/Wound Management 41:80S–87S

Clinical Aspects

5 Pathophysiology

G.W. Cherry and T.J. Ryan

Decubitus ulcers are the end result of an inadequate nutrient blood supply to the tissues. In discussing the pathophysiology of these lesions, it is important to distinguish between the cause, which is usually pressure on the skin, usually over bony prominences, and other factors that contribute to non-healing once the ulcer has formed. Numerous factors have been postulated to be important in the causation of decubitus ulcers (Table 1), and those factors that lead to a delay in healing have also been the subject of a number of studies. Factors that occlude capillary flow and those that delay healing overlap, of course, to some extent, but the pathophysiology of decubitus ulcers is usually blamed correctly on occlusion of capillary flow by pressures greater than mean capillary pressure (25 mmHg), along with shearing forces, infection, and a lack of cutaneous sensation [2-9]. Repetitive injury and prolonged pressure are especially important.

Table 1. Factors delaying wound healing

Global	General	Local
Building inadequate	Age	Inadequate blood supply
No access	Malnutrition	Hematoma formation
Transport	Cancer	Foreign body implantation
Health care worker	Anemia	Necrotic tissue
Knowledge	Systemic infection	Wound infection
Availability	Steroid treatment	Radiation therapy
Patient complaints	Vitamin and trace metal deficiency	Recurrent trauma
Management support	Cancer chemotherapy	Duration of surgery
	Diabetes	Experience of surgeon
	Jaundice	Suture material
	Uremia	Wound tension
	Obesity	Absence of nature's secret remedy
	Hypothermia	
	Anti-inflammatory drugs	
	Gender	
	Genetic defects–skeletal or adhesion proteins	

Blood Supply to the Skin

To understand the etiology of pressure sores, it is important to appreciate the anatomic and functional distribution of the blood supply to different regions of the skin. Claude Manchot (1889) is given credit for one of the more detailed descriptions of regional cutaneous blood supplies (Fig.1) [9]. It is also necessary to keep in mind the role of the perforating arteries and veins that supply the skin from skeletal muscles. External pressure can restrict the blood supply to soft tissue and muscle when these tissues are compressed between underlying bone structure and the skin.

The aim of this chapter is to examine the relationship between the blood supply of muscle and skin under normal conditions and to demonstrate the ways in which ischemic injury from pressure to these tissues along with repetitive stress can lead to abnormal tissue metabolism, which in all probability predisposes these structures to breakdown and ulcer formation.

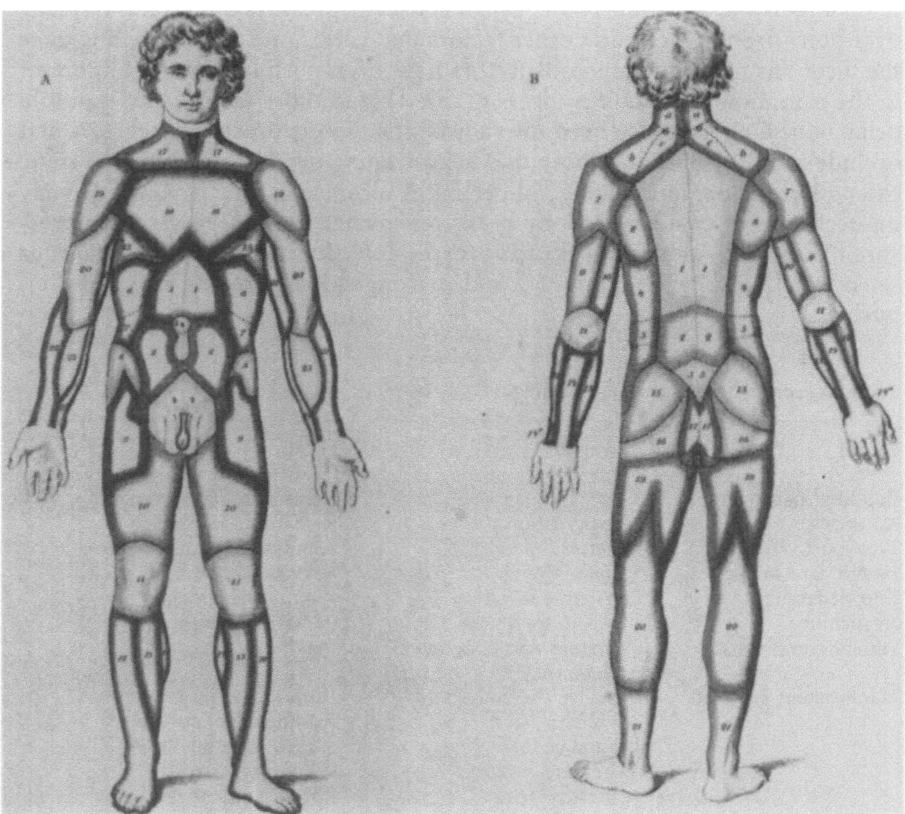

Fig. 1. Manchot's detailed anatomical distribution of different regions of the skin supplied by specific vessels

Daniel and Kerrigan [10], in an excellent review of the anatomic and hemodynamic characteristics of skin flaps, divide the vascular circulation into three distinct systems: segmental, perforator, and cutaneous. The segmental system includes the body's main distributing vessels stemming from the aorta. The perforator system provides nutritional blood supply to muscle and interchange of supply to the skin. The cutaneous system consists of supply arteries, capillary beds, and draining veins at different levels. On the basis of anatomic, embryologic, and physiologic evidence, the supplying arteries are further classified by these authors into musculocutaneous and direct cutaneous arteries. The clinical significance of this anatomic classification has been recognized in experience gained over the last few years in plastic surgical procedures dealing with musculocutaneous flaps that involve a specific cutaneous territory dependant on the distribution of arteries from the muscle component of the flap. Interruption of the blood supply to the muscle can lead to necrosis of the skin. It is reasonable to suspect that the same type of necrosis could result from muscle ischemia induced by pressure in bedridden patients. Cutaneous lesions in these patients would be secondary to impairment in muscle circulation.

Blood Supply Characteristics and Breakdown of Skin

When examining nutritional blood supply, it is important to recognize that regional and age variations as well as gross changes may be reflected in the pathology. The nutritional capillary bed varies in the richness of its provision, as does the blood flow, the density of the vasculature per unit area, and the distance of the nutritional blood supply from the peripheral skin. Regional variations are fixed at birth or in early stages of development. Regional differences exist in the capillary density of normal human dermis, with a notable paucity of arteriolar vasculature at certain sites, particularly over the long bones of the lower leg [12]. Many elderly legs lose not only elements of the capillary bed supplying the epidermis, but also hair , sweat glands, and adipose tissue. Adipose and adnexal tissues usually have a rich capillary bed that is important in the recruitment of endothelium for vessel formation. The morphology of the capillary bed is severely disturbed in patients with arteriosclerosis, and clinically ischemic skin often shows evidence of abnormal vascular patterns that contribute to the vulnerability of tissues exposed to external trauma such as pressure (Fig. 2) [13]. Cutaneous blood flow is also more likely to be obstructed by shearing strains in patients who show evidence of the tortuous proliferating vessels characteristic of ischemic skin (Fig. 2c) [14]. Ischemic injury is a summation of demand and supply.

Normal skin requires very little oxygen, and it has always been supposed that the relative richness of its blood supply is concerned more with thermoregulation than nutrition. Ryan [15] has emphasized that blood supply also contributes to the swelling pressures of the ground substance, so necessary to maintenance of the protective resilience and turgor of the skin. Cool skin is less

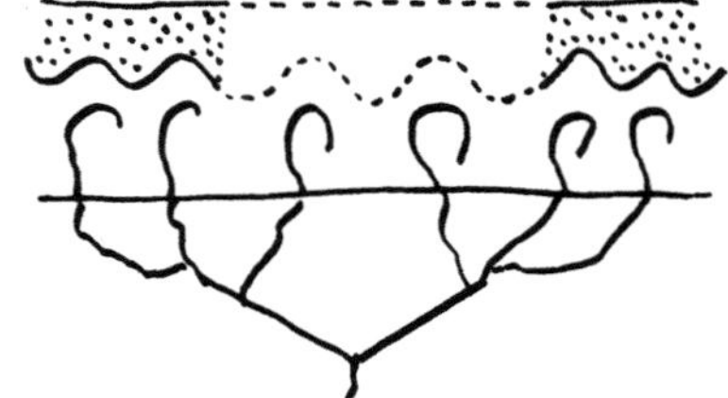

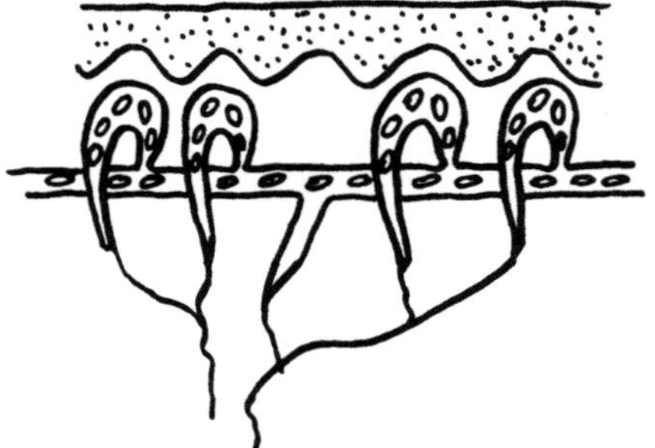

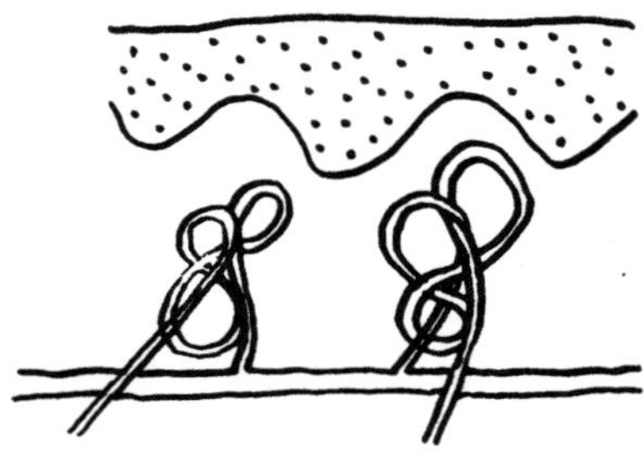

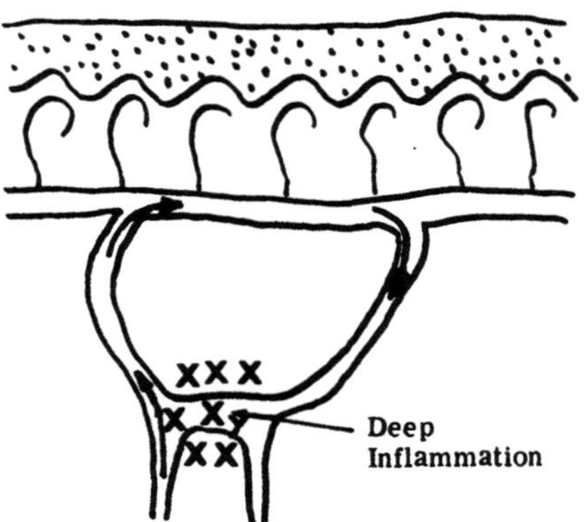

Fig. 2. Causes of redness and factors influencing repair. Within 1 mm from the skin surface there is a nutritional blood supply. It is in close (less than 0.1 mm from the surface) apposition to the epithelium, with perpendicular capillary loops, only found in health and repair. Thinning and increased transparency with atrophy of the vasculature is a feature of ageing, and it is associated with impaired nutrition with loss of loops. Increased vulnerability, pin point bleeding or thrombosis, with early healing as a consequence of epidermal damage, is a feature of skin that is well endowed with loop-shaped vessels in the upper portion of the dermis. Dermal injury to the horizontal vessels, especially when there is an absence of upper dermal loops, is more likely from shearing stresses in atrophic skin – senile purpura; not pin point – there is usually a lag phase before such vessels repair. Much of the upper portion of the dermis in white skin is sufficiently transparent for colour to be observed from deeper tissues, but in such skin, redness is less easily transmitted than blueness. Hence, deep dilated vessels often appear to be blue. The color can be further influenced by the presence of other pigments such as hemosiderin or melanin

demanding than warm, inflamed skin, and atrophic skin in turn is less demanding than repairing or hypertrophic skin.

Immobility as a factor contributing to the formation of decubitus ulcers is emphasized in many places in this text. However, it is not blood supply alone that is affected by this factor. Lymphatic flow is also impaired by immobility, and decubitus care should include massage of tissues to facilitate lymphatic dispersal of wastes and excess inflammatory products. Another factor of importance is nutrition. Takeda et al. [16], studying experimentally induced decubitus ulcers in malnourished rabbits, found that malnutrition of a degree sufficient to produce hypoproteinemia did not change red cell numbers or hemoglobin concentration, but nevertheless had a profound effect on the initiation of ulcers.

Some parallels exist between the problem of non-healing leg ulcers due to venous disease and ulcers caused by pressure. The pathogenesis of leg ulcers associated with venous hypertension is believed now to include leakage of agents into capillary walls, cuffing of vessels, stiffness of vessels, a tendency for white cells to sequestrate, and an inflammatory process that upgrades the adhesion of white cells to endothelium. Ultimately, lymphocytes and macrophage are attracted to the site and contribute a battery of lymphokines that may promote or delay healing [17]. While much of this has been well worked out in leg ulcer research and could easily apply to decubitus ulcers, such studies remain to be done.

One of the concepts popular in recent years contends that impaired perfusion and reperfusion introduces into tissue, after a period of ischemia, oxygen free radicals capable of producing damage. While this concept is of interest, the most important factor contributing to the pathogenesis of decubitus ulcers is the obliteration of blood supply. The capacity of human skin to resist such compression and deformity from shearing forces has also been studied, particularly by Bader et al. [18]. Compliance of tissues depends, among other things, on water content. It has been observed that the skin of young individuals is stiffer and less elastic in the morning, a feature not observed in the elderly [19]. Factors important in clearing fluid are related mainly to the lymphatics. The lymphatic system is perhaps compromised more than any other by immobility and by excessive mechanical stress [20].

The remodeling of tissues, let us say the healing of wounds, includes the control of proteases and their inhibitors. In human decubitus ulcers, levels of the serum protease inhibitor α_2-macroglobulin was lower than in acute wounds and, in one experiment, wound fluid from ulcers degraded transforming growth factor β_1 (TGF-β_1),making it unavailable for its supposedly beneficial effects in the promotion of wound healing [21].

Skin Tolerance to Ischemia

Surprisingly little work has been done on the effect of ischemia on the survival of skin. Most information available has been obtained indirectly from studies concerned with the pathogenesis of decubitus ulcers. In these investigations, much attention has been devoted to the influence of pressure on underlying muscle degeneration. In a study by Husain [16] on rats, it was found that an external pressure of 100 mmHg applied to the skin for 2 h produced ischemic histologic changes in underlying muscle. When the same pressure was applied for 6 h, complete muscle degeneration occurred. Husain also noted that localized pressure obliterated more vessels in the skin and subcutaneous tissue than in the muscle. This is one of the few studies in which the effect of a previous vascular insult on tissue survival was assessed when another episode of ischemia was applied. In this case, pressure was applied to a limb 3 days after ligation of the femoral artery. Degeneration of muscle fibers occurred at a pressure as low as 50 mmHg for 1 h. In other words, the threshold tolerance to the amount of pressure and length of ischemia caused by pressure was drastically lowered by a previous vascular insult that did not cause necrosis initially. This finding is important in clinical vascular pathology, where the majority of occlusions that occur in organs that are usually supplied by arteriosclerotic vessels and have probably been subjected to previous sublethal amounts of ischemia [17].

In most studies devoted to ischemia and tissue survival, experiments have been performed on animals with healthy organs that have not suffered earlier vascular insults. In the work of Kosiak [18] on dogs, a pressure of 100–550 mmHg was applied to the skin for periods of 1–12 h. He found that ulceration of the skin occurred after a shorter period when the pressure was raised, i.e., the time–pressure relationship is inverse and follows a parabolic curve.

Lindan [19] found that 100 mmHg pressure applied with a special clip to the ears of rabbits for 7 h did not produce ulceration of the skin, although healing was retarded and hair failed to grow in the area exposed to pressure. When the period of pressure was extended to 13–15 h, necrosis occurred. Pressures less than 100 mmHg (20, 40, 60 mmHg) for the same length of time failed to produce ulceration.

In other words, pressures capable of producing venous occlusion did not result in necrosis. This is not surprising as it has been shown in skin flap research that venous obstruction by itself seldom causes necrosis [20].

A study on normal and paraplegic swine by Dinsdale [6] demonstrated that external pressure above 150 mmHg applied to the skin for 3.5 h in conjuction with friction resulted in superficial epidermal necrosis 7 days later. No differences were noted between paraplegic and control pigs. Although Dinsdale stated that friction in conjuction with ischemia was necessary to produce ulceration, he did not speculate on the mechanisms involved.

Skin Survival After Ischemia: Reperfusion and Previous Injury

In vivo studies have demonstrated that skin can withstand periods of ischemia for as long as 9 h at normothermic conditions before irreversible damage takes place. Selye [22] found that the resistance of rat skin to ischemia could be increased if the animals were subjected to a form of stress prior to occlusion of the blood supply. In control animals, 9 h of compression of a fold of skin by means of an umbilical clamp led to necrosis after reperfusion. When animals were pretreated with stress (starvation for 48 h, hypothermia, spinal cord transection, or epinephrine administration) little or no necrosis occurred with 9 h of ischemia. When rats were pretreated with cortisol acetate and cortisol succinate, the same amount of necrosis occurred as in the controls. Selye postulated that this protective mechanism might be chemical in nature, provided perhaps by systemic catecholamines released during stress.

Palmer [23] found that survival of freshly raised skin flaps in rats was reduced when the animals were subjected to stress by restraint. The clinical implications of this finding are important in dealing with immobilized patients. When Palmer pretreated rats with an adrenergic α-receptor-blocking agent, surviving lengths of skin flaps increased. In an earlier study he had demonstrated that the vessels of the skin flap became innervated within 18–30 h after surgery [24]. Myers and Cherry [25] demonstrated that skin flap survival could be increased by the administration of phenoxybenzamine, an adrenergic α-receptor-blocking agent. An increase in blood flow in the tube pedicles and flaps in patients has been described with the administration of thymoxamine, another α-receptor-blocking agent [26].

Stefani [27] observed as early as 1886 that gangrene of an extremity following ligation of the axillary artery in the salamander occurred only if the limb were denervated. Denervation has been shown by several investigators to increase the sensitivity of vessels to circulating catecholamines [28, 29]. Selye worked with normally innervated skin, while Palmer's experiments were conducted on skin flaps that had been denervated and were therefore more sensitive to circulating catecholamines.

In a study by Willms-Kretschmer and Majno [30], more attention is paid to the histologic changes that occur during the period of ischemia before necrosis occurs. A fold of skin on the back of a rat was occluded with a pressure device for varying periods of time. Skin that had been ischemic for 2 h and reperfused for 24 h showed no abnormalities. After 4–6 h of ischemia, muscle and fat necrosis occurred; 8 h of occlusion resulted in complete necrosis of the compressed skin. In the same study, a similar experiment was conducted on the ears of rabbits. Unlike the results in the rat experiments, 8 h of ischemia produced no significant necrosis. The authors furnished no explanation for this species difference, but pointed out that the rabbit's ear has relatively little fat and muscle, the latter tissues being more susceptible to ischemia than skin.

Neither of the above studies attempted to quantify the amount of tissue that survived after periods of temporary ischemia. In his work on the effect of ischemia on tissue survival in delayed and control island skin flaps, Milton [31] was the first to quantify the effects of ischemia and reperfusion on skin survival. He found that control island skin flaps could tolerate an average of 8 h of ischemia. This was surprisingly similar to the findings of Selye, and Willms-Kretschmer and Majno. An unexpected finding was that skin (delayed flaps) with augmented vascularity could withstand only an average of 4 h of ischemia. This result was not anticipated, as delaying the raising of a skin flap in stages has been shown to increase the vascularity of the skin and increase surviving lengths up to 100% [32, 33]. The discrepancy between increased vascularity and tissue survival in the skin has been noted by other investigators. With respect to metabolic needs, skin is oversupplied with blood. The mean blood flow in the skin of digits is 20–30 times greater than the minimum flow needed for nutrition [34]. A flow rate of 0.8 ml blood/min per 100g has been stated to be adequate for oxygen requirements [35].

Muscle Tolerance to Ischemia

Dependence of the blood supply to the skin on perforating vessels from the underlying muscle can be compromised when the muscle is damaged by excessive external pressure. Gordon and colleagues [36] found that rat quadriceps subjected to different periods of ischemia for up to 5 h and then reperfused showed severe histologic changes when ischemia periods exceeded 1 h. Cherry and coworkers [37] demonstrated ultrastructural ischemic changes in the endothelium of sartorius muscle flaps when the blood supply was reduced by simple surgical elevation. These studies imply that the tolerance of muscle to ischemia is considerably less than skin and may explain why muscle damage underlying decubitus ulcers is usually more extensive than the damage to overlying skin.

Role of Tissue Fibrinolysins in Decubitus Ulcer Formation

Fibrin deposition and removal are important processes in normal wound physiology. Impaired fibrinolysis can lead to an increase in susceptibility to micro-thrombus formation with subsequent tissue necrosis. On the other hand, Teh [38] has shown that slowly healing chronic ulcers that are infected are characterized by the presence of excessive fibrinolysis and excessive amounts of fibrin degradation products. Cherry and Ryan [39], studying the effect of ischemia on skin, found that occlusion of vessels by clotting was not an immediate effect of ischemia, but followed shedding of the damaged endothelium on reperfusion. Klenerman [40] observed that a period of ischemia resulted in increased blood fibrinolysis; but Larsson and Risberg [41], studying the human leg following ischemia and reperfusion during meniscectomy, noted that release of factor VIII from endothelial cells and, still later, impairment of tissue fibrinolysis occurred during the reperfusion phase. If exhaustion of fibrinolytic activators from endothelial cells explains to some extent the changes in decubitus ulcers, then other factors contributing to such exhaustion may be important. Damage to the epidermis results in a complete loss of fibrinolysis in the upper dermis some 6–12 h later; abrasion is particularly harmful [42].

The endothelial cell is normally equipped to control platelet aggregation by the generation of prostacyclin. Study of this and related phenomena is a rapidly growing field. It is clear that the interaction of mast cells, epithelial cells, and endothelial cells is an important element in this process. The provision of substrate by the epidermis for prostaglandin formation and the role of oxygen in determining which prostaglandin-like substance will be produced are matters not yet adequately studied. Similarly, the effect of these agents on the secretion of fibrinolytic enzymes by the endothelial cell, and heparin or other agents by the mast cell are also subjects to be explored in the future.

The leakiness of vessels damaged by ischemia enhances the localization of noxious circulating agents and leads in turn to damage induced by bacteria, immune complexes, and platelet aggregations. It is not surprising, therefore, that diseases such as septicemia and rheumatoid arthritis have a higher incidence of complicated decubitus ulcers [43].

Studies on repetitive injury highlight the heightened vulnerability of tissues that have experienced previous injury sufficient to cause exhaustion of fibrinolysis, an increase in vascular permeability, and blood stasis. The Shwartzmann phenomenon, gravitational stasis, the delayed skin flap, cold, and other types of injury qualify in this respect. Microcirculation of the skin is often considered in the context of blood flow alone, but interstitial fluid and lymphatic flow are also a part of the microcirculation. The metabolism of skin cells depends on these mechanisms as well, and failure to clear protein from tissue can cause great irritation and changes in interstitial osmotic pressure and cellular hydration. The manner in which the blood vascular system handles blood protein clearance when the lymphatics are impaired is also relevant to decubitus ulcers [15]. Lymphatic drainage from the skin depends on the orientation of the connective tissue fibers, and movement of solid elements between tissues is particularly important. Blood flow is rarely completely static in immobilized skin, but lymphatic flow is often completely so, especially when arterial pulsation is diminished as in the elderly, hypotensive, and atherosclerotic limb.

Conclusions

In the final analysis, decubitus ulcers result from an enormous failure of the blood supply. In young, healthy skin, this failure is almost all that is relevant. In the sick and aged, who are more susceptible to the development of decubitus ulcers, other more subtle factors contribute to the increased susceptibility. An understanding of these factors is more than an interesting academic exercise; it is in fact essential to success in the management of the patient.

References

1. Ryan TJ (1993) Wound healing in the developing world. Dermatol Clin 11:791–799
2. Groth KE (1942) Klinische Beobachtungen und exerimentelle Studien über die Entstehung des Dekubitus. Acta Chir Scand 87 [Suppl 77]:1
3. Daniel RK, Hall EJ, Macleod MK (1979) Pressure sores – a reappraisal. Ann Plast Surg 3:53–63
4. Constantian MB (1980) Aetiology: gross effects of pressure. In: Constantian MB (ed) Pressure ulcers: principles and techniques of management. Little Brown, Boston, pp 15–24
5. Kosiak M (1959) Aetiology and pathology of ischaemic ulcers. Arch Phys Med 40:62
6. Dinsdale SM (1973) Decubitus ulcers in swine: light and electron microscopy study of pathogenesis. Arch Phys Med Rehabil 54:51–59
7. Barton AA (1976) The pathogenesis of skin wounds due to pressure. In: Kenedi RM, Cowden JM, Scales JT (eds) Bedsore biomechanics University Park Press, Baltimore, pp 55–62
8. Larsen B, Holstein P, Lassen NA (1979) On the pathogenesis of bedsores. Scand J Plast Reconstr Surg 13:347–350
9. Manchot C (1889) Die Hautarterien des Menschlichen Körpers. Vogel, Leipzig

10. Daniel RK, Kerrigan CL (1979) Skin flaps: an anatomical and hemodynamic approach. Clin Plast Surg 6:181–200
11. Marinov G, Tzvetkova TZ (1976) About the microvascularization of the inferior limb skin in the cast of obliterating diseases. Folio Morphol 25:209
12. Marinov G, Tzvetkova TZ (1976) Age-related differentiation in the local peculiarities of the terminal vascular bed of the lower limb skin. Vert Anat Ges 71:689
13. Fagrell B (1977) The skin microcirculation and pathogenesis of ischemic necrosis and gangrene. Scand J Lab Clin Invest 37:473–476
14. Ryan TJ (1975) The lymphatics of the skin. In: Jarrett A (ed) Physiology and pathophysiology of the skin, vol 5. Academic, London
15. Ryan TJ (1995) Exchange and the mechanical properties of the skin; oncotic and hydrostatic forces controlled by blood supply and lymphatic drainage. Wound Repair Regen 3:258–264
16. Takeda T, Koyama T, Izawa Y, Makita T, Nakamura N (1992) Effects of malnutrition on development of experimental pressure sores. J Dermatol (Tokyo) 19:602–609
17. Telek G, Sinclair R, Ryan TJ, Cherry GW, Arnold F (1994) Do lymphocyte products contribute to wound failure? (Abstract) Wound Repair Regen 2:226
18. Bader DL, Barnhill RL, Ryan TJ (1986) Effect of externally applied skin surface forces on tissue vasculature. Arch Phys Med Rehabil 67:807–811
19. Gniadecka M, Gniadecki R, Serup J, Søndergaard J (1994) Skin mechanical properties present adaptation to man's upright position: in vitro studies of young and aged individuals. Acta Derm Venereol (Stockh) 74:188–190
20. Reddy NP (1990) Effects of mechanical stresses on lymph and interstitial fluid flows. In: Bader DL (ed) Pressure sores – clinical practice and scientific approach. Macmillan Scientific and Medical, London
21. Yager DR, Chen S, Diegelmann RF, Cohen IK (1995) Human pressure ulcers: levels of α_2-macroglobulin is inversely related to the ability to degrade exogenous peptide growth factors (abstract). Wound Repair Regen 3:108
22. Selye H (1967) Ischaemic necrosis; prevention by stress. Science 156:1262
23. Palmer B (1972) The influence of stress on the survival of experimental skin flaps. Scand J Plast Reconstr Surg 6:110–113
24. Palmer B (1970) Sympathetic denervation and reinnervation of cutaneous blood vessels following surgery. Scand J Plast Reconstr Surg 4:93–99
25. Myers M, Cherry G (1968) Enhancement of survival in devascularised pedicles by the use of phenoxybenzamine. Plast Reconstr Surg 41:254–260
26. Barron J, Veall N, Arnott DG (1951) The measurement of the local clearance of radioactive sodium in tubed skin pedicles. Br J Plast Surg 4:16–27
27. Liebow AA (1963) Collateral circulation. Handbook of physiology: circulation II. American Physiological Society, Bethesda, p 1257
28. Trendelenberg U (1963) Supersensitivity and subsensitivity of sympathetic amines. Pharmacol Rev 15:225
29. Malfros T, Sachs C (1965) Direct studies on the disappearance of the transmitter and the changes in the uptake storage mechanisms of degenerating adrenergic nerves. Acta Physiol Scand 64:211–223
30. Willms-Kretschmer K, Majno G (1969) Ischemia of the skin – electron microscopic study of vascular injury. Am J Pathol 54:327–353
31. Milton SH (1972) Experimental studies on island flaps. II. Ischaemia and delay. Plast Reconstr Surg 49:444–447
32. Milton SH (1969) The effects of "delay" on the survival of experimental pedicled skin flaps. Br J Plast Reconst Surg 22:244–252
33. Myers M, Cherry G (1971) Differences in the delay phenomenon in the rabbit, rat and pig. Plast Reconstr Surg 47:73–78
34. Burton AC (1939) The range and variation of the blood flow in the human fingers. Am J Physiol 127:437–443
35. Feigl E (1974) The arterial system. In: Ruch T, Patton H (eds) Physiology and biophysics. Saunders, Philadelphia, pp 117–128

36. Gordon L, Buncke JJ, Townsend JJ (1976) Histological changes in skeletal muscle after temporary independent occlusion of arterial and venous supply. Plast Reconstr Surg 57:133–143
37. Cherry G, Faller R, Manders E, Grabb WC (1980) Functional microcirculatory changes after flap elevation – possible factor in flap failure. Plast Surg Forum 3:206
38. Teh BT (1979) Why do skin grafts fail? Plast Reconstr Surg 63:323–332
39. Cherry GW, Ryan TJ, Ellis J (1974) Decreased fibrolysis in reperfused ischemic tissue. Thromb Diathes Haemorrh 32:559–664
40. Klenermann K (1977) Prophylaxis against deep vein thrombosis. Lancet I:970
41. Larsson J, Risberg B (1977) Ischemia-induced changes in tissue fibrinolysis in human legs. Biblio Anat 15:556
42. Ryan TJ, Nighioka K, Dawber RPR (1971) Epithelial-endothelial interactions in the control of inflammation through fibrinolysis. Br J Dermatol 84:501–515
43. Kanan MW, Ryan TJ (1976) The localization of granulomatous diseases and vasculitis in the nasal mucosa. Maj Probl Dermatol 7:195

6 Clinical Picture

The decubitus spectrum extends from an innocent-appearing reddened cutaneous area to a catastrophic ulcer that involves destruction of skin, subcutaneous tissue, muscle, and bone [1]. Whether the lesion is referred to as a decubitus ulcer, pressure sore, bedsore, or even euphemistically as a torsion stress injury, it is evidence that a significant interruption in the integrity of the skin has occurred [2].

The decubitus ulcer is a definitive entity, *sui generis*, and is not to be regarded as some ill-defined hodgepodge of necrosis and debris contained in a hole in the skin. With practice, the clinician can learn to identify each step in the ulcer development pathway. Mastery of the elementary dermatologic skills essential to the identification of these steps will often permit timely intervention and allow healing to take place with little or no permanent damage. Alleviation of pressure is essential. Clinicians should be aware that significant pressure operational for any length of time may result in damage not readily recognizable at first and that deceptively small cutaneous defects may be associated with massive destruction of underlying tissue (the volcano effect) [3].

The decubitus pathway begins with blanchable erythema which, unchecked, progresses step by step to nonblanchable erythema, decubitus dermatitis, early ulcer, and chronic ulcer. Eschar/gangrene presentations belong to a special destruction category to be considered separately. The morphology of each phase of the decubitus pathway is a reflection of the nature and extent of tissue damage. Typical presentations can be rendered atypical when secondary bacterial infections [4] or allergic contact dermatitis from topical medications complicate the picture [5], or the patient's immune system has been compromised [6, 7] (Fig. 1).

Patient Types

Patients most susceptible to decubitus development fall into four categories:
1. The spinal cord injury patient: in good health prior to the injury, this individual usually retains adequate regeneration capability and will heal once bed and chair pressure alleviation measures are in place [8].

Fig. 1. Decubitus ulcer pathway

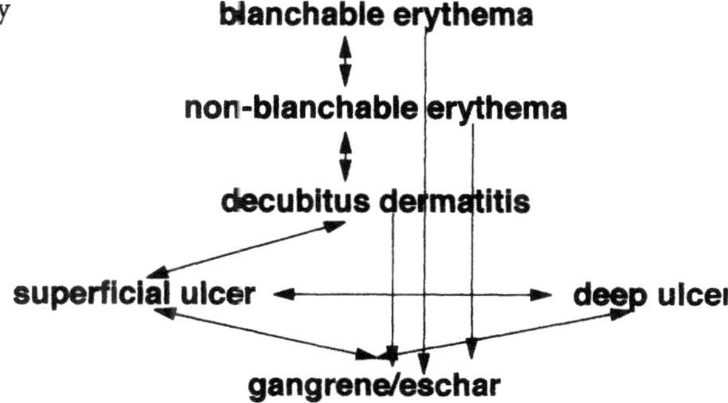

2. The neurologic patient: aside from the neurologic impediment, bodily functions and wound healing capabilities are largely intact.
3. The elderly or immune-depressed patient: multiple organ systems are failing; wound healing capacity is significantly or profoundly diminished [5, 6, 9, 10].
4. The surgical patient: patients undergoing lengthy surgical operations, particularly cardiac and neurologic procedures, sometimes develop decubitus ulcers, particularly in the area over the sacrum. Differentiation between decubitus and an electrical burn is difficult in these cases [11–13]. In rare instances a decubitus ulcer may be associated in situ with a thermal burn [14].

Areas at Risk

Decubitus ulcers can occur on any area of the body. The position of the patient in the bed or the chair will usually determine the location of the ulcer.

Common Locations

1. In supine patients, areas overlying the sacrum, ischial tuberosities, dorsal thorax, the C7 prominence, elbows, heels, posterior aspects of the calf, and the occiput are the usual sites for development of decubitus ulcers. The sacral area ranks number one [15, 16].
2. In the prone patient, the common sites are the iliac crest, elbows, knees, anterior aspects of the thighs, anterior chest, and dorsum of the feet and ankles.
3. In patients in the lateral position, sites most often affected are the area over the greater trochanter of the femur, the lateral surface of the knee, the ischium, the external malleolus, the shoulder, ear, and side of the head.
4. In patients in the sitting position, the usual locations are the areas over the ischial tuberosities, the sacrum, coccyx, scapulae, popliteal areas, heels, and the plantar surfaces of the feet.

Less Common Locations

Patients on support systems are susceptible to the development of ulcers on the heels and occiput. Levitation is an unachievable goal; pressure has to be allocated to some area [17, 18].

Ulcers may also occur at the site of application of a doughnut cushion. This outmoded device is unable to distribute pressure over an area wide enough to prevent damage.

Unusual locations such as the temple, mastoid area, or inner aspect of the thigh suggest pressure from extraneous objects – the frames of glasses, hearing aids, catheters, surgical appliances, and the like. A continually clenched fist may result in an ulcer on the palm [19].

The Decubitus Ulcer Spectrum

Blanchable Erythema

The initial phase in the decubitus ulcer spectrum is blanchable erythema. It begins as an ill-defined erythematous patch at the point of pressure and varies in color from pale pink to bright red. Digital compression produces total blanching, and the erythema reappears promptly when the finger is lifted. Occasionally a slight edematous elevation can be seen when the lesion is cross-lighted. Temperature elevation may be perceived with the back of the examiner's hand, an observation of considerable importance in dealing with dark-skinned patients in whom milder degrees of redness may be masked by cutaneous pigment. Tenderness and pain may be prominent when the patient is alert and/or sensory innervation is intact.

When pressure is removed from areas of blanchable erythema the skin usually returns to normal within 24 h. Failure to relieve pressure leads to nonblanchable erythema, phase II in the decubitus ulcer spectrum.

Nonblanchable Erythema

Nonblanchable erythema is a sequel to the initial phase and represents a more profound alteration in the underlying cutaneous vessels. The color of the disease site is more intense, more saturated, and varies from bright red to cyanotic while in darkly pigmented patients, the localized area may become bluish or purplish. Borders of the area are usually sharply defined; configuration is irregular, sometimes conforming to the shape of an underlying bony prominence, or to the outlines of an external object that has exerted pressure on the skin. The characteristic feature of this phase is the failure of the erythema to fade to any extent on digital pressure. When sensory innervation is functional, which is unusual in these cases, the lesion is painful and tender. It is often cool to the touch, and the skin in the area may be soft, edematous, or slightly indurated.

When treatment is instituted without delay, the changes are reversible, clearing in 1–3 weeks. If pressure is not relieved, progress to the ulcer or eschar/gangrene phase may occur. Cyanotic lesions usually progress directly to eschar/gangrene without passing through the phase of decubitus dermatitis.

Decubitus Dermatitis

Decubitus dermatitis represents a further deterioration in tissue at the nonblanchable erythema site. Scaling appears and sometimes vesiculation. Bullae may form and, when broken, may be accompanied by serous and hemorrhagic crusting. Initially, vesicles may be small and easily overlooked. Bullae may be oval or oddly configured, conforming to the shape of an object in contact with the skin – a catheter, for example. A bulla that occupies the entire area of a pre-existing nonblanchable erythema may appear to be arising from normal skin. The bullae of decubitus are not easily broken, an indication of their deep subepidermal location. When sensory innervation is functional, pain and tenderness are prominent.

Two to four weeks are normally required for healing, which can occur without permanent damage, although a favorable outcome – failure to progress to ulceration – is less certain than in the earlier phases.

Decubitus Ulcer

It is convenient to subdivide the ulcer phase into superficial and deep.

The superficial ulcer is an erosion, an area of nonblanchable erythema or decubitus dermatitis from which the epidermis has been lost. Vesicles or bullae have ruptured or have been rubbed off, exposing the dermis. The ulcer is shallow, with indistinct borders and an irregular shape. Fresh lesions often display a glistening erythematous base, while older examples are covered by a thin, adherent, yellowish membrane. The ulcer is characteristically surrounded by a zone of decubitus dermatitis or nonblanchable erythema that varies considerably in width.

Failure to relieve pressure over an early ulcer results inevitably in the development of the true pressure sore, the deep decubitus ulcer. The skin surrounding an established ulcer is erythematous, blanches very little on pressure, and sometimes exhibits a mottled pigmentation intermixed with redness. It is warm, indurated, and fixed to underlying tissue.

The average decubitus ulcer is 5–12 cm in diameter. Borders may be overhanging or thickened to form a fibrous ring. The size of the ulcer visible at the skin surface can be most deceiving; a small ulcer sometimes opens into a much larger necrotic cavity beneath (the "volcano effect"). The base of the deep ulcer is usually flat and dusky red in color; it does not bleed easily. Decubitus ulcers vary in depth, from destruction at the level of subcutaneous fat to destruction deep enough to include muscle, tendons, joint capsules, and sometimes bone. Wide undermining with extensive fat necrosis is common.

Nonblanchable erythema in the skin surrounding an ulcer indicates that the lesion is enlarging.

Eschar/Gangrene

A black eschar develops as the result of full thickness (skin to muscle or bone) tissue death within a relatively short space of time. It is a sharply marginated, tough, adherent, black membranous form of dry gangrene that is fixed to the structures beneath. Characteristically the black eschar is painless and non-tender, regardless of the patient's mentation or neurologic status. The gangrenous area may be surrounded by a zone of nonblanchable erythema, which may in turn be ringed by an outer zone of blanchable erythema.

Differential Diagnosis

Blanchable Erythema

- First-degree burn
- Contact dermatitis
- Cutaneous candidiasis
- Miliaria

Decubitus Dermatitis

- Second-degree burn
- Herpes simplex
- Immune bullous disease
- Diabetic bullosis
- Contact dermatitis

Black Eschar

- Septicemia
- Coumarin skin necrosis

Ulcer

- Ischiorectal abscess
- Pilonidal cyst
- Neoplasm
- Vasculitits, rheumatoid nodule
- Deep mycosis
- Pyoderma gangrenosum
- Venous stasis
- Arteriosclerosis
- Factitial

The diagnosis of a decubitus ulcer is usually straightforward. Blanchable and nonblanchable erythema may be confused with a fixed drug eruption, first-degree burn, miliaria rubra, contact dermatitis, candidosis, or herpes simplex. Decubitus dermatitis may resemble contact or nummular dermatitis. Bullous forms may suggest bullous pemphigoid, diabetic bullosis, or contact dermatitis. The bullae and subsequent ulceration characteristic of carbon monoxide poisoning would also have to be considered [20].

The decubitus ulcer itself may resemble ulcers of venous stasis, arteriolar compromise, pilonidal cyst, neoplasms, rheumatoid nodules, vasculitis, or pyoderma gangrenosum. The diagnosis of decubitus ulcer depends on the recognition and assessment by the clinician of the role played by pressure in the induction of the lesion [21]. Atypical ulcers suggest malignancy or factitial causes [22, 23]. In eschar/gangrene presentations, septicemia, coumadin- or heparin-induced necrosis, calciphylaxis, and ecthyma gangrenosum should be considered.

Complications

The much-feared development of squamous cell carcinoma in decubitus ulcers is in fact rare [23].

The most significant complication is infection, and the diagnosis is sometimes difficult to make. Infections usually present with purulent, foul-smelling drainage from an ulcer surrounded by erythematous, indurated, tender tissue, but in some cases changes are more subtle, with the typical signs much diminished. Fever and leukocytosis are usually restricted to severe infections [4].

Unusually destructive ulcers may be associated with gas gangrene or sepsis [24]. The infected area may erode into adjacent tissue, with the development of fistulae to the skin surface or into neighboring organs [25]. Osteomyelitis can occur [26]. Computed tomographic (CT) scans or magnetic resonance imaging (MRI) may be necessary to confirm the diagnosis. Bone biopsy is useful, both for diagnostic confirmation and for identification of the bacteria involved.

References

1. Yarkony GM (1994) Pressure ulcers: a review. Arch Phys Med Rehabil 75:908–917
2. Parish LC, Witkowski JA, Millikan LE (1988) Cutaneous torsion stress alias the decubitus ulcer: a felony. Int J Dermatol 27:375–376
3. Witkowski JA, Parish LC (1992) Diagnosis and management of pressure ulcers. In: Moschella S, Hurley HJ (eds) Dermatology. Saunders, Philadelphia, pp 2237–2250
4. Parish LC, Witkowski JA (1989) The infected decubitus ulcer. Int J Dermatol 28:643–647
5. Parish LC, Witkowski JA (1994) Chronic wounds: myths about decubitus ulcers. Int J Dermatol 33:623–624
6. Witkowski JA, Parish LC (1993) Skin failure and the pressure ulcer. Decubitus 6(5):4
7. Mawson AR, Siddiqui FH, Biundo JJ Jr (1993) Enhancing host resistance to pressure ulcers: a new approach to prevention. Prev Med 22:433–450
8. Ditunno JF Jr, Formal CS (1994) Chronic spinal cord injury. N Engl J Med 330:550–556

9. De Conno F, Ventafridda V, Saita L (1991) Skin problems in advanced and terminal cancer patients. J Pain Symptom Manage 6:247–256

10. Spoelhof GD, Ide K (1993) Pressure ulcers in nursing home patients. Am Fam Physician 47:1207–1215

11. Steward TP, Magnano SJ (1988) Burns or pressure ulcers in the surgical patient? Decubitus 1:36–40

12. Papantonio CT, Wallop JM, Kolodner KB (1994) Sacral ulcers following cardiac surgery: incidence and risks. Adv Wound Care 7:24–36

13. Kemp MG, Keithley JK, Smith DW, Morreal B (1990) Factors that contribute to pressure ulcer in surgical patients. Res Nursing Health 13:293–301

14. Calvin M (1995) Thermal burns in the elderly: classification and pathophysiology. J Geriatr Dermatol 3:149–157

15. Versluysen M (1986) How elderly patients with femoral fracture develop pressure ulcer in hospital. BMJ 292:1311–1313

16. Teasell R, Dittmer DK (1993) Complications of immobilization and bed rest. Part 2: other complications. Can Fam Physician 39:1440–1442, 1445–1446

17. Parish LC, Witkowski JA (1980) Clinitron therapy and the decubitus ulcer: preliminary dermatologic studies. Int J Dermatol 19:517–518

18. Pase MN (1994) Pressure relief devices, risk factors, and development of pressure ulcers in elderly patients with limited mobility. Adv Wound Care 7:38–42

19. Parish LC, Witkowksi JA, Crissey JT (1989) Unusual aspects of the decubitus ulcer. Decubitus 1:22–24

20. Arndt KA, Mihm MC, Parrish JA (1973) Bullae: a cutaneous sign of a variety of neurologic diseases. J Invest Dermatol 60:312–320

21. Parish LC, Witkowski JA (1990) Leg ulcers due to miscellaneous causes. Clin Dermatol 8(3,4):150–156

22. Lyell A (1979) Cutaneous artifactual disease. J Am Acad Dermatol 1:391–407

23. Grotting JC, Bunkis J, Vasconzez LO (1987) Pressure sore carcinoma. Ann Plast Surg 18:527–532

24. Shibuya H, Terashi H, Kurata S et al. (1994) Gas gangrene following sacral pressure sores. J Dermatol 21:518–523

25. Muburak SJ, Owen CA, Hargens AR et al. (1978) Acute compartment syndromes: diagnosis and treatment with the aid of the wick catheter. J Bone Joint Surg 60:1091–1095

26. Darouiche RO, Landon GC, Klima M, Musher DM, Markowski J (1994) Osteomyelitis associated with pressure sores (see comments). Arch Intern Med 154:753–758

7 Atlas

Decubitus Ulcer Pathway

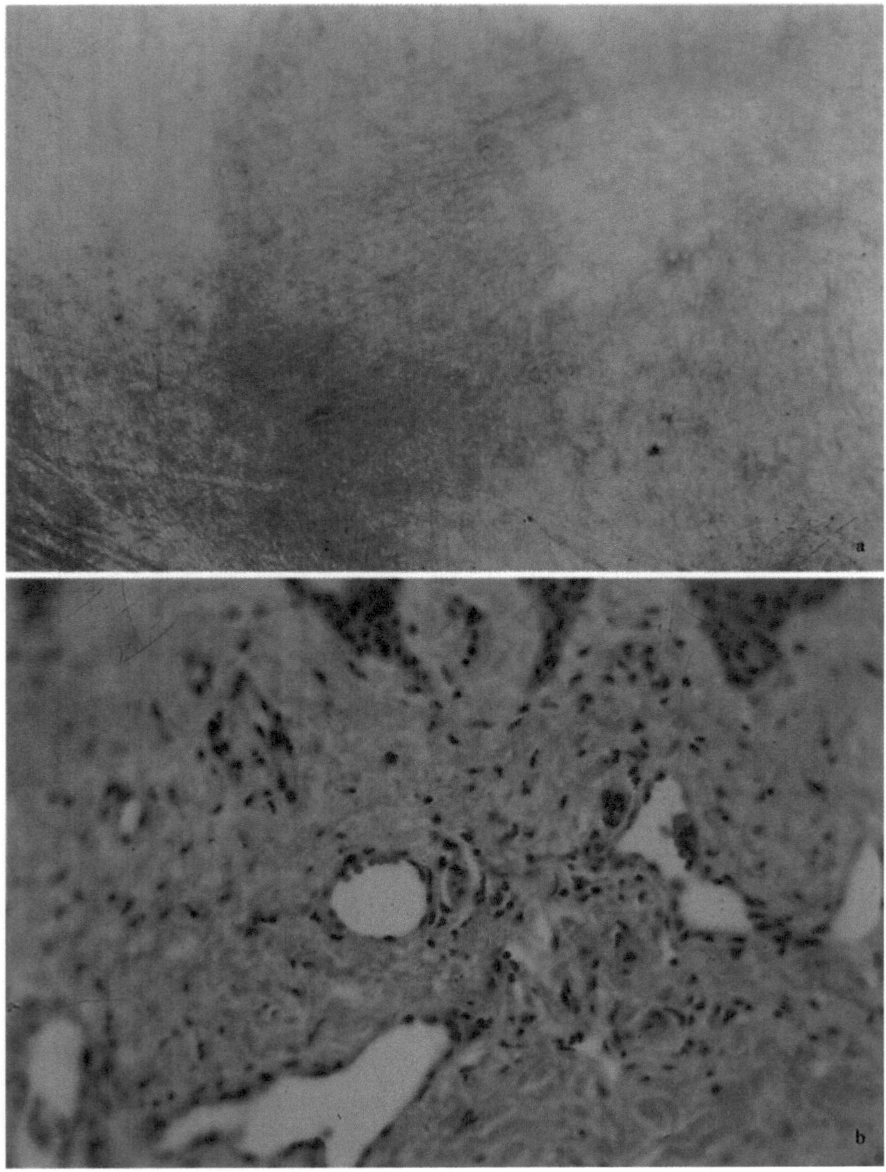

Fig. 1a–d. Blanchable erythema – redness which disappears on finger pressure. **a** Reappearance of normal skin within 24 h; **b** edema, vascular dilatation, and perivascular round cell infiltrate

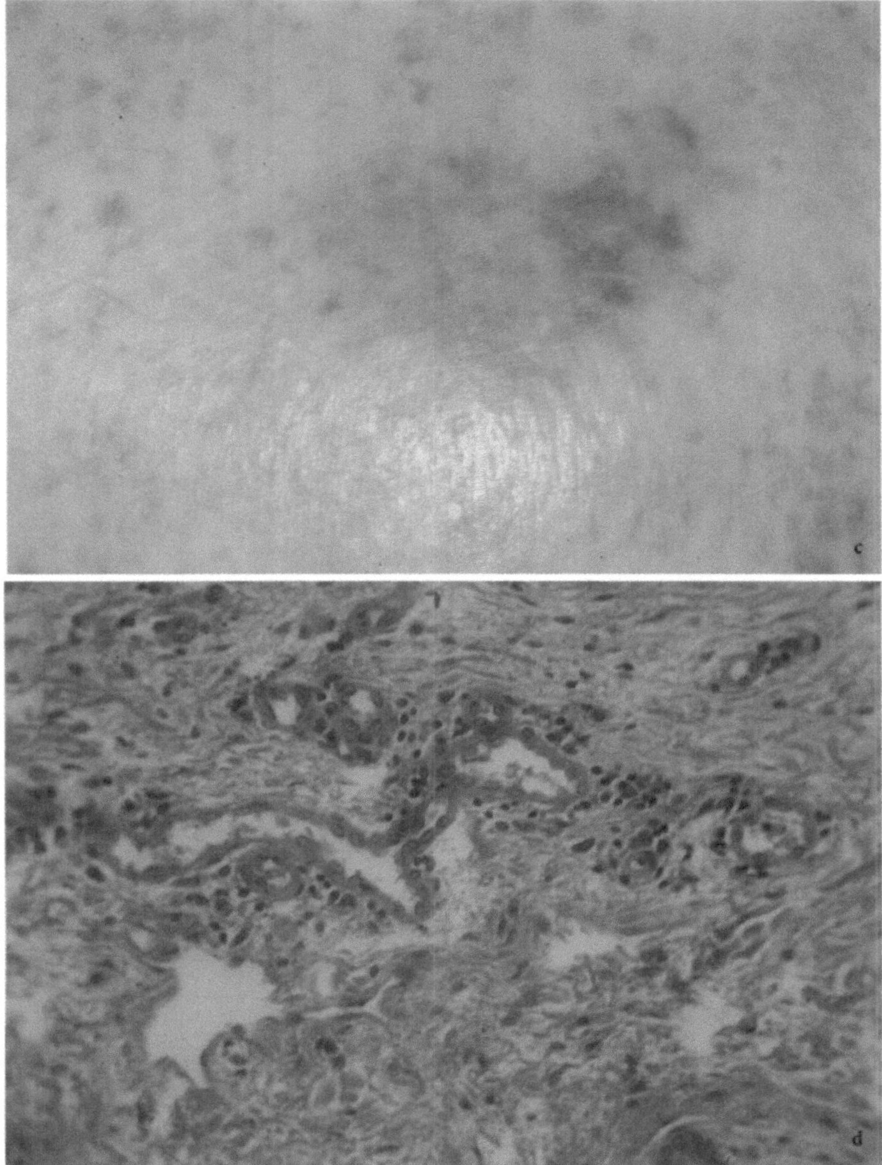

Fig. 1. c Lack of return to normalcy within 24 h; d edema, vascular dilatation, swollen endothelial cells, platelet aggregate, and fibrin thrombi, and perivascular round cell infiltrate

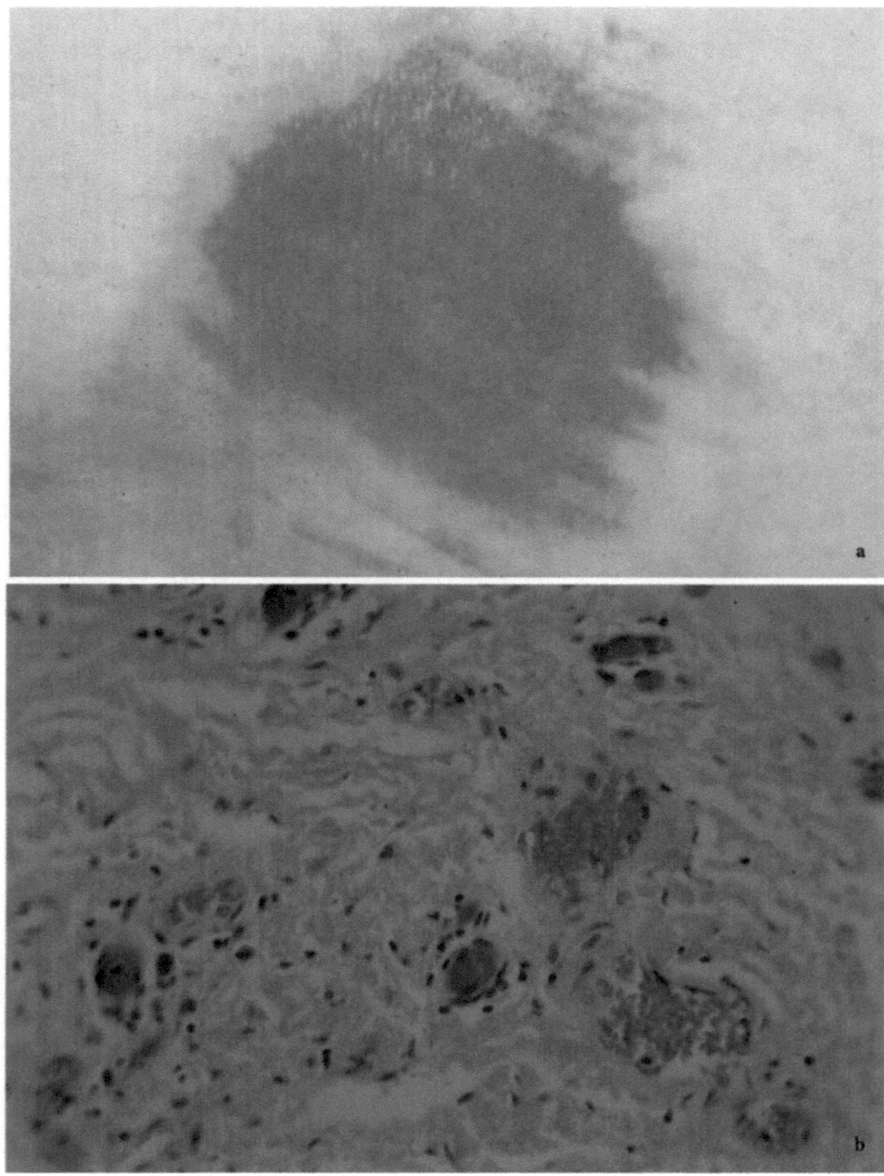

Fig. 2a–d. Nonblanchable erythema – redness which does not disappear on finger pressure. **a** Bright red color; **b** erythrocyte engorgement, vascular dilatation, edema and perivascular round cell infiltrate

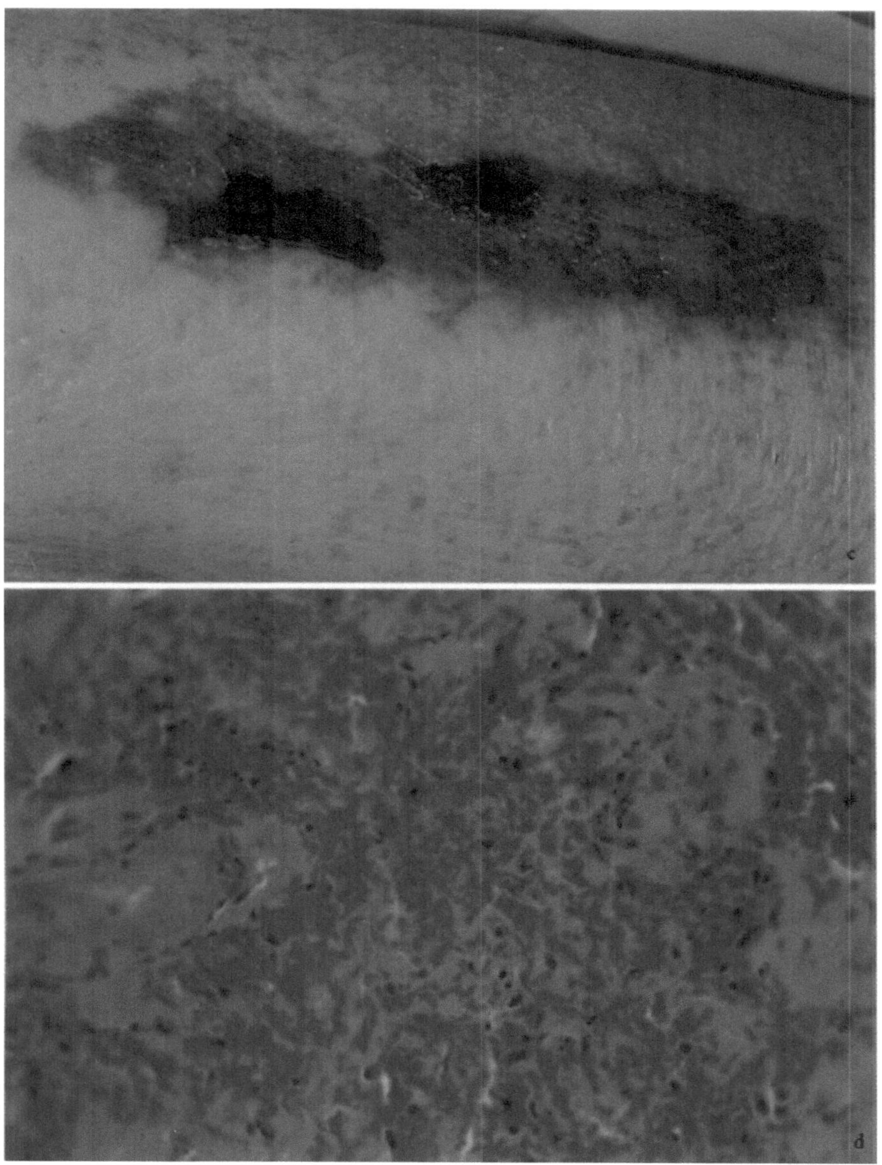

Fig. 2. c Purple color; **d** hemorrhage, erythrocyte engorgement and perivascular round cell infiltrate

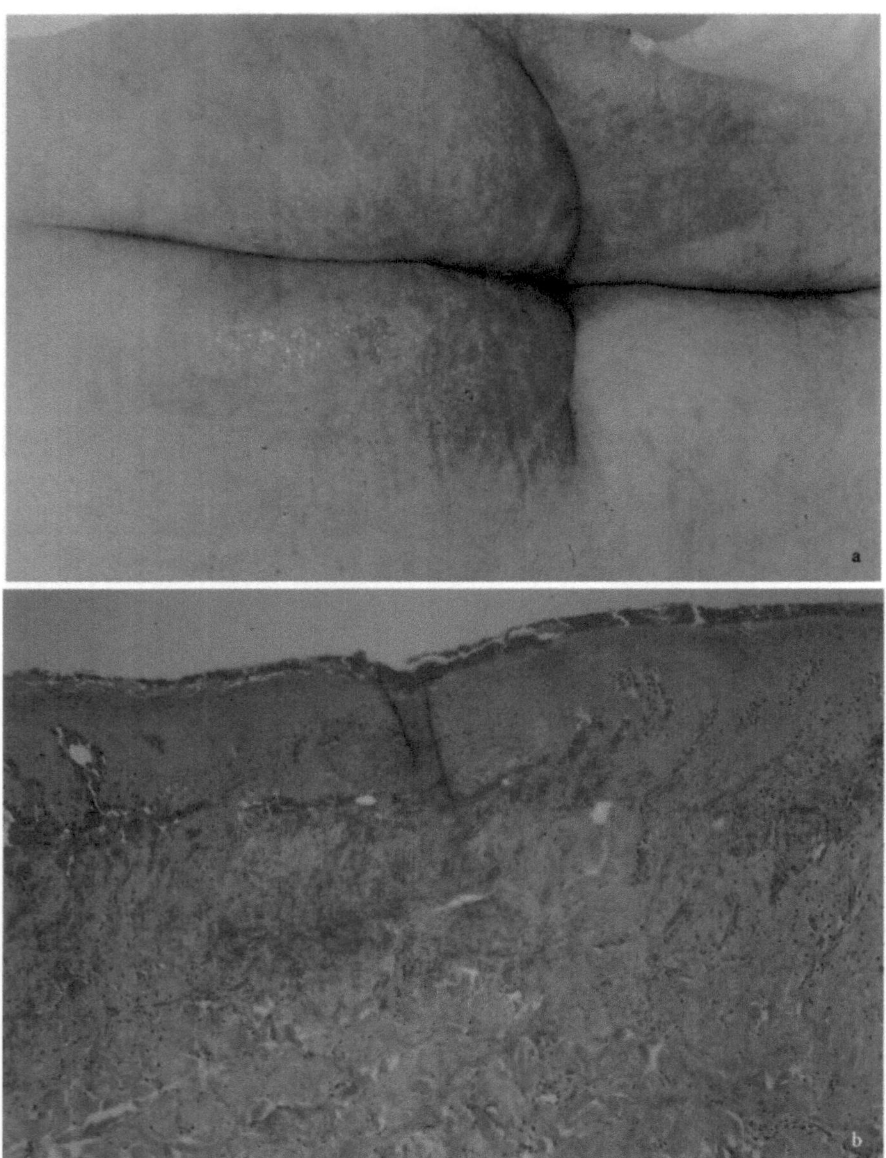

Fig. 3 a–d. Decubitus dermatitis – various inflammatory responses. **a** Erythema and scaling; **b** epidermal necrosis, edema, and hemorrhage

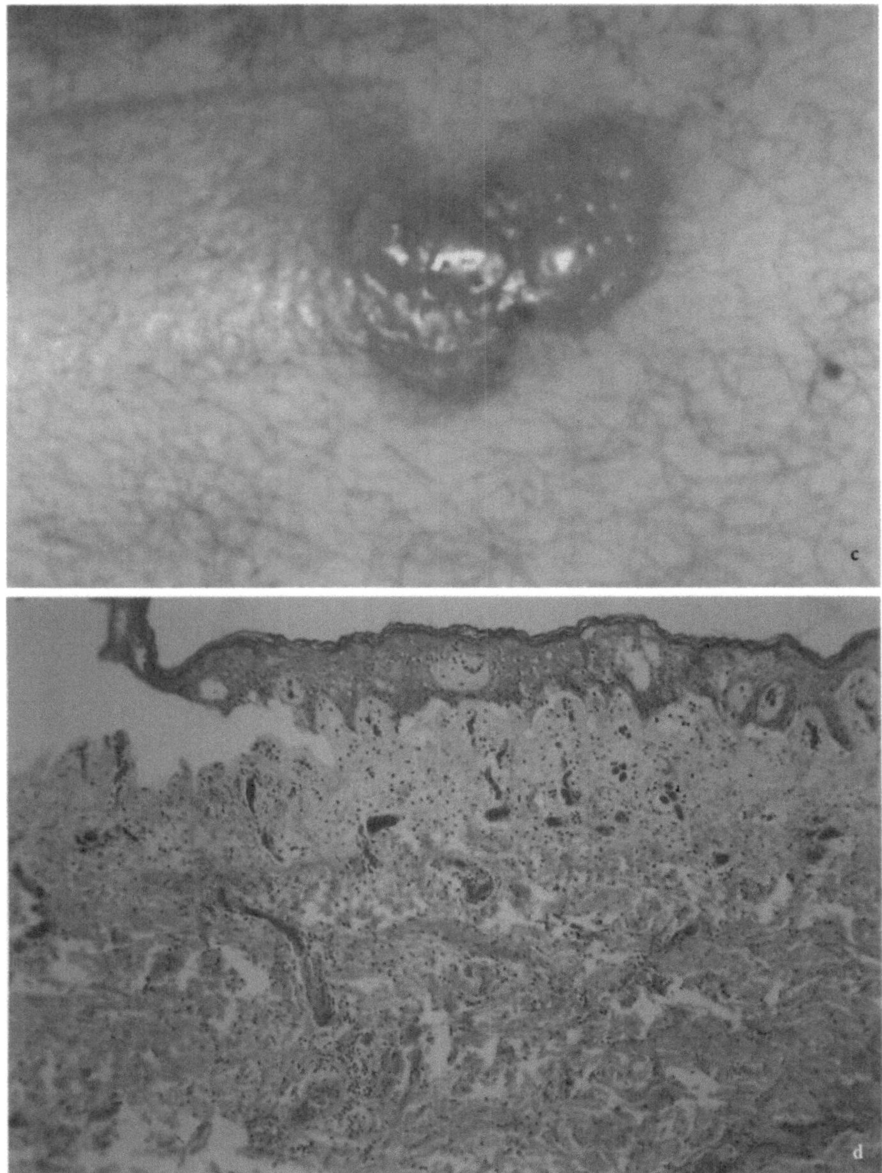

Fig. 3.c Vesicular and bullous formation; **d** focal necrosis of the epidermis, dermal–epidermal separation and erythrocyte engorgement

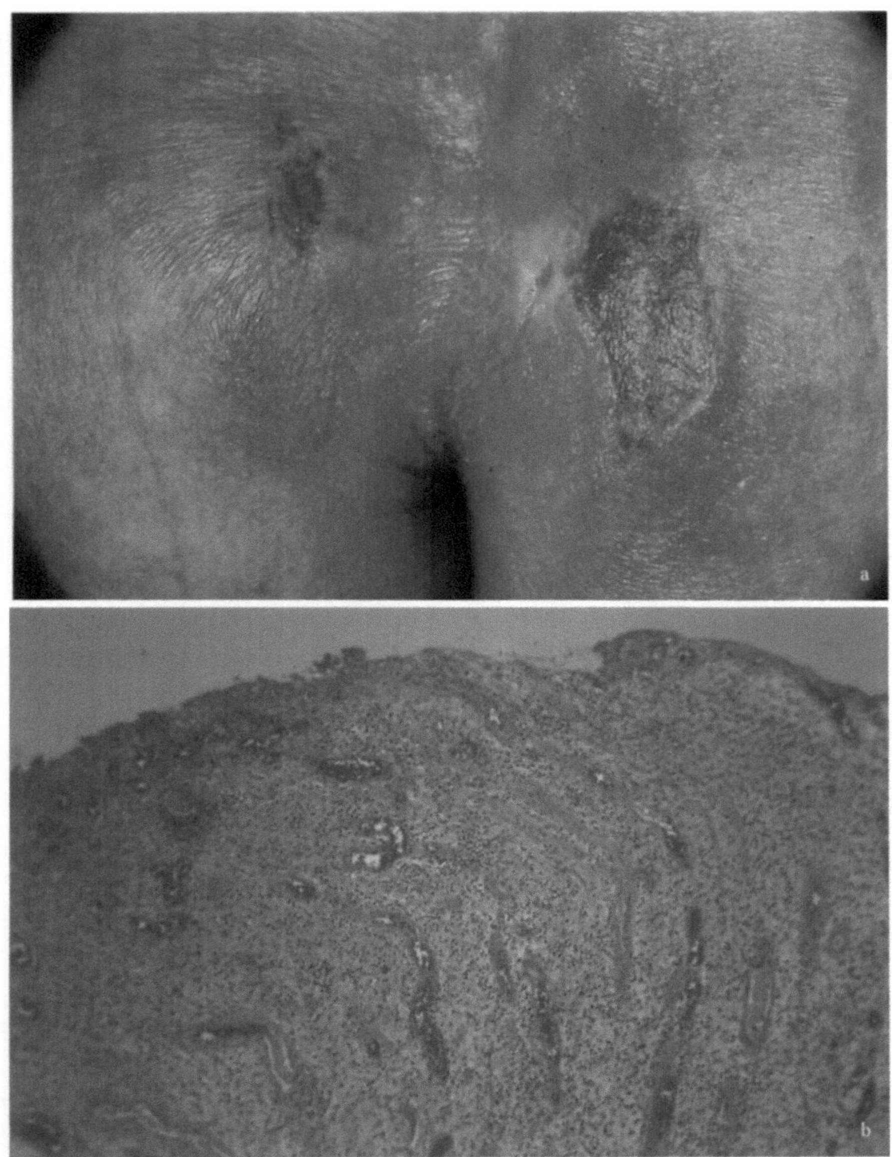

Fig. 4a–f. Decubitus ulcer – superficial to deep ulcerations. **a** Superficial ulcer (early) – loss of epidermis; **b** loss of epidermis, erythrocyte engorgement, vascular dilatation, and polymorpholeukocyte and lymphocyte infiltration

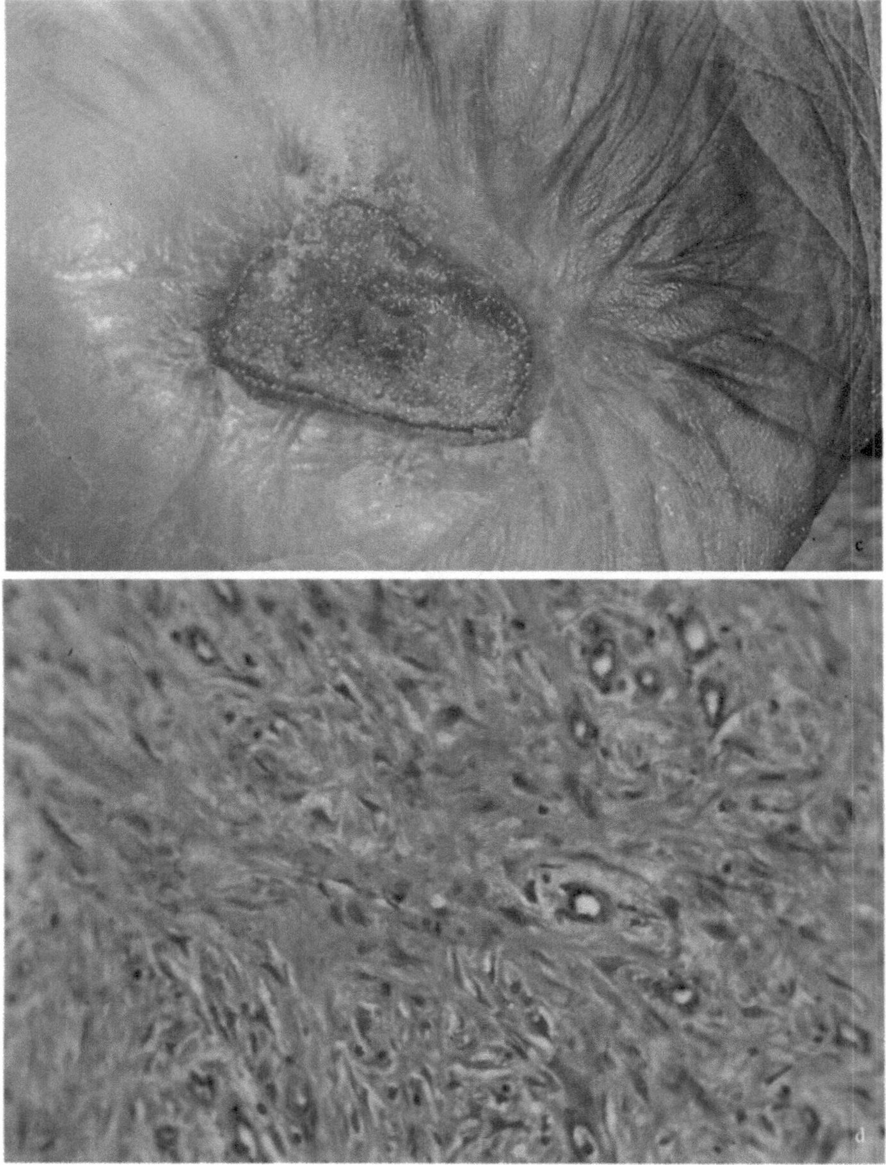

Fig. 4. c Chronic ulcer – dried-out ulcer bed; d extensive fibrosis surrounding groups of capillaries

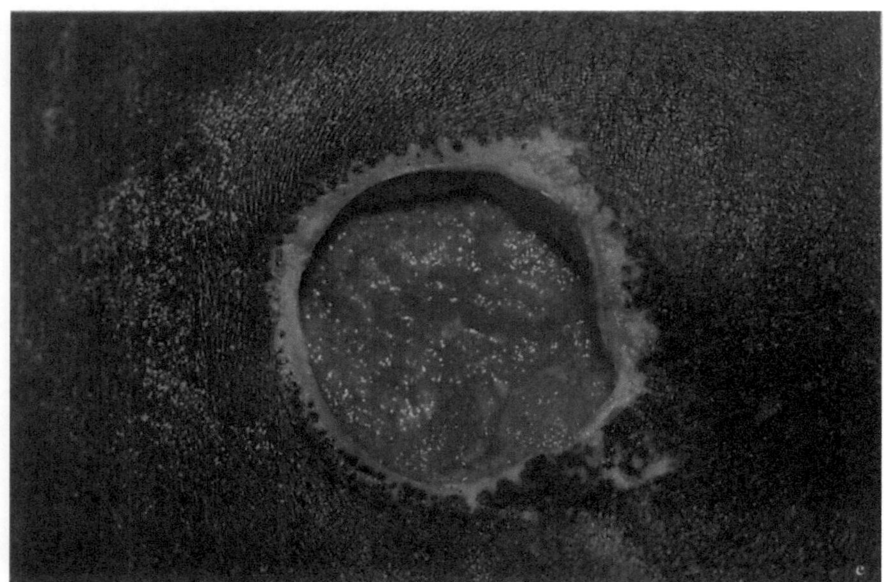

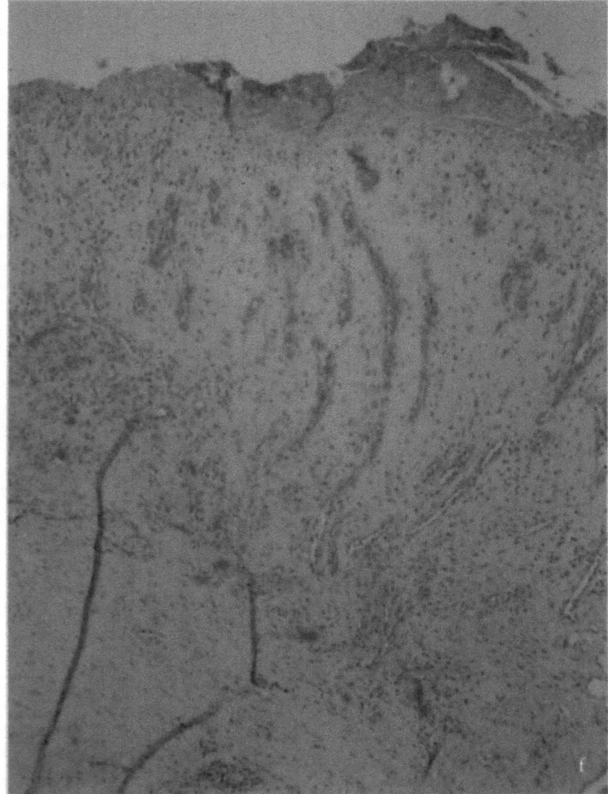

Fig. 4. e Healing ulcer – clean granulation base; **f** vertically oriented capillaries

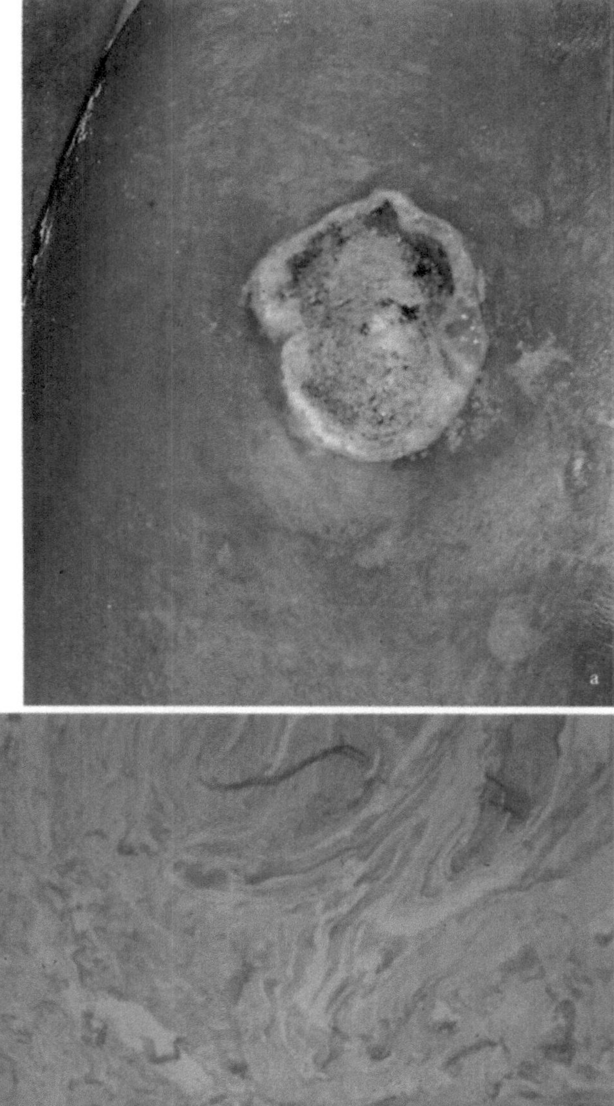

Fig. 5a,b. Eschar/gangrene – marked tissue necrosis. **a** Adherent black membrane; **b** coagulation necrosis

Unusual Observations

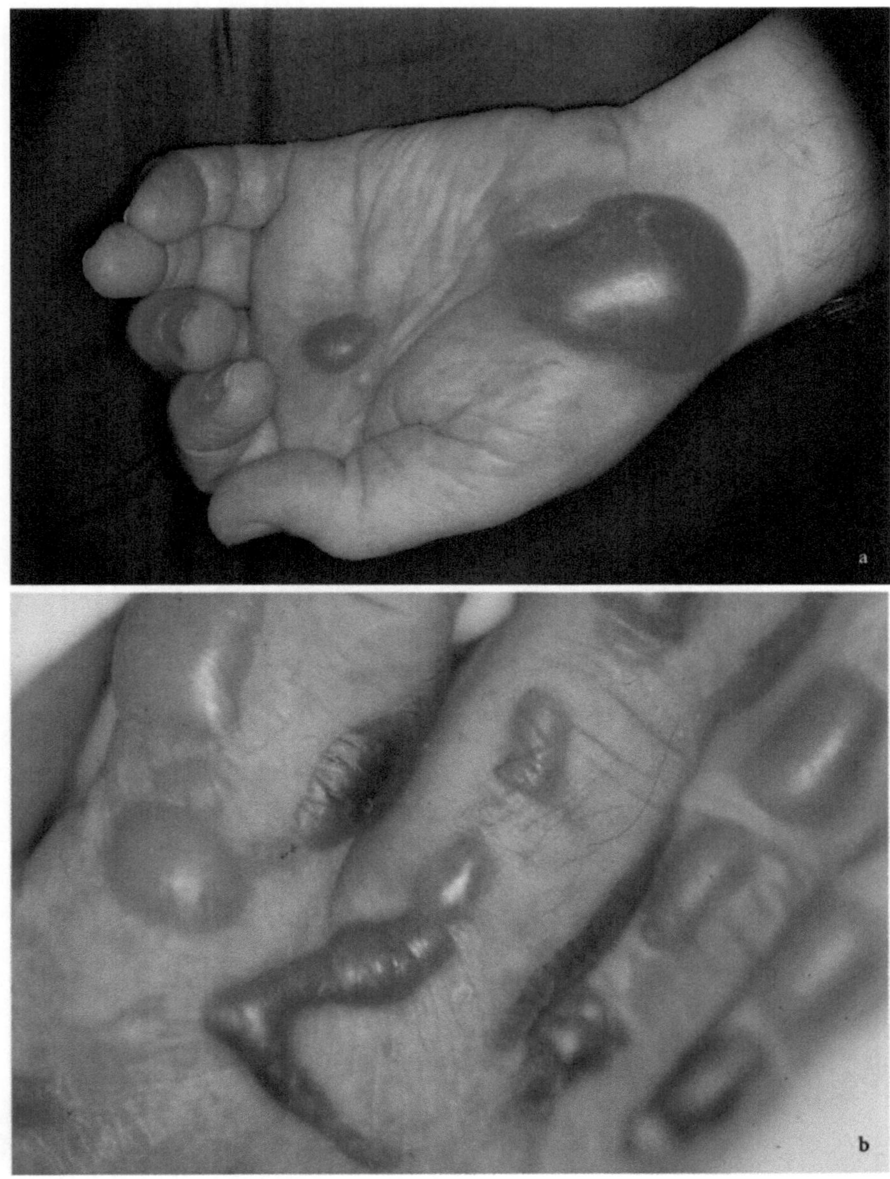

Fig. 6a,b. Pressure bullae. **a** Palm; **b** fingers

Fig. 7a-c. Eschar/gangrene. **a** Nose;
b scalp

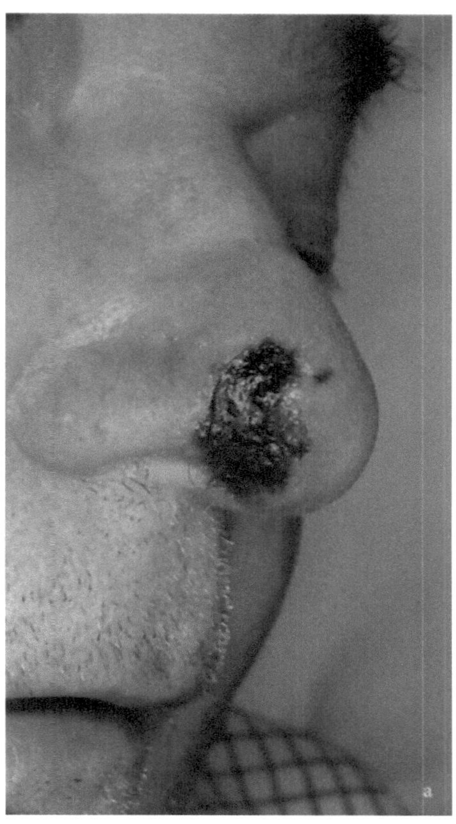

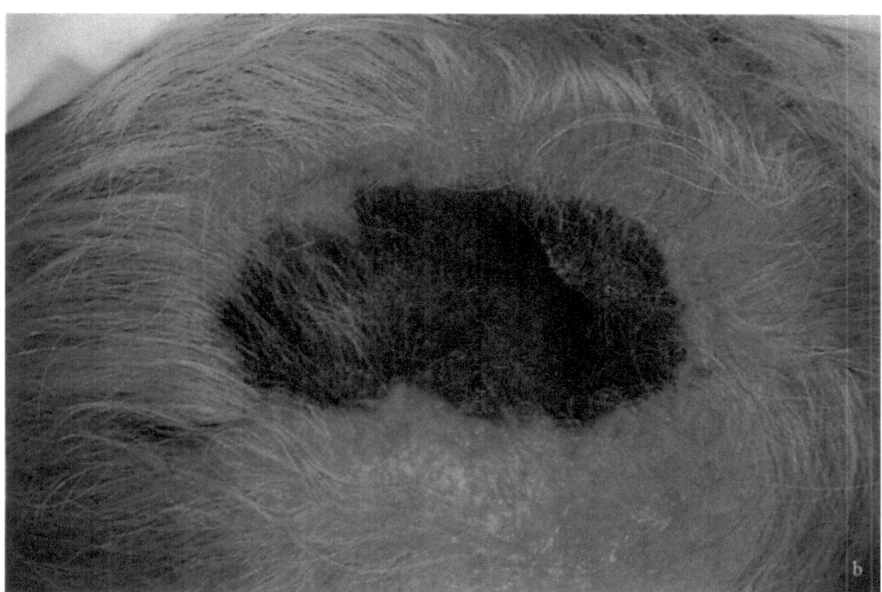

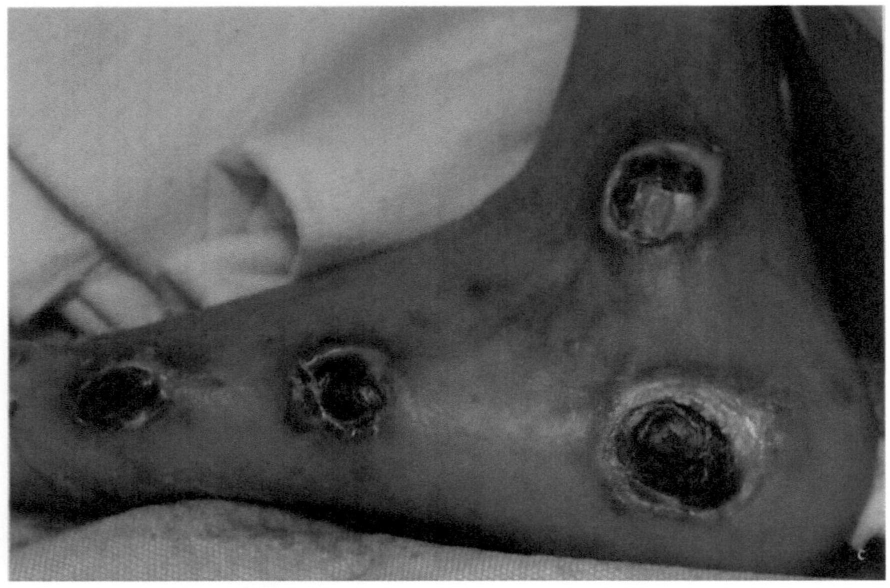

Fig. 7. c Foot and ankle

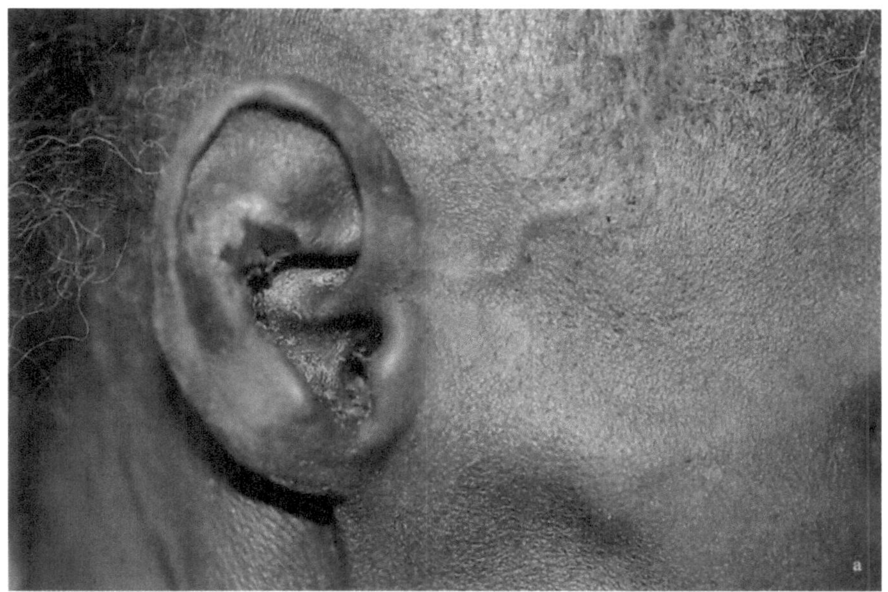

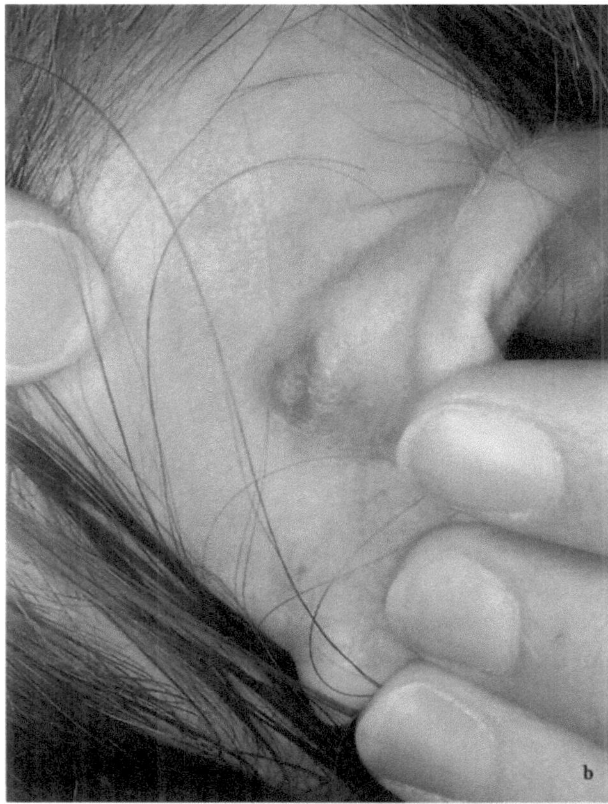

Fig. 8a,b. Decubitus ulcer, superficial. **a** Ear – helix; **b** ear – posterior aspect

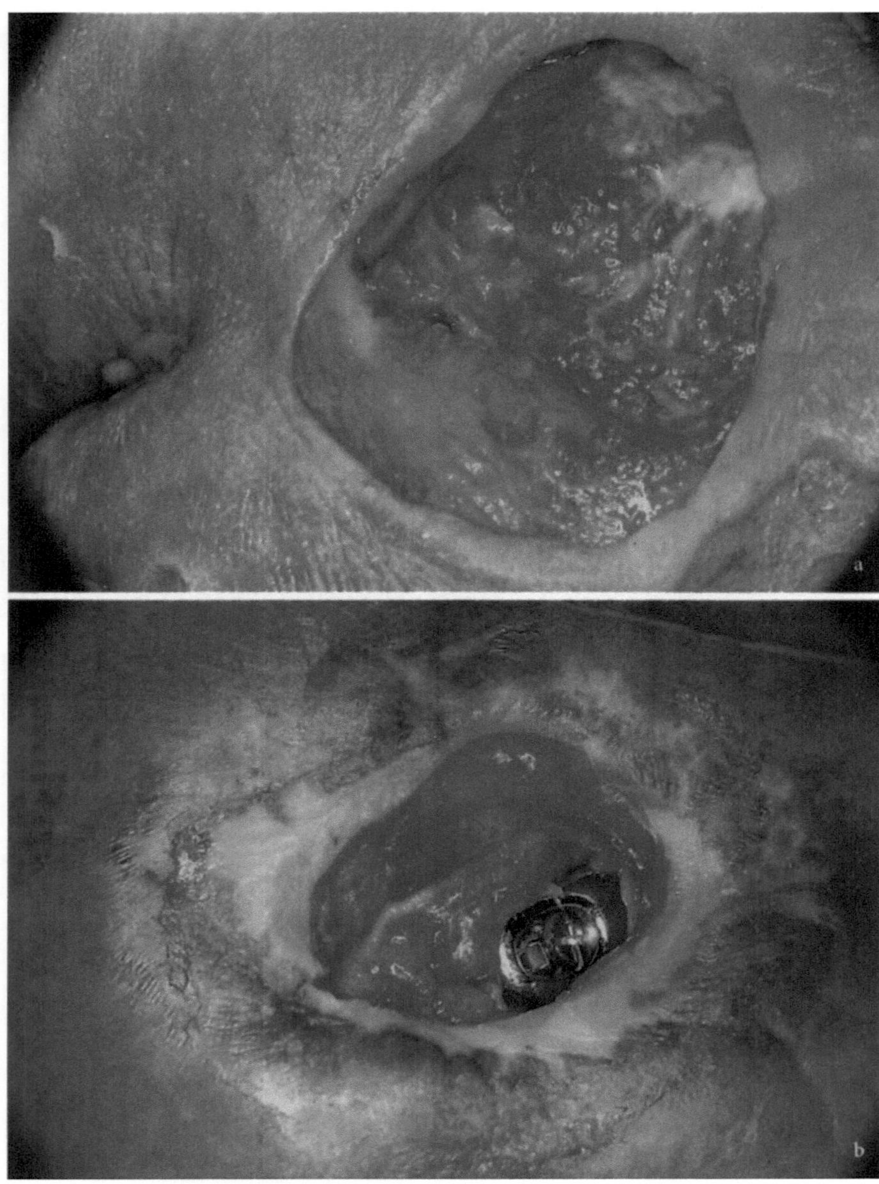

Fig. 9a,b. Decubitus ulcer, deep. **a** Rectal fistula appearance; **b** orthopedic implant revealed

8 Histopathology

The exchange process necessary for life takes place in the capillaries at a pressure of 13–32 mmHg. Pressure on the tissue which partially or completely occludes the capillaries impedes the inflow and outflow of blood. When this occurs for an extended period of time, tissue ischemia and hypoxia result. The lack of oxygen causes a shift from aerobic to anaerobic metabolism. As the lactate concentration increases, the pH decreases [1]. The amounts of histamine, bradykinin, prostaglandins, carbon dioxide, lysosomal enzymes, collagenase, hyaluronic acid, and hypoxanthine increase. Following the relief of pressure, during the reflow phase, there are increases in superoxide anion hydrogen peroxide and hydroxyl radicals [2], factor VIII, and uric acid. Fibrinolytic activity decreases. These changes lead to increased capillary permeability, edema, and finally cell death. Necrosis appears first in the secretory cells and ducts of the eccrine sweat glands and in the subcutaneous fat, and progresses to involve the sebaceous glands. The epidermis and the hair follicles are the last structures to be affected by ischemia and hypoxia.

Blanchable Erythema

The papillary dermis is the site of the most characteristic histologic change seen in blanchable erythema. The capillaries and venules are dilated with prominent endothelial cells. Following this, mild to moderate edema appears along with a mild perivascular, predominantly lymphocytic infiltrate. Blanchable erythema of long duration shows platelet aggregates and fibrin thrombi in the ectatic vessels with similar findings in the reticular dermis. Degenerative changes begin to appear in the eccrine sweat gland unit and the subcutaneous fat. The nuclei of the cells of the secretory coil and then the duct become ghost-like. The cytoplasm becomes granular or vacuolated and eosinophilic. Cell membranes become indistinct and finally periglandular hyalinization appears. Neutrophils are seen surrounding and invading the necrotic sweat glands. The subcutaneous fat shows foci necrosis with a loss of cell membranes and an infiltrate of neutrophils. Complete destruction of the adipose tissue is the end result.

If pressure is removed to permit perfusion of the tissue and removal of accumulated toxic products, these initial changes are completely reversible. The initial vasodilatation is a reactive hypermia due to vasodilatation caused by vasoactive substances and tissue metabolites. The cutaneous structures most sensitive to hypoxemia are the eccrine sweat glands and the subcutaneous fat cells [3]. The tendency for adipose tissue to become necrotic early probably accounts for the extensive undermining and tunnelling often seen in decubitus ulcers when the ulcer bed reaches the level of the subcutaneous fat.

Nonblanchable Erythema

The histologic change which characterizes this phase of the decubitus ulcer pathway also occurs in the papillary dermis. The most constant feature is erythrocyte engorgement of the capillaries and venules. This is followed by perivascular and later by diffuse extravasation of erythrocytes. Similar vascular changes are occasionally seen in the reticular dermis. The destructive changes in the eccrine sweat glands and adipose tissue described in blanchable erythema occur more frequently and are more pronounced. In this phase, the sebaceous glands begin to show evidence of degeneration. There is loss of cell membranes and an inflammatory infiltrate.

The presence of platelet aggregates in specimens taken from the earliest phase of nonblanchable erythema suggests a possible therapeutic role for prostaglandin inhibitors [4]. When used in an experimental model, however, ibuprofen was not effective in preventing decubitus ulcers [5]. Histologically, the bright red variety of nonblanchable erythema corresponds to the stage of red blood cell engorgement of the capillaries and venules. Histologically, the deep red or purple variety corresponds to the hemorrhagic phase. This usually progresses to a black eschar.

Decubitus Dermatitis

The histologic hallmark of this phase is centered on the epidermal changes. Four types of epidermal alterations are seen: (a) focal eosinophilia and necrosis with or without dermo-epidermal separation; (b) diffuse eosinophilia with erosions and crust formation; (c) epidermal atrophy with a subepidermal blister; and (d) subepidermal bulla with a relatively normal-appearing epidermis. In addition, the follicle shows evidence of necrosis in this phase. There is degeneration of the internal and external root sheaths and occasionally hemorrhage in the hair papilla. The other changes in the dermis, the epidermal appendages, and subcutaneous fat described in blanchable and nonblanchable erythema occur more frequently and are more pronounced.

The different types of epidermal alterations described above probably reflect the speed with which the necrotic process occurred. The subepidermal bulla formation beneath a relatively normal epidermis indicates an acute process, while the diffuse epidermal eosinophilia picture represents a more chronic process. The diffusely atrophic epidermis accompanied by dermo-epidermal separation probably represents a recurrent process, a new episode of decubitus dermatitis occurring in a scar.

Friction does not appear to play a primary role in the genesis of the decubitus ulcer. All of the bullae seen in decubitus dermatitis are subepidermal, in contrast to friction blisters, which are characteristically located in the epidermis just below the granular cell layer [6]. It is more likely that friction plays a secondary role by removing already devitalized epidermis. In addition, friction can remove the stratum corneum. This has been reported to decrease the fibrinolytic activity of the dermis, making the skin more susceptible to pressure necrosis [7]. Loss of the stratum corneum also increases transepidermal water loss, allowing the accumulation of moisture on the skin surface with resultant increased susceptibility to friction.

Decubitus Ulcer

Early Ulcer/Superficial Ulcer

This is essentially a decubitus dermatitis without the epidermis. The dermal papillae may still be visualized. There is a diffuse infiltrate of polymorphonuclear leukocytes. In addition to the perivascular round cell infiltrate and the erythrocyte engorged vessels, all the epidermal appendages are necrotic.

Healing Ulcer

Histologically, new blood vessels and fibroblast proliferation characterize the healing ulcer. The new blood vessels are oriented vertically, perpendicular to the plane of the ulcer bed. There is diffuse edema of the dermis. All the previously described changes in the blood vessels and adnexae have disappeared.

Chronic Ulcer

The ulcer base may be covered by a crust consisting of red blood cells and acute inflammatory cells, a layer of coagulation necrosis or fibrin. The ulcer bed consists of diffuse fibrosis with isolated collections of capillaries.

Eschar/Gangrene

The tissue appears basophilic. Although the general architecture is discernable, the cellular details are lost. Shearing force injury is probably responsible for this cutaneous change. A frequent precursor of the eschar/gangrene is the dark red or purple variety of nonblanchable erythema. Shearing force is a mechanical force operating parallel to the skin surface. It interrupts the blood supply to the skin by stretching or tearing the large blood vessels at the level of the subcutaneous fat and the superficial fascia [8]. The subcutaneous fatty layer is especially vulnerable to this type of injury as it lacks sufficient tensile strength to withstand such distortion. Vascular occlusion is complete, reperfusion of the tissue does not occur, and coagulation necrosis occurs.

Conclusion

Histologic examination of the various phases of the decubitus ulcer spectrum of changes shows that not all the structures in the skin are equally susceptible to the effects of ischemia and hypoxia. The most sensitive structures are the blood vessels, followed by the eccrine sweat gland unit, the subcutaneous fat, the sebaceous glands, the hair follicles, and the epidermis. This knowledge is significant at the clinical level in that, although the skin may appear normal on the surface, structures within may show evidence of damage[9].

References

1. Meehan SE, Walker WF (1979) Measurement of tissue pH in skin by glass microelectrodes. Lancet II:70–71
2. McCord JM (1985) Oxygen-derived free radicals in post ischemic tissue injury. N Engl J Med 312:159–163
3. Arndt KA, Mihm MC, Parrish JA (1973) Bullae: a cutaneous sign of a variety of neurological diseases. J Invest Dermatol 60:312–320
4. Ehrlich HP, MacGarvey U, McGrane WL, White ME (1987) Ibuprofen as an antagonist of inhibitors of fibrinolysis in wound fluid. Thrombasis Res 45:17–28
5. Salcido R, Donofrio JC, Fisher SB et al. (1995) Evaluation of ibuprofen for pressure ulcer prevention: application of a rat pressure ulcer model. Adv Wound Care 8(4):30–55
6. Sulzberger MB, Cortese TA Jr, Fishman L, Wiley HS (1966) Studies of blisters producted by friction: results of linear rubbing and twisting techniques. J Invest Dermatol 47:456–465
7. Turner RH, Kurban AK, Ryan TJ (1969) Fibrinolytic activity in human skin following epidermal injury. J Invest Dermatol 53:458–462
8. Reichel SM (1958) Shearing force as a factor in decubitus ulcers in paraplegics. JAMA 166:762–763
9. Witkowski JA, Parish LC (1982) Histopathology of the decubitus ulcer. J Am Acad Dermatol 6:1014–1021

9 Bacteriology

Bacterial infection has been recognized as a sometimes serious complication of decubitus ulcers since the nineteenth century. Only in recent years, however, has the spectrum of potential invaders been fully appreciated. The role played by *Staphylococcus aureus, Enterococcus faecalis*, and the coliform bacilli was stressed in the past, while the importance of anaerobes in sepsis was overlooked, largely because investigators failed to utilize the special technics necessary to isolate these fastidious organisms. Recognition of the presence of anaerobic bacteria in decubitus infections is of the utmost importance. Invasion by these organisms often results in a bacteremia with a high mortality rate. Prompt surgical debridement and the careful selection of appropriate antibiotics is essential if a fatal outcome is to be avoided.

Aerobic Infection

Decubitus ulcers are colonized continuously by a wide variety of bacteria – aerobes, anaerobes, and facultative organisms. In the absence of clinical signs of infection, the significance of routine culture results is therefore difficult to evaluate. When signs of infection are present, aerobes are the most common isolates, exceeding anaerobes in ratios as high as 5 to 1 [1]. Organisms most frequently encountered are shown in Table 1. Ordinary cellulitis, which manifests itself as erythema, heat, and swelling at the periphery of the ulcer, is usually caused by *S. aureus*, especially when satellite follicular lesions are also

Table 1. Aerobic bacteria isolated from sepsis associated with decubitus ulcers (adapted from [1])

From the ulcer	From the blood
Staphylococcus species, especially *S. aureus*	*Proteus mirabilis*
Streptococcus, group A	*Escherichia coli*
Streptococcus, group D	*Klebsiella species*
Proteus species	*Citrobacter* species
Escherichia coli	*Staphylococcus aureus*
Pseudomonas	*Streptococcus*, group A
Klebsiella	*Streptococcus*, group D

present and systemic symptoms are minimal. Deeper abscess formation with malaise, chills, and fever may also occur. When redness and edema at the periphery of the ulcer are intense, extension of the lesion is rapid, and vesicles or bullae appear, the organism responsible is usually a group A *Streptococcus*. Other streptococcal groups can produce a similar picture, however, and it would be especially important to identify group D representatives. These enterococcal bacteria are generally resistant to the penicillin and penicillinase – resistant penicillins ordinarily prescribed for cellulitis. There is, however, little evidence that group D *Streptococci* play a significant role in sepsis associated with decubitus ulcers [2].

It should be remembered that in the presence of extreme debilitation, as is often the case in decubitus situations, signs and symptoms pointing to infection may be diminished or absent.

When bacteremia occurs in association with decubitus infections, *Proteus mirabilis* is the most common aerobic isolate, followed closely by *S. aureus* and *Streptococci*. *Escherichia coli*, *Klebsiella* species, and *Citrobacter* species are occasionally encountered.

Anaerobic Infection

From the clinical standpoint, anaerobic infection in decubitus ulcers can be suspected when:

1. The ulcer is foul smelling.
2. Necrosis, gangrene, or pseudomembrane formation is evident.
3. Bloody exudates show a blackish discoloration.
4. Crepitus is present in tissue areas around the ulcer.
5. Systemic signs of infection occur in the presence of negative aerobic cultures.
6. Systemic signs of infection persist despite treatment with antibiotics routinely prescribed for aerobic infection.

Infection of decubitus ulcers by anaerobes is usually polymicrobic, with several species of anaerobes or combinations of anaerobes and facultative organisms multiplying simultaneously. In these situations, the key to isolation success lies in the collection and transport of the specimen itself. The finest laboratory may fail to isolate fastidious anaerobes if initial tasks are not carried out properly.

While cotton swab specimens are useful for the detection of aerobes such as *S. aureus*, they may be unreliable indicators of the deeper tissue infections characteristic of the anaerobes. Deep tissue biospy specimens are to be preferred in these situations and are superior to needle aspirates as well [3]. Tissue collected by curettage also yields satisfactory results.

Whether obtained by aspiration, surgical drainage, curettage of tissue, biopsy, or cotton swab, specimens should be transferred immediately to containers designed specifically for anaerobic culture and transported to the laboratory without delay. Good laboratory practice includes transfer of clinical

Table 2. Anaerobic bacteria isolated from sepsis associated with decubitus ulcers (adapted from [1])

From the ulcer	From the blood
Bacteroides species, especially *B. fragilis*	*Bacteroides* species, especially *B. fragilis*
Peptococcus and *Peptostreptococcus*	*Peptococcus* and *Peptostreptococcus*
Clostridium species	*Fusobacterium*
Eubacterium	
Propionibacterium	
Microaerophilic *Streptococcus*	

material expeditiously – certainly in less than 24 h – to anaerobic culture media. Whether the roll tube system or anaerobic chamber technics are used will depend on the training and experience of the laboratory personnel, and the equipment and space available. Differences of opinion exist on the relative efficiency of these methods, but the consensus is that, carefully done, both are effective in the isolation of clinically significant anaerobic bacteria from clinical specimens [4].

Anaerobic bacteria commonly isolated from patients with infected decubitus ulcers are shown in Table 2.

The importance of the non-clostridial anaerobes – *Bacteroides* species, and especially *B. fragilis* – in sepsis associated with decubitus ulcers has been pointed out by a number of investigators [1, 5–7]. The anaerobic bacteremia, which occurs in nearly four out of five of the cases in which these organisms are implicated, carried with it in one study [1] a mortality rate of 75%, when therapy was judged to be inadequate. Even when treatment was judged to be ideal, 14% of patients failed to survive. Signs and symptoms of anaerobic bacteremia include fever, chills, profuse sweating, jaundice, and in some cases the classic picture of toxic shock.

A new spot test technic for the rapid identification of *B. fragilis* shows promise [8].

References

1. Chow AW, Galpin JE, Guze LB (1977) Clindamycin for treatment of sepsis caused by decubitus ulcers. J Infect Dis 135:565–568
2. Galpin JE, Chow AW, Bayer AS, Guze LB (1976) Sepsis associated with decubitus ulcers. Am J Med 61:346–350
3. Rudensky B, Lipschits M, Isaacsohn M, Sonnenblick M (1992) Infected pressure sores: comparison of methods for bacterial identification. South Med J 85:901–903
4. Edelstein MAC (1990) Processing clinical specimens for anaerobic bacteria: isolation and identification procedures. In: Baron EJ, Finegold SM (eds) Bailey and Scott's diagnostic microbiology. Mosby, St Louis, pp 477–507
5. Brook I (1995) Anaerobic infections in children with neurologic impairments. Am J Mental Retard 99:579–594

6. Rissing JP, Crowder JG, Dunfee T et al. (1974) Bacteroides bacteremia from decubitus ulcers. South Med J 67:1179–1182
7. Shibuya H, Terashi H, Kurata S et al. (1994) Gas gangrene following sacral pressure sores. J Dermatol (Jpn) 21:518–523
8. Mangels J, Edvalson I, Cox M (1993) Rapid presumptive identification of Bacteroides fragilis group organisms with use of 4-methylumbelliferone-derivative substrates. Clin Infect Dis 16 [Suppl 4]:S319–321

Therapy – General

10 Medical Management

The medical management of the decubitus ulcer has been placed on a firmer scientific footing in recent years. Current treatments are more effective and yet, because the ulcers frequently coexist with debilitating disease, healing can still be significantly delayed or entirely impaired [1, 2].

Many decubitus ulcer patients suffer from diminished mentation or severe neurologic impairment; these individuals may be unaware of their predicament, registering neither pain nor discomfort. Others, alert and equipped with an intact neurologic system, will naturally be alarmed at the destruction of a part of the body. Along with physical pain, reactive depression, feelings of hopelessness, and even suicidal ideation may be prominent.

Therapy selection should be made on a rational basis. The use of a detergent on tissue already injured will only worsen the condition [3]. Topical application of a contact sensitizer can add yet another disease to the mix, and substances of this type may even be toxic to fibroblasts [4].

At least 2200 remedies have been recommended for the treatment of decubitus ulcers. Table 1 provides a representative listing of therapeutic agents for which no efficacy has been demonstrated and which may in fact add to the destruction of tissue [5]. These remedies should be avoided [6].

Local Measures

Treatment is most effective when keyed to the clinical phase of the decubitus ulcer pathway. Determination of the phase of the disease is an arbitrary clinical decision, to be sure, but it provides a useful guide for selecting the medications to be used. When several ulcers coexist, it is better to choose a modality that can be used on all of them. The selection of ulcer A for one treatment and ulcer B for another only leads to confusion with little increase in efficacy.

In accordance with modern and well-established wound healing concepts, treatments are now directed towards keeping the ulcer moist to facilitate re-epithelialization. Lesions should not be dried out indefinitely by agents such as dextranomer isomer (Debrisan), a preparation we previously recommended, as healing will be delayed [7].

Table 1. Topical preparations not recommended: these preparations have not been shown to be efficacious and in some instances are injurious to wound healing

Allantoin
Balsam of Peru
Benzoin compound
Betadine
Bismuth
Blood (dried)
Boric acid
Brilliant green
Brine baths
Carfucsin paint
Caroid
Castor oil
Charcoal
Coal tar paste
Cocoa butter
Cod liver oil
Dakin's solution
Diethylstilbestrol
Egg whites
Electric lights
Epsom salts
Eusal
Formaldehyde tissue
Gentian violet
Granulex powder
Honey
Insulin
Karaya powder or gum
Maalox and merthiolate
Madecassol
Mutton tallow
Pectin
Plasma
Potassium permanganate
Red blood cell powder
Scarlet red
Silicone
Starch poultices
Sugar
Sugar and egg white
Tannic acid
Titanium
Tragacanth paste
Vegetable poultices (carrots, turnips, bread, and charcoal)
Vitamins A and E
Ultraviolet light
Urea paste
Urine
Zinc
Various combinations of the above

Blanchable and Nonblanchable Erythema

Because these initial phases resemble dermatitis, anti-inflammatory agents may be helpful. Fluorinated steroid cream or gel applied to the diseased area acts through its pharmacologic properties to counteract vasodilatation, reduce edema, and decrease local reaction to accumulated metabolic waste products. The cream or gel should be applied three times a day and gently massaged into the affected area to increase transepidermal absorption.

In the bright red form of nonblanchable erythema, nitroglycerin ointment (2%) may be applied, 0.25–1.0 cm of the ointment is placed on the lesion and occluded by an impermeable plastic wrap. Application should be limited to 12 h per day to prevent the development of tolerance. Nitroglycerin appears to cause local vasoconstriction and a reduction in the inflammatory process.

Zinc oxide paste (Lassar's paste), applied three times a day, provides a protective barrier against fecal or urinary incontinence. It also has some anti-inflammatory qualities [8].

An occlusive dressing, Duoderm for example, can be useful, both as a protector of the area and as an anti-inflammatory agent [9] (see Chap. 13).

Pressure relief is essential; blanchable and nonblanchable erythema are reversible processes.

Decubitus Dermatitis

This more intense dermatitic process often responds to cool compresses of aluminum subacetate (Burow's) 1:40 or normal saline, applied for 30 min three times a day. Heat is to be avoided; it adds to the vasodilatation and increases the metabolic requirements. Topical steroids may be applied after the compresses.

Occlusive dressings are also helpful. They promote re-epithelization and are particularly recommended when erosions are present. Unless clinical evidence of infection is present, vesicles and bullae should be left intact to minimize bacterial contamination and to expedite wound healing.

Superficial and Deep Ulcers

Eschar/Gangrene

Debridement. Decubitus ulcers will not heal unless necrotic debris is first removed [10]. Necrotic tissue creates a physical barrier that prevents tissue repair and provides an ideal medium for bacterial colonization. In eschar/gangrene presentations, it may be wise to wait several days for the eschar to demarcate from viable tissue before intensive debridement. An eschar may provide a protective barrier against infection, but if it overlies an area of fluctuation, it should be removed.

Occlusive Dressings. Occlusive dressings can be used to macerate necrotic tissue. With autolytical debridement, the material liquefies and comes away when the dressing is changed, provided wound fluid is present.

Wet to Dry Dressings. In this technique, which is effective in the removal of small amounts of necrotic tissue, coarse gauze rolls or gauze sponges are dampened with saline or aluminum subacetate (Burow's solution) and packed into the recesses of the ulcer. The area is then covered with a nonocclusive dry dressing; 4–6 h later, the relatively dry packing is removed, carrying with it loosened dead tissue. The procedure is repeated every 6–8 h until the ulcer is clean. Because it can inhibit spontaneous closure by interrupting epithelialization, prolonged use of this form of debridement is to be avoided.

Antimetabolites. Topically applied, 5-fluoruracil 5% cream (Efudex) is effective in separating viable from nonviable tissue. It is particularly useful in removing the black eschar. The cream is applied twice daily to the edge of necrotic tissue. It is believed that the antimetabolite interferes with cell division in the actively proliferating fibroblasts at the junction of viable and nonviable tissue.

Enzymes. The enzymatic agents would appear to be the ideal way to digest away unwanted tissue. Unfortunately, the efficacy of the agents available is variable and they are often of limited usefulness [11]. An ideal agent would digest necrotic material completely, spare normal tissue, be nontoxic, and non-sensitizing. None approaches this ideal. When using one of the enzymes, care should be taken to avoid the concomitant application of antagonistic agents. Aluminum subacetate (Burow's solution) and heavy metals interfere with the action of collagenase, for example, while hydrogen peroxide negates the effectiveness of papain. Table 2 lists the agents available.

Hydrotherapy. The whirlpool or Hubbard tank provides a relatively painless method for the removal of loosened necrotic debris. The major disadvantage is logistical, namely, the transportation of patients to and from the treatment facility.

Surgery. Surgery is covered in detail in Chap. 11. Scissors, scalpel, and forceps can be used at the bedside. Necrotic tissue is cut away until there is pinpoint bleeding or pain. Debridement of deep and severely undermined ulcers can

Table 2. Enzymatic agents

Enzyme	Brand name	Substrate
Collagenase	Santyl	Collagen
Sutilains	Travase	Protein in general
Trypsin	Granulex	Muscle
Fibrinolysin and desoxyribronuclease	Elase	Purulent material
Papain	Panafil	Protein

lead to significant hemorrhaging. Caution and commonsense should be exercised in removing tissue not completely visualized.

Cleansing. Ulcers containing purulent and loose necrotic tissue may be cleaned with aluminum subacetate (Burow's solution), saline, or even an antiseptic such as chlorhexidine gluconate (Hibilcens) or polyvinyl pyrrolidone (Betadine). The antiseptics should be used for only a few days. Beyond that they begin to interfere with granulation tissue formation [12]. Wounds that ooze a great deal can be treated with dextranomer isomer (Debrisan) or calcium alginate packing (Sorbisan). Both agents will absorb and adsorb the unwanted material. Dakin's solution (sodium hypochlorite) is a relic of the post-World War I era, best elevated now to emeritus status and left on the shelf. Similarly, hydrogen peroxide has outlived its usefulness and may in fact be destructive to epithelial cells.

Anti-infective Measures. When the ulcer and surrounding tissue show signs of infection, systemic antimicrobial agents are indicated. These medications are discussed in detail in Chap. 15. Topical antimicrobial agents often fail to penetrate sufficiently into ulcers to reduce bacterial loads [13]. Metronidazole gel (Metrogel) has been found useful in eliminating the odor caused by anaerobic bacteria [14]. Some authorities recommend mafenide acetate cream (Sulfamylon) or silver sulfadiazine cream (Silvadene), the active ingredients of which have been shown to penetrate into necrotic tissue and even into eschars. Like other topical sulfonamides, these agents are capable of producing severe forms of contact dermatitis and systemic allergic reactions. Less commonly used today, but still effective, are iodoform gauze and acetic acid. Iodoform gauze is packed into the ulcer, removed, and replaced very 8–12 h for a period of several days. Along with its modest ability to inhibit bacterial growth, iodoform gauze also acts as a gentle debriding agent. Acetic acid compresses (0.25%–1.0%) or irrigations may also be useful, particularly when Gram-negative infections are suspected.

Healing Promotion. Current wound healing concepts point towards keeping the wound moist [15]. Occlusive dressings create a liquor that allows the epithelial cells to proliferate. These dressings are covered in more detail in Chap. 13. Absorbable gelatins such as Gelfoam were formerly recommended to accelerate the healing of decubitus ulcers, but they are no longer in favor. Similarly, topical benzoyl peroxide preparations, believed at one time to stimulate the formation of granulation tissue, are not currently recommended. Several experimental wound-promoting agents, growth hormone and peptide preparations, for example, are currently being evaluated.

Ancillary Measures

Theoretically, turning the patient every 2 h will decrease the chances for the development of a decubitus ulcer. It is likely that this schedule will even help in healing lesions already present, although scientific data to support this concept are surprisingly sparse. It is reasonable and desirable to turn patients frequently, to be sure, but there is no way to eliminate pressure from all parts of the body. Neither levitation nor suspended animation is possible [16, 17].

Support systems are highly effective means for reducing pressure. They are discussed in detail in Chap. 14.

Complications

Osteomyelitis and sinus tract formation are dealt with by the administration of appropriate antimicrobial agents and, in selected cases, by surgical elimination of the infected bone or fistulae [18].

The most serious problem is the septicemia, often fatal, that occurs most frequently with *Bacteroides fragilis* infection. Antimicrobial agents and supportive measures are required [19, 20].

Systemic Measures

Decubitus ulcer patients often have other diseases that require attention if treatment is to be successful [22, 23].

Anemias of all types interfere with the healing process. Therapy appropriate to the type discovered should be instituted promptly, with the goal of maintaining a hemoglobin of 10 mg/100 ml or better.

Diabetes mellitus can also delay wound healing. All decubitus patients should be checked for this disease [23, 24].

Nutrition and incontinence are issues of paramount importance in the management of decubitus. These matters are considered in depth in Chaps. 16 and 17.

References

1. Parish LC, Witkowski JA (1994) Chronic wounds: myths about decubitus ulcers. Int J Dermatol 33:623–624
2. Witkowski JA, Parish LC (1993) Skin failure and the pressure ulcer. Decubitus 6(5):4
3. Thompson W, Herschman B, Unthank P et al. (1990) Toxicity of cleaning agents for removal of grease from wounds. Ann Plast Surg 24:40–44
4. Johnson AR, White AC, McAnalley B (1989) Comparison of common topical agents for wound treatment: cytotoxicity for human fibroblasts in culture. Wounds 1:186–192
5. Parish LC, Witkowski JA (1994) Dos and don'ts of wound healing. Clin Dermatol 12:129–131
6. Parish LC, Witkowski JA (1982) The decubitus ulcer. Int J Dermatol 21:259
7. Weber DE, Parish LC, Witkowski JA (1984) Dextranomer in chronic wound healing. Clin Dermatol 2(3):116–120
8. Ågren MS, Söderberg TA, Reuterving C et al. (1991) Effect of topical zinc oxide on bacterial growth and inflammation in full-thickness skin wounds in normal and diabetic rats. Eur J Surg 157:97–101

9. Helfman T, Ovington L, Falanga V (1994) Occlusive dressing and wound healing. Clin Dermatol 12:121–127
10. Witkowski JA, Parish LC (1991) Debridement of cutaneous ulcer: medical and surgical aspects. Clin Dermatol 9:585–593
11. Habekbäck B, Lundborg H (1982) Studies on the cytotoxic effect of enzyme preparations. Eur Surg Res 14:386–392
12. Rodeheaver G, Ballamy W, Kody M et al. (1982) Bactericidal activity and toxicity of iodine-containing solutions in wounds. Arch Surg 117:181–186
13. Berger BA, Barza M, Haher J et al. (1981) Penetration of antibiotics in decubitus ulcers. J Antimicrob Chemother 7:193–195
14. Witkowski JA, Parish LC (1991) Topical metronidazole gel – the bacteriology of the decubitus ulcer. Int J Dermatol 20:660–661
15. Bolton L, Fattu A-F (1994) Topical agents and wound healing. Clin Dermatol 12:95–120
16. Barbenel JC (1991) Pressure Management. Prosthet Orthot Int 15:225–231
17. Frantz R, Xakellis GD, Arteaga MD (1993) The effects of prolonged pressure on skin blood flow in elderly patients at risk for pressure ulcers. Decubitus 6(6):16–20
18. Sugarman B (1987) Pressure sores and underlying bone infection. Arch Inter Med 147:553–555
19. Galpin JE, Chow AW, Bayer AS, Guze LB (1976) Sepsis associated with decubitus ulcers. Am J Med 61:346–350
20. Bryan CS, Dew CE, Reynolds KL (1983) Bacteremia associated with decubitus ulcers. Arch Intern Med 143:2093–2095
21. Starer P, Libow LS (1992) Medical care of the elderly in the nursing home. J Gen Intern Med 7:350–362
22. De Conno F, Ventafridda V, Saita L (1991) Skin problems in advanced and terminal cancer patients. J Pain Symptom Manage 6:247–256
23. Jelinek JE (1994) Cutaneous manifestations of diabetes mellitus. Int J Dermatol 33:605–617
24. Kertesz D, Chow AW (1992) Infected pressure and diabetic ulcers. Clin Geriatr Med 8:835–852

11 Surgical Management

D. LaRossa and L.P. Bucky

The ultimate goal in the treatment of decubitus ulcers is to obtain a closed, healed wound that resists recurrence. The surgical means to this end evolved in the period during and following World War II when surgeons were faced with large numbers of casualties with spinal cord injuries. Prior to that time, the treatment was essentially nonsurgical. This evolution in our modern concept of the surgery of decubitus ulcers occurred in three overlapping but relatively distinct phases:

Phase 1. Techniques to obtain wound closure were devised. These included the use of skin grafts and flaps alone or in combination with the eventual recognition that a large padded flap would be most reliable and suitable for wound coverage and long-term durability.

Phase 2. The role played by the underlying bony prominence in the pathophysiology of the ulceration was recognized. Ostectomy was added to the procedures in an attempt to reduce the risk of continued pressure or retained foci of infection.

Phase 3. The design of flaps became more sophisticated through a clearer understanding of their vascular anatomy and physiology producing a second generation of flaps, the arterialized flaps.

Davis, in 1938 [1], is usually credited with the first suggestion that pedicle flaps be used for the treatment of pressure sores. He used the method to resurface areas of scar epithelium from "bed sores," initiating the concept that padded, well-vascularized tissue was needed. The first report of excision and closure of decubitus ulcers occurred in 1945 by Lamon and Alexander [2]. Penicillin prophylaxis was used in their patients. It was Scoville, however, in 1944 (cited in [3]), who is credited with suggesting surgical treatment for pressure sores. A cascade of reports of successful methods of closure using skin grafts and skin flaps followed in the mid 1940s. White et al. used rotation flaps [4]. Barker reported a 70% success rate using direct closure, skin grafts, and rotation flaps [5]. Multiple sacral flaps were used by Croce et al. [6], while Gibbon and Freeman treated 65 ulcers with S-type flaps [7]. Additional reports by Barker et al. [8] White and Hamm [9], and Croce and Beakes [10] followed. The reliability of these techniques is illustrated by a report of 298 decubitus ulcer closures by Conway et al. [11] using a variety of techniques: direct closure, z-plasties, and combinations of rotation flaps with and without skin grafts.

The recognition of the contribution of the underlying bony prominence in the pathophysiology of the decubitus ulcer marks an important milestone in their surgery. Reports began appearing in the late 1940s emphasizing the importance of ostectomy. Kostrubala and Greeley [12] advised reduction of bony prominences, and later extended this to include excision of the ischium [13]. Conway et al. [14] increased their success rate when ischiectomy was added (47%–81%). Comarr and Bors [15] went so far as to recommend total ischiectomy. Caution with radical bone removal was later recommended because of the high incidence of urethral fistulae [16, 17].

The third phase, which is still continuing, reflects sophistication in flap design based on an accumulating knowledge of the micro- and macrovasculature of the body's soft tissues. Bigger flaps were emphasized by Gordon in 1947 [18]. Campbell and Converse [19] published their experience with the large medially based thigh flap for closure of ischial ulcers in 1954.

The introduction of muscle flaps in the surgery of decubitus ulcers was an important event. Kostrubala and Greeley, (in 1947 [12]), suggested the use of muscle for padding. Bors and Comarr, in 1948 [20], utilized portions of the gluteus maximus muscle along with primary excision and closure of ischial ulcers. Muscle flaps of obturator internus for coverage of ischial ulcers were used in 1949 [13] and the biceps femoris in 1956 [21] to fill dead space left by excision and to provide padding. A major thrust in the use of muscle flaps for ulcerations was provided by Ger [22, 23], who adopted their use for the management of leg and heel ulcerations. Adaptation of these principles for sacral ulcerations was reported by Stallings et al. in 1974 [24] and by Ger and Levine in 1976 [25]. The vastus lateralis muscle was used for successful closure of trochanteric sores by Minami et al. in 1977 [26].

The more recent major advance in the management of decubitus ulcers by surgery is the use of skin–muscle, myocutaneous, or musculocutaneous flaps. Although their usage dates back to 1896 when Tansini [27] used a latissimus dorsi skin–muscle flap to reconstruct the breast, it is only recently that a better knowledge of the vascular anatomy of the skin and muscles has generated a myriad of flaps usable for many coverage problems. Much of our current understanding of skin–muscle flaps has been consolidated by McCraw et al. [28, 29]. The tensor fasciae latae [30], gluteus maximus [31], and gracilis [28] skin–muscle flaps are now in common usage. The ultimate skin–muscle flaps – the total thigh and leg flaps – have been used to salvage patients with massive decubitus ulcers [32–38].

Further sophistication of the surgical armamentarium is evolving. Neurovascular sensory island flaps have been used in small numbers of selected patients to provide a sensory pad in insensate areas [39, 40]. Tissue expansion has also been reported to provide additional sensate tissue while decreasing the donor site deformity. Microvascular free tissue transfers have provided additional solutions in the management of the difficult and challenging problem of decubitus ulcers.

The concurrent parallel advances in collaborative medical disciplines that have facilitated these surgical gains are also of great importance.

The importance of surgical nutrition was emphasized early by Mulholland et al. [43] who noted rapid healing of pressure sores with restoration of positive nitrogen balance through supplemental feedings. The evolution of total parenteral hyperalimentation from the early work of Dudrick et al. [44] has implemented our ability to restore health to these unfortunate patients. Likewise, advances in nursing, rehabilitation, anesthesia, psychiatry, dermatology, urology, and bioengineering specifically directed toward the care of the bedridden or paraplegic patient have facilitated more successful surgery. The surgeon treating such patients should be familiar with these resources and should be able to draw freely from them to optimize care.

Selection of Patients for Surgery

Every patient with a decubitus ulcer is a potential surgical candidate. Most lesions, however, are superficial and respond to local measures without surgical intervention. All patients with full–thickness loss of soft tissue will require varying degrees of surgical wound care. This may be limited to debridement and local wound care with the goal of obtaining a stable, clean wound that will not worsen or significantly threaten their lives. In selected patients, however, the goal will be restoration of a soft tissue cover at the ulcer site. The surgery necessary is often formidable in terms of blood loss, operative time, and risk. Postoperatively, prolonged periods of immobilization and assiduous nursing care to prevent pressure on the operative site or additional secondary areas of breakdown are imperative for success. A constellation of factors for each patient in making a judgement regarding major surgical intervention must therefore be reviewed. The following guidelines may be helpful and should be considered.

What Is the Patient's Rehabilitation Potential?

Those patients who are young, basically healthy, motivated, and who have spinal cord injuries are usually the best surgical candidates. On the contrary, elderly, terminally ill patients are not usually suitable candidates. Age alone is not a criterion, however, nor is a specific disease process. The patient should be able to expect a reasonable improvement for the expenditure in time and risk.

Can the Patient's Comfort, Management, and Quality of Life Be Improved?

Although decubitus ulcers are not commonly a source of pain, they can be a source of esthetic discomfort to the patient, friends, and family. The presence of an ulcer may condemn the patient to a hospitalized or nursing home status because of the inability or reluctance of the family to care for him or her in such a condition. Recurrent sepsis from an uncared-for ulcer is not only a threat to the patient's life but adds to the misery. Surgery may be valuable in subtracting at least one problem with which the patient must contend.

Does the Patient's General Medical Condition and Underlying State of Health Permit Such a Procedure?

Surgery should be reserved for those patients physically able to withstand and benefit from the procedure. This would include those whose health can be restored by ancillary measures to make them surgical candidates. The magnitude of routine ulcer excision or flap closure can hasten the death of a debilitated patient. In some instances, however, well-timed surgical intervention can be life saving. Those patients with sepsis and/or massive ulcerations may need early debridement and coverage to prevent further deterioration, malnutrition, wasting, and death.

A careful assessment of the patient and the goals hoped for must be made by all the members of the treatment team. The surgeon's input is crucial to the decision since s/he must perform the surgery and can best judge the risk to the patient. Nonetheless, the patient's motivation, potential need for long-term psychiatric support, prolonged nursing care, chronic urinary attention, etc., must be considered and amalgamated into planning for the patient. In this way, the best candidates for surgery can be selected and the desired outcome achieved.

Incidence and Location of Decubitus Ulcers

Decubitus ulcers occur at sites of bony prominence. They are commonly seen in the lower torso, hips, buttocks, and lower extremities. However, their distribution is influenced by several factors: positioning, patient size, soft tissue cover, state of consciousness, state of paralysis (spastic versus flaccid), underlying medical diseases, the presence of medical devices, etc. Any area overlying a bony prominence is at risk. Table 1 is representative of the incidence and distribution of pressure sores.

Principles of Wound Care and Patient Preparation

The goal of wound care in the patient with decubitus ulcer is conversion of a region of tissue necrosis to a clean, closed wound as quickly and safely as possible. The number of intervening stages is dependent on the condition of the wound when the surgeon intercedes, but the process is similar – debridement of devitalized tissue, followed by wound closure.

The aim of the care of superficial wounds is to prevent deterioration into a deeper ulceration. Surgical debridement, frequent cleansing, and protection from further insult will usually permit the wound to close by contraction and re-epithelialization.

Early in the evolution of a deep decubitus ulcer, a surface area of demarcation appears. Initially, the surface is sealed by an eschar, contiguous with

Table 1. Incidence and distribution of decubitus ulcers

Site	1954 Yeoman and Hardy [45] 240 decubitus ulcers %	1964 Dansereau and Conway [46] 1604 decubitus ulcers %
Ischium	28	28
Sacrum	27	17
Trochanter	12	19
Heel	18	9
Malleolus	8	5
Tibial crest	4	
Anterosuperior spine	2	2.5
Pretibial		5
Patellar		4
Elbow		1.5
Foot		3
Costal margin	1	
Miscellaneous		6
	100	100

surrounding normal skin. The wound at this stage is either sterile or has a low bacterial content. A stage of liquefaction then occurs with separation of the necrotic tissue from surrounding viable tissue. In this process, bacterial counts rise, often producing sepsis from the undrained wound. At this time, the wound may drain spontaneously or, more often, is debrided surgically. A crater-form wound results with walls of granulation tissue and, usually, a bony base which eventually also develops a granulation tissue cover. With this process, bacterial counts decrease. The entire sequence is not unlike the evolution of a full-thickness burn. The rate at which the wound attains the state of a granulating ulcer depends upon the methods of wound management. There appear to be two phases at which surgical excision of the ulcer with subsequent coverage can be done with relative safety:

1. A primary excision and closure may be warranted shortly after the insult occurs (5–7 days) and a demarcated, dry eschar appears. The devitalized tissue can be excised to the margin of normal tissue and covered immediately by a flap. Intravenous fluorescein, 20 mg/kg, may be helpful in assessing tissue viability during the operative procedure since only vascularized tissue will be fluorescent under Wood's lamp illumination 20 min following intravenous injection [47]. Since tissue bacterial counts are low during this period, the risk of postoperative infectious complications should be reduced.

2. More commonly, patients are treated by delayed primary closure with periodic debridement until a "healthy" wound is obtained. The ulcer bed is then excised and the wound closed with an appropriate soft tissue cover. The procedure should not be delayed for too long a time since continued collagen deposition will gradually render the granulation tissue less vascular, and a concurrent increase in bacterial contamination may occur.

Adequate debridement is the foundation for successful closure. Periodic sharp debridement is usually done at the bedside and is carried out until bleeding, obviously viable tissue is reached, or to the point of pain in patients with sensation. It may be necessary to perform debridement in the operating room for those patients in whom major debridements are planned. The advantage of sharp debridement lies on the speed at which nonviable tissues can be removed. Between debridements, one needs to provide an environment that promotes healing and maintains bacterial control of the wound. This can take the form of moist gauze dressing changes, or the application of moisture-retentive dressings like polymers or hydrocolloids.

These are various alternatives to bedside or intraoperative debridement. The use of autolytic, osmotic, enzymatic, and chemical debridement techniques are reserved for those patients that do not require early surgical intervention. These techniques balance selective tissue removal with preservation of epithelialization to promote wound healing. These forms of debridement can be performed over prolonged periods of time and do not require a hospital setting.

A helpful adjunct to determining the "health" of a wound is periodic quantitative bacterial cultures [49]. A safe level of contamination is below 10^5 bacteria per gram of tissue. Other clinical parameters are: decreasing wound size, reduction of exudates, color of granulation tissue, and the appearance of an advancing epithelial margin. Systemic antibiotics are used by some workers. Septic episodes are treated with antibiotics dictated by wound and blood cultures. Culture data are helpful in selecting "prophylactic" antibiotic coverage during the operative treatment of the ulcer.

Radiographic examination of the involved area can be valuable in assessing the status of underlying bones and joints. Soft tissue calcification is commonly seen as a result of disuse. Localized areas of osteitis and even osteomyelitis may be in evidence. This should not be treated with long-term systemic antibiotics with an aim to cure since, without debridement of bone and coverage with vascularized soft tissue, a "cure" cannot be effected. Septic episodes should be treated with appropriate antimicrobials and debridement of sequestrae.

Sinograms may be helpful in delineating the extent of ulceration, joint involvement, or rare communication with the bowel [50]. With extensive trochanteric ulceration, the hip joint is not uncommonly involved by a septic pyarthrosis. Excision of the femoral head and involved proximal femur (Girdleston procedure) may be a necessary part of treatment. Consultation with the orthopedic service should be considered. An essential and often overlooked part of wound management is the patient's nutritional status. A careful and complete assessment should be made including skin fold thickness, serum proteins, hemoglobin and transferrin levels, and anergy testing. Consultation by a nutritional support service can be rewarding. Caloric intake should be augmented enterally (or parenterally) during this period of protein loss, periodic sepsis, and debilitation. The hemoglobin level should be restored to 12–15 g by transfusion and administration of iron preoperatively. Every attempt should be made to restore the patient to a high-grade nutritional status prior to definitive surgery. This will enhance the patient's immunologic capacities and his/her ability to withstand the trauma of surgery and promote a favorable outcome.

Other sources of sepsis must be searched for and excluded. The urinary tract is particularly vulnerable in the spine-injured patient. Urologic consultation and treatment of existing infection is imperative not only to prevent sepsis in the patient, but to prevent secondary seeding of newly operated sites following definitive surgery.

In patients with massive ulcerations and/or contiguous ulcers of the buttocks and hips, fecal contamination may make wound care difficult or impossible. Such patients may be candidates for temporary diverting colostomies prior to definitive surgery. It is important to get all patients into a regular schedule of bowel evacuation. This will facilitate pre- and postoperative care. To prevent soilage following surgery, a modified bowel preparation is used preoperatively. This consists of a low-residue diet 2 days prior to surgery and liquid diet only the day prior to surgery. A mild laxative and cleansing enemas are given up to 24 h prior to surgery to prevent accidental fecal contamination during the procedure.

Control of spasms is the final preoperative detail to be addressed. Most patients respond well to a regular program of diazepam. Occasionally, patients will require the more permanent effects of rhizotomy, femoral nerve crush, or obturator neurectomy. Neglecting this important detail may invite an early postoperative wound catastrophe.

Anesthesia

Although patients with impaired sensation may be operated upon with sedation only, a general anesthetic is usually a better choice. Having a patient anesthetized often provides a more controlled, comfortable atmosphere for both patient and surgeon. When sedation alone is used, careful monitoring by an attendant anesthesiologist is very useful.

A number of possible anesthetic problems have been encountered [51]. Wide fluctuations in pulse and blood pressure, often with severe hypertension, are evidence of autonomic hyperreflexia. This is reportedly seen when a spinal injury in the region of the fifth thoracic segment has occurred. It is triggered by a stimulus in the denervated area and is relieved by removal of the stimulus.

Psychiatric difficulties are sometimes seen, especially in patients with paraplegia of short duration. They may be associated with unrecognized drug or alcohol dependence.

Hyperthemia may occur, especially if a closed anesthetic system is used. Normal thermoregulatory signals from the thalamus fail to effect an end-organ response in the region of denervation.

Secondary amyloidosis is a not infrequent complication of prolonged infection sometimes seen in paraplegic patients. A potential for adrenal insufficiency exists in patients with an established diagnosis, and one must consider prophylactic hydrocortisone coverage, if not preoperative evaluation of adrenal function.

Positioning problems during anesthesia can result in complications of hypotension, respiratory embarrassment, and new decubitus ulcers. Paraplegic patients seem to bleed excessively despite normal clotting parameters. This may be related to poor vascular tone and a generally poor nutritional level. In addition to preoperative transfusion, one should be prepared to replace blood to normal or above-normal levels. Airway management and adequate ventilation can be significant problems in high spinal injuries.

The use of succinylcholine in paralyzed patients is controversial. Some workers feel that it is safe to use in the immediate postinjury phase. However, it is in the period from 2 weeks to 6 months post injury, the hyperreflexive period, that one must be concerned about abnormal potassium release [52]. Cardiac standstill can occur in patients with severely reduced muscle mass [53].

Principles of Wound Closure

Two basic modalities are used for definitive closure of decubitus ulcers: (a) skin grafts; or (b) flaps. Skin grafting is of limited usefulness because of the lack of durability and padding provided by this "parasitic" cover. It is often useful in obtaining a closed wound quickly in patients who are expected to ambulate when recovered and will therefore not subject the graft site to repeated trauma. Grafts can also be used as a temporary cover and as an aid in restoring positive nitrogen balance prior to definitive coverage with flaps.

Overgrafting and reversed dermal grafting can also be used to thicken the cover [54]. In this method, a reversed graft of dermis is covered by a split thickness skin graft which either "takes" or is replaced by a thick, split-thickness graft. This results in a cover two to three times thicker than the split-thickness graft alone. Skin grafts 0.35–0.45 mm thick should be harvested from nonweight-bearing areas with a mechanical dermatone and are usually meshed at 1.5:1 and applied unexpanded to facilitate drainage and to conform to topographical irregularities. Grafts may be secured at the recipient site by a tie-over dressing of cotton soaked in glycerine or other bulky material. They are examined 4 days postoperatively or earlier if there is a suspicion of infection or impaired "graft take." Donor areas heal spontaneously in 10–14 days by re-epithelialization from adnexal structures.

Flap coverage is generally preferred for the definitive closure of decubitus ulcers because flaps provide padding, "nonparasitic" vascularity, and, in some instances, sensation. A knowledge of the blood supply of the skin as it pertains to flaps is a prerequisite to reliable flap design.

The skin vasculature conforms to one of two major patterns (Fig. 1). The majority of skin is supplied through a musculocutaneous perforator system where one or more major, but often unnamed, arteries supply a muscle and a rather well-defined area of underlying skin through numerous small perforating vessels (vascular territory) [55]. This skin is said to have "random pattern" circulation [56]. The dimensions of a skin flap raised in such an area is usually 1:1 or, at most, 1.5:1 in clinical practice.

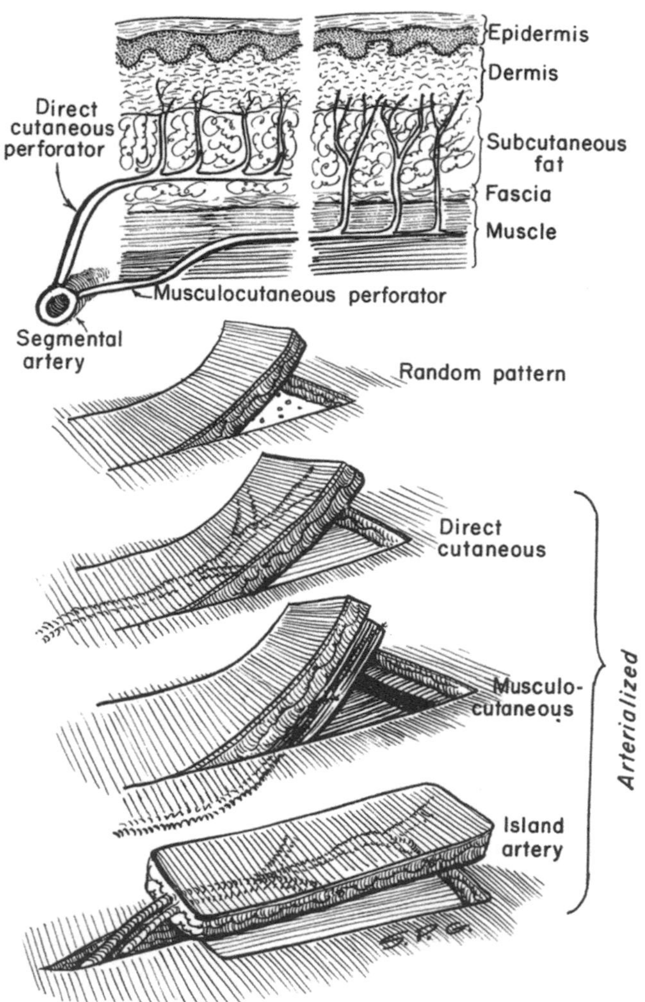

Fig. 1. The blood supply of the skin conforms to two major patterns: musculocutaneous perforator system and direct cutaneous perforator system. Elevation of a nonarterialized skin flap results in a random pattern flap

The muscle alone can be used as a flap. Those muscles supplied by a single vascular pedicle (or leash) are more useful for flaps than those with a segmental supply. The principles involved in the use of muscle flaps have been well described by Ger [22, 23, 25].

Elevation of the muscle with its overlying vascular territory of skin creates a skin–muscle, or musculocutaneous flap. It is possible to raise the entire vascular territory, a portion of it, or to include an adjacent "random territory" depending upon the vascular architecture of the muscle and skin in that region. Ideal skin-muscle flaps have a single major neurovascular pedicle at one end. These will be illustrated later as they apply to the management of decubitus ulcers.

The other major supply of the skin comes through the direct cutaneous perforator system [55]. Examples of these are the forehead, deltopectoral, and groin flaps. The length of the skin flap raised on such an arterial system is determined by the course and length of the artery and may be 3–4:1.

Flaps designed on the direct cutaneous perforator and musculocutaneous perforator systems are "arterialized" flaps, and hence can be converted to "island flaps" by severing all tissue connections except the neurovascular bundle, or "free flaps" capable of being transferred to a recipient area by microvascular and microneural anastomosis [57, 58].

An important axiom in decubitus ulcer surgery is tissue conservation. Unless a patient's recovery excludes the possibility of recurrence, one must assume that the patient will have a recurrent ulceration at some time in the future. Soft tissue of possible future usefulness must be saved. Traditional skin flaps are often the best method of closure for a first occurrence depending upon the location of the ulceration. In this way, the use of a muscle or skin-muscle flap at a later time is not precluded.

A corollary to this axiom is to design flaps large enough so they can be "readvanced" should recurrent ulceration occur. The large size of flaps will occasionally permit closure of the entire wound, but one should not hesitate to use a skin graft to permit a "tension-free" closure.

Thirdly, incision lines should be designed to avoid areas of repeated trauma or pressure where they could form sites of future ulcerations.

Bony prominences should be reduced when:

1. They are involved in the destructive process and have periostitis, osteitis, or osteomyelitis.
2. They do not create an imbalance of pressure as will occur when a unilateral partial or total ischiectomy is done.

Ostectomy of the sacral prominence and articular crests and the greater trochanters of the femur is generally recommended as part of the definitive surgical procedure for ulcers at these sites. Conservatism is recommended in the treatment of ischial ulcerations. Involved bone should be excised, but subtotal or total ischiectomy should be reserved for patients with significant bone involvement, bilateral disease, or following contralateral ischiectomy.

Excision of the ulcer should be to healthy, unaffected tissue. Determination of the extent of the cavity and completeness of excision is often aided by staining with methylene blue dye-soaked sponges packed into the ulcer. Not all undermined skin need by excised, but scarred, discolored, and hypovascular tissue is included. An attempt is made to remove the affected bony prominence en bloc with the ulcer bed (Fig. 2).

Hemostasis should be meticulous. This is often difficult because of the noncontractile nature of blood vessels in paralyzed patients. Accumulation of hematoma or seroma will almost guarantee failure. The use of electrocautery for excision and hemostasis is helpful. The CO_2 laser has been helpful in those

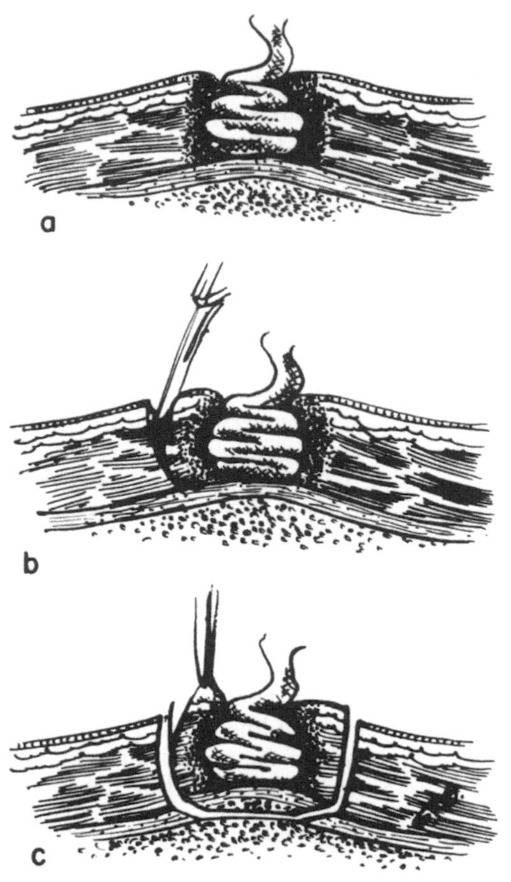

Fig. 2a-c. Packing of the ulcer cavity with gauze sponges soaked in methylene blue dye permits en bloc excision of the ulcer

institutions with access to one [59]. Bone bleeding can be controlled by mechanical compression of the bleeding marrow by a mallet. Bone wax is not recommended because of its reactivity.

Prolonged postoperative suction should be used and continued for 5-10 days despite the small return of drainage fluid. Soft catheters such as Snyder drains (Zimmer, Dover, Ohio, USA) are preferred, as are multiple catheters should one fail. They should parallel the axis of the flap to prevent embarrassment of the flap's blood supply. De-epithelialization of the tip of the flap and "tucking" it in, or use of a portion of muscle to fill any residual cavity may be used to obliterate any dead space (Fig. 3).

Intravenous fluorescein 5-10 mg/kg may be of aid in determining flap viability during the operative procedure [47]. Twice this dosage may be used in darkly pigmented patients. Vascularity is assessed with a Wood's lamp in a darkened room 20 min following slow injection. Nausea occurs not uncommonly. Anaphylaxis is rare, but reported, as is cardiac arrest [60, 61]. Areas of poor or nonfluorescence can be excised.

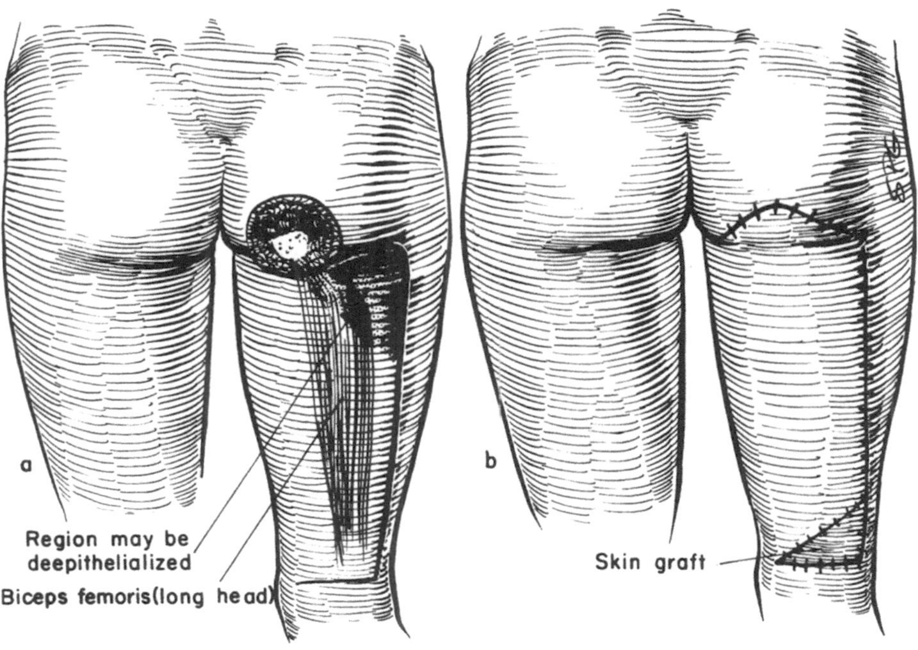

Fig. 3a,b. The dead space left from ischial ulcer excision can be filled with muscle or the deepithelialized tip of the skin flap

Careful closure in layers is then performed. Skin sutures may be tied over bolsters to protect the skin and prevent erosion. Surface sutures are removed 3 weeks postoperatively.

The operated area should be immobilized by careful patient positioning and control of spasms to prevent shearing forces from separating the flap from its bed or placing undue tension on suture lines. Avoidance of prolonged pressure on other potential ulcer sites is essential during and after the operative procedure. Limited weight bearing is permitted 3 weeks following surgery and is gradually increased thereafter.

As in most surgery, careful attention to details does most to insure a successful outcome.

Coverage Techniques for Specific Decubitus Ulcers

Sacral Decubitus Ulcers

Anatomy

The floor is the sacral promontory and small medial portions of the gluteus maximus muscles. The walls are the subcutaneous fat of the buttocks.

Skin Grafts

On rare occasions, a skin graft is useful for a patient expected to ambulate following recovery or as a temporary cover prior to flap closure.

Skin Flaps

A large inferiorly based rotation flap works well in this instance (Fig. 4). S-shaped and bilateral flaps can be used but have the disadvantage of placing the final scar directly over the pressure point. A superiorly based flap does not have as good a blood supply as one based inferiorly. These are random flaps whose dimensions should not exceed 1:1.

The transverse back flap described in Vasconez et al. [42] contradicts our traditional concepts of crossing the midline "watershed" with flaps. However, the crossover of vessels in this location makes it generally reliable. The flap is elevated at the fascial level (Fig. 5). A transverse, bipedicle back flap has limited usefulness because of the lack of mobility of the flap.

Muscle Flaps

Gluteus Maximus Turnover Flaps. The flap is based on the inferior and superior gluteal vessels and is elevated in the plane between the gluteus medius and

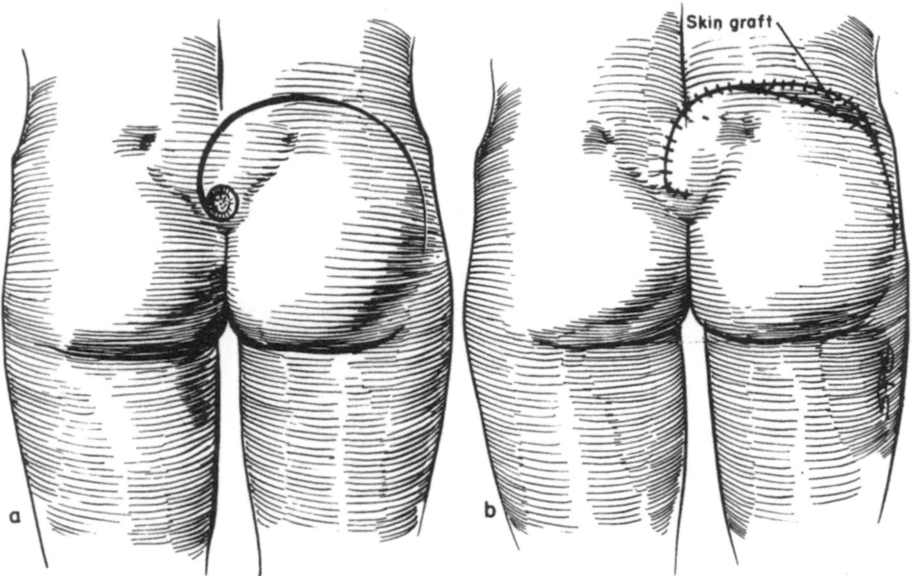

Fig. 4a,b. Coverage of an excised sacral decubitus ulcer by a large, inferiorly based, random pattern rotation skin flap. A skin graft fills the donor defect

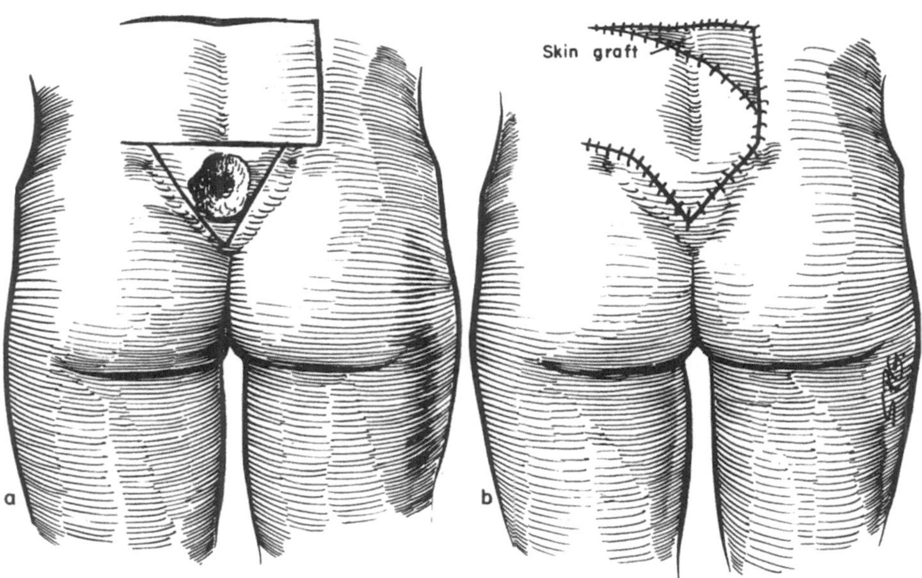

Fig. 5a,b. The transverse back flap used for coverage of a sacral decubitus ulcer

maximus. The flap, hinged medially, is brought across the ulcer bed and covered with a skin graft [24, 25] (Fig. 6). Bilateral flaps can be used to cover very large defects.

Skin–Muscle Flaps

Gluteus Maximus Skin–Muscle Flap. A composite of gluteus maximus muscle and overlying buttock skin (vascular territory), based inferomedially on the gluteal vessels, is rotated superomedially to fill the defect [31] (Fig. 7).

Ischial Decubitus Ulcers

Anatomy

The ulcer's floor is the ischial tuberosity. Along its superior wall are the lower fibers of the gluteus maximus muscle. Inferiorly and medially the walls are subcutaneous fat.

Skin Flaps

Medially Based Posterior Thigh Flap. This random pattern flap has the advantages of reliability, places the resultant scars away from pressure sites, and

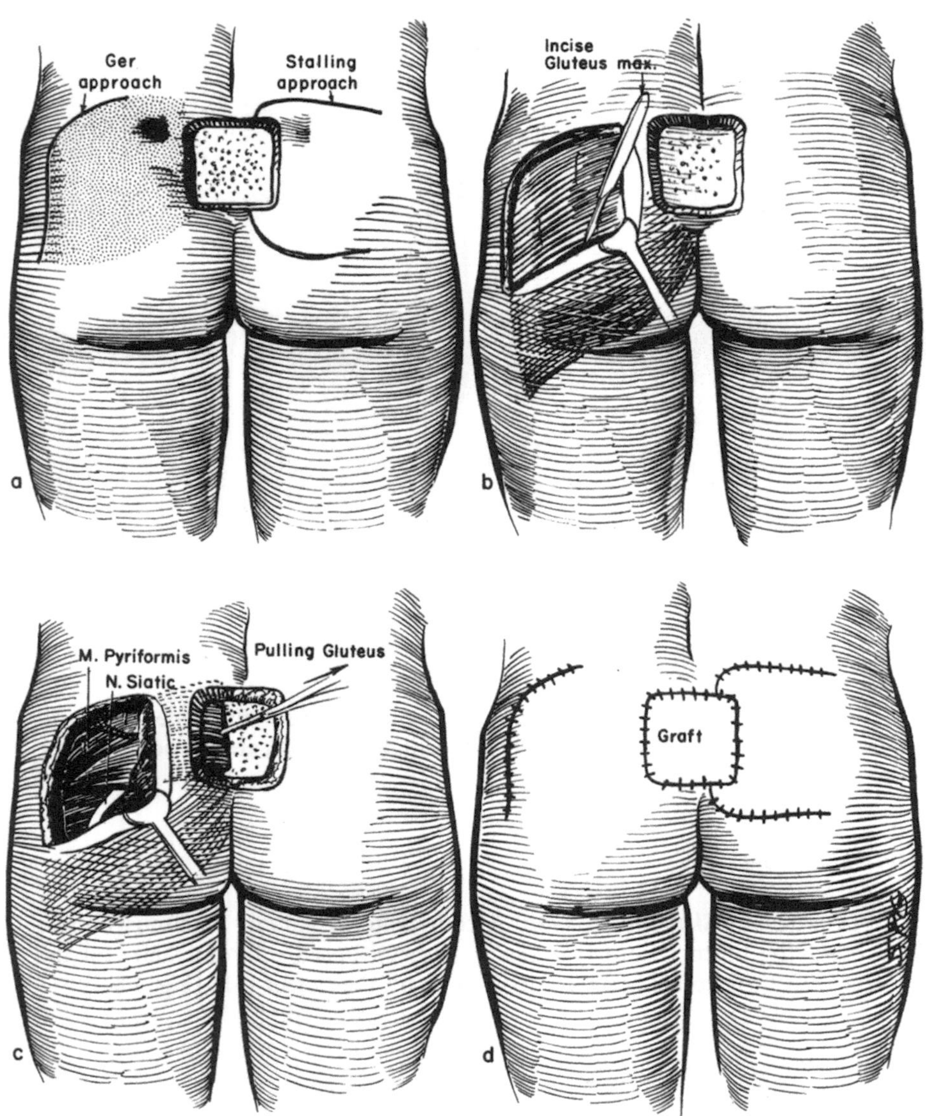

Fig. 6a–d. Coverage of a sacral decubitus ulcer by gluteus maximus muscle turnover flaps. The Ger and Stalling approaches to the muscle are shown (**a**) Upper fibers of the gluteus maximus are elevated and folded medially (**b, c**). Final coverage is by a split thickness skin graft (**d**)

permits readvancement should the ulcer recur. It can be modified by filling the dead space resulting from ulcer excision with buried dermis and fat from the deepithelialized tip [62] or the biceps femoris muscle detached at its insertion and folded upward (Fig. 3).

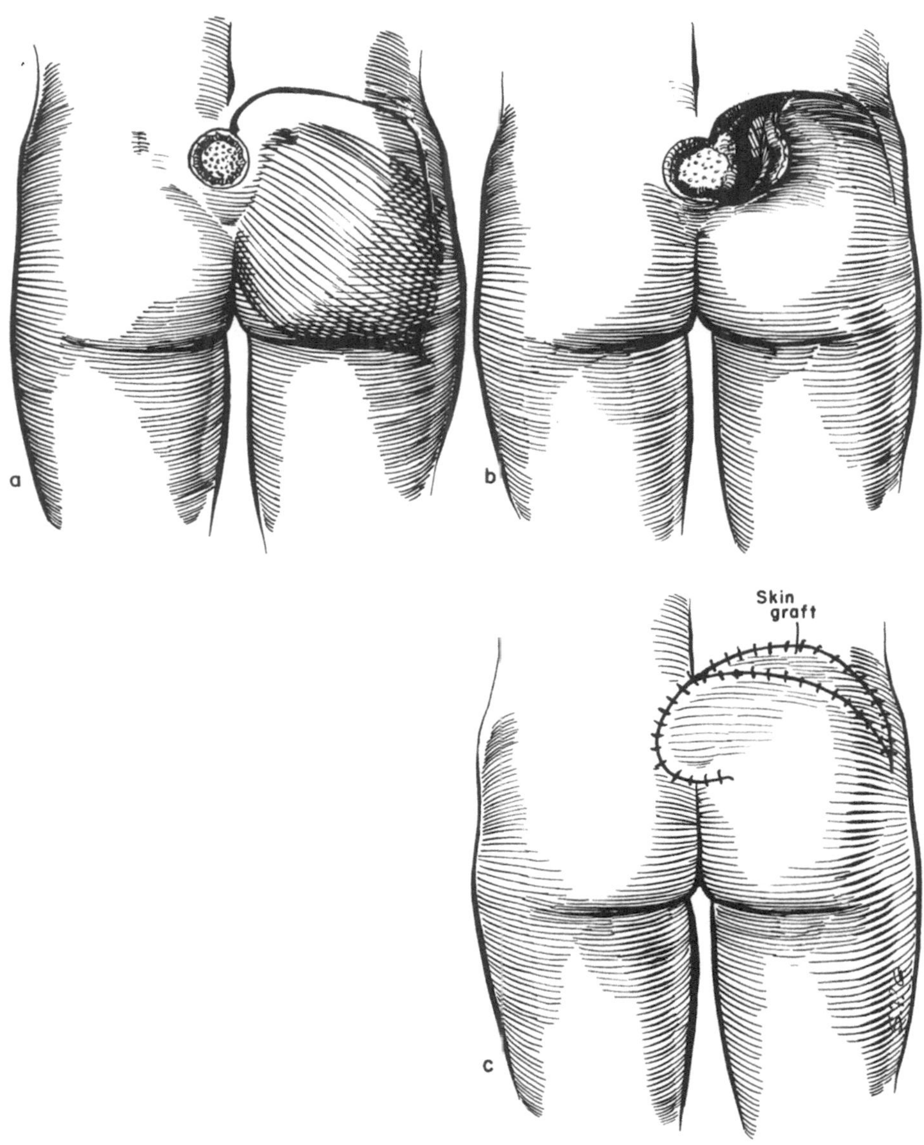

Fig. 7a–c. A gluteus maximus skin–muscle flap is used to cover a sacral decubitus ulcer (**a, b**). A skin graft resurfaces the donor defect (**c**)

Muscle Flaps

Lower Gluteus Maximus. The gluteus maximus muscle can be split in the direction of its fibers and the lower portion, vascularized by the inferior gluteal

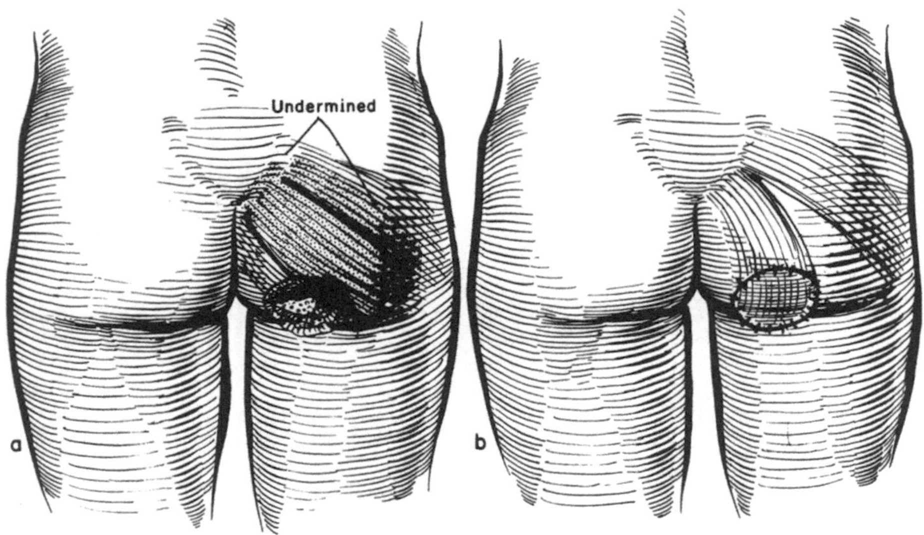

Fig. 8a,b. The lower fibers of the gluteus maximus muscle, vascularized by the inferior gluteal vessels, is used to cover an ischial decubitus ulcer. The muscle is exposed by extending the decubitus ulcer laterally. Final coverage is with a skin graft

vessels, used to cover the ischial area [24, 25] (Fig. 8). The upper portion may be used simultaneously to cover a sacral decubitus ulcer. Skin grafts complete the closure.

Saddle Flap. A smaller version of the above flap [19]. The disadvantages of this flap are its small size and the location of resultant scars where they may be subjected to trauma in the sitting patient.

Skin–Muscle Flaps

Lower Gluteus Maximus Skin–Muscle Flap. This medially based flap utilizes the lower portion of the gluteus maximus and overlying skin [31] (Fig. 9). Its disadvantage is the resultant scar on the buttock.

Gracilis Skin–Muscle Flap. A skin island based on the upper and middle thirds of the gracilis muscle can be introduced into the ulcer excision site beneath the intervening skin bridge [28, 63] (Fig. 10). This technique has been useful and reliable in our hands, but some surgeons have found it unreliable because of muscle atrophy and a somewhat precarious blood supply to the skin. The muscle usually has a major vascular pedicle from the superficial femoral at its superior end, but has variable contributions from minor pedicles distally. Patients are positioned in lithotomy with the legs in a "ski position." The flap is elevated posterior to a line from the pubic tubercle to the tendon of the

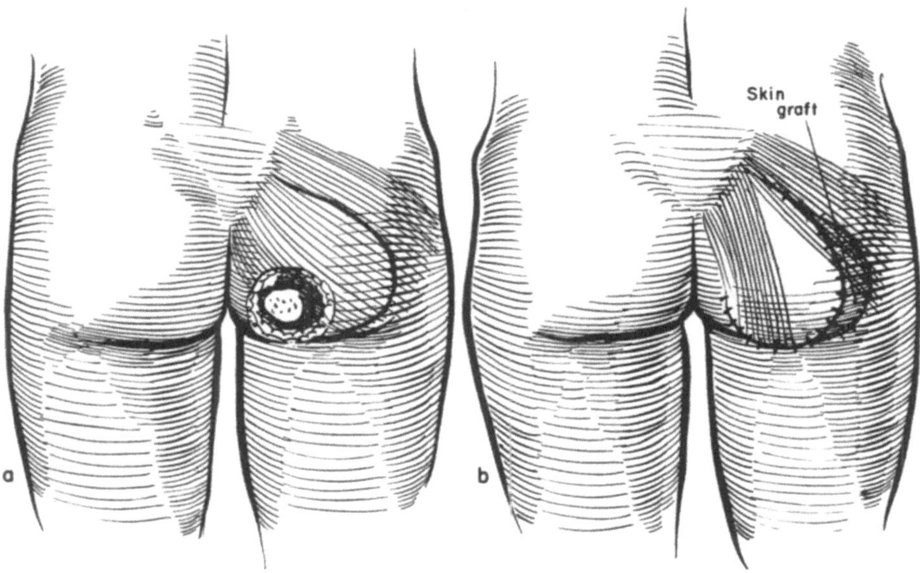

Fig. 9a,b. The lower portion of the gluteus maximus muscle and overlying skin territory is used to cover an ischial decubitus ulcer

semitendinosus muscle. The donor site can be closed primarily in the vast majority of cases with excision of a skin is-and 7–10 cm in width.

Tensor Fasciae Latae Skin–Muscle Flap. This very reliable, easy to elevate flap is based on the lateral femoral circumflex artery which enters the flap (tensor fasciae latae muscle) just below the trochanter, emerging between the rectus femoris and vastus lateralis muscles [30] (Fig. 11). It has an extensive arc of rotation that can reach the ischium and sacrum. Its vascular territory extends to at least 5 cm above the knee and may include virtually the entire lateral thigh (M.J. Jurkiewicz 1979, personal communication). Donor sites can often be closed primarily with flap widths up to 10 cm depending on the laxity of the thigh skin. Patients are operated upon in the lateral position to facilitate exposure to both donor and ulcer site.

Sliding Posterior Thigh Skin–Muscle Flap. A recently described flap of hamstring muscles and overlying skin [64]. The composite is detached except for its vascular leash and moved superiorly as an island. Since it is innervated by the lateral femoral cutaneous nerve, it can provide protective sensation in patients with low meningomyeloceles. The nerve originates at the L1,2,3 level.

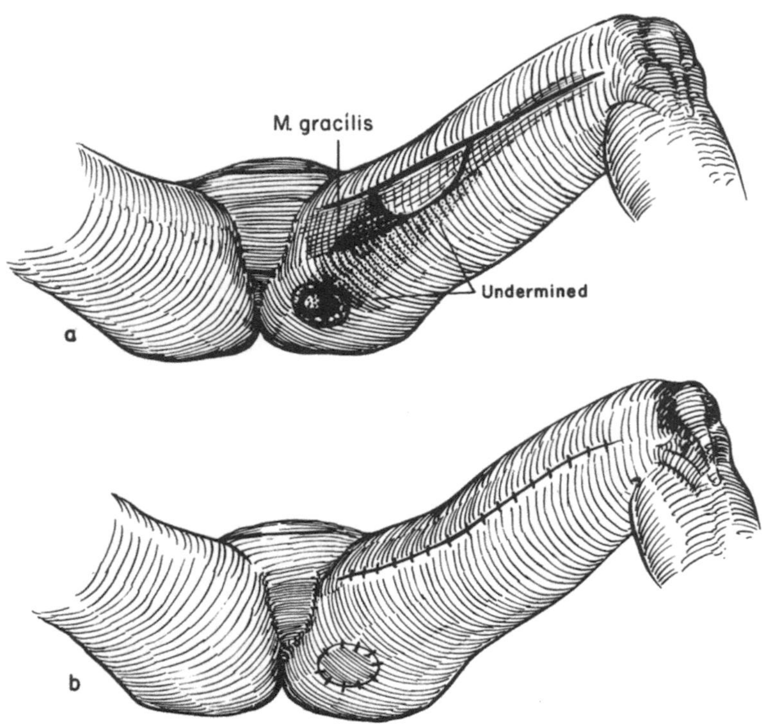

Fig. 10a,b. Coverage of an ischial decubitus ulcer with gracilis skin–muscle island flap. The patient is operated in the ski position

Trochanteric Decubitus Ulcers

Anatomy

The base of this ulcer is the greater trochanter of the femur. The walls are composed of the subcutaneous fat and fascia lata of the thigh. A portion of its anterior margin includes the thickened iliotibial tract of the fascia lata and the posterior fibers of the tensor fasciae latae muscle – posteriorly and inferiorly the fibers of the gluteus maximus and medius.

Skin Flaps

Bipedicle Longitudinal Thigh Flap. The limited mobility of this flap limits its usefulness for all but the smallest ulcers. It is not recommended.

Spiral Thigh Flap. Anteriorly based and probably arterialized by an unnamed branch of the femoral artery, this flap is raised below the level of the fascia lata [42] (Fig. 12).

Fig. 11. The tensor fasciae latae skin–muscle flap used to resurface an ischial decubitus ulcer. A large vascular territory on the lateral thigh is supplied by its musculocutaneous perforator system which enters the tensor fasciae latae muscle below the trochanter of the femur

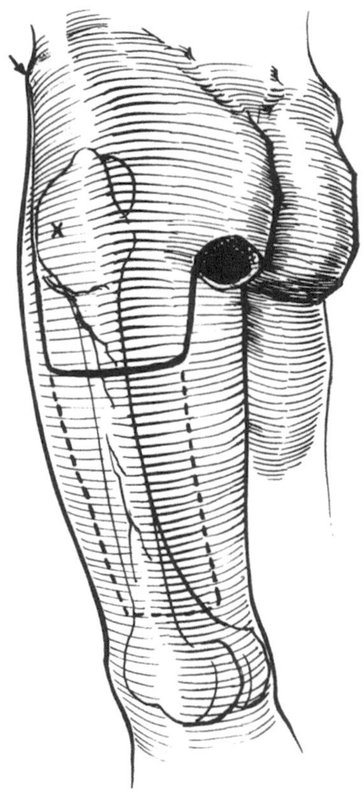

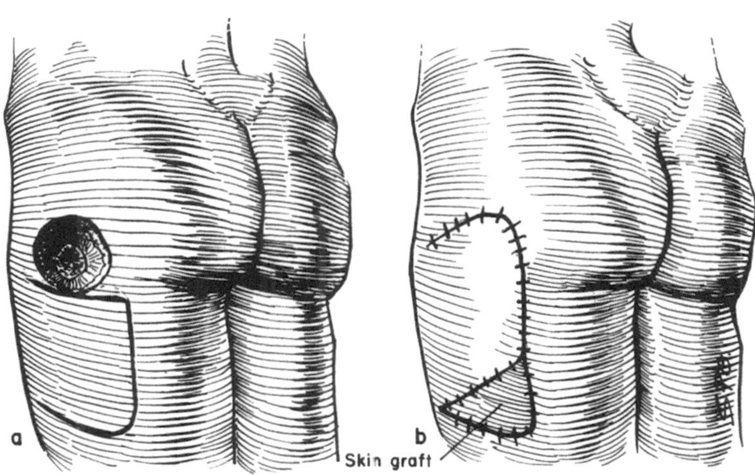

Fig. 12a,b. The anteriorly based spiral thigh flap, raised at the level of the fascia lata, is used to resurface a trochanteric decubitus ulcer

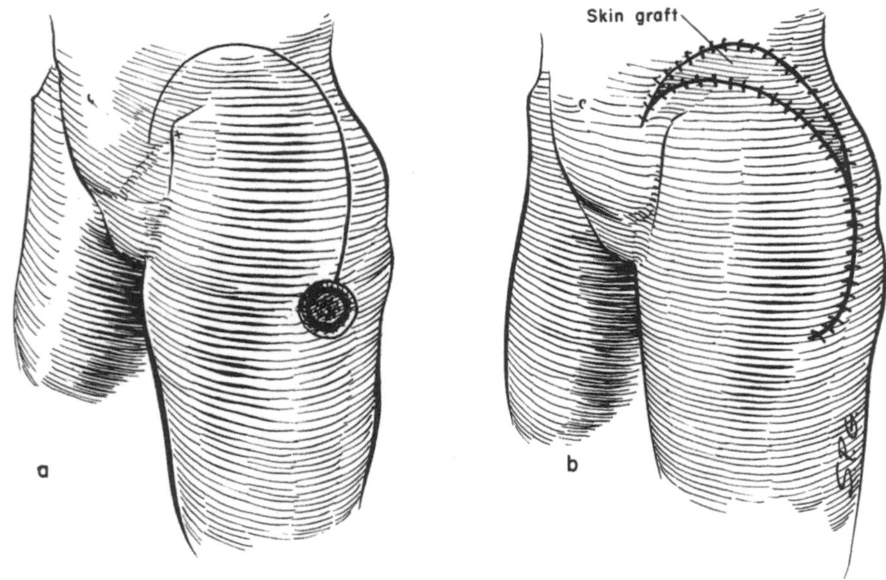

Fig. 13a,b. An extended groin flap can be rotated downward to cover a trochanteric decubitus ulcer. This arterialized skin flap, based on the superficial circumflex iliac vessels, gives a reliable cover. The donor defect is covered with a skin graft

Groin Flap. Based on the superficial circumflex iliac artery and vein, this arterialized flap can be elevated to the posterior axillary line without delay [65] (Fig. 13). The flap is raised above the fascia laterally until the sartorius is reached. The dissection proceeds beneath the muscular fascia to protect the vessels. The territory can be enlarged by including the superficial inferior epigastric circulation. A drawback is the suture line over the iliac crest.

Skin–Muscle Flap

Gluteus Maximus Skin–Muscle Flap. Based on the lower fibers of the gluteus maximus muscle and based posteriorly, this arterialized flap is rotated downward to cover the trochanteric site [31] (Fig. 14). Questions about the adequacy of flap size and complication rate (28%) have been raised [31].

Muscle Flaps

Vastus Lateralis Muscle Flap. Supported by a proximal leash of lateral and femoral circumflex vessels, the vastus lateralis can be moved as an island to cover trochanteric ulcers [26] (Fig. 15). A skin graft completes the closure. The initial incision is the same as for the tensor fasciae latae flap – along a line from the anterior superior iliac spine to the outer angle of the patella (Henry's approach).

Fig. 14. The posteriorly based thigh flap, based on the lower fibers of the gluteus maximus muscle and inferior gluteal vessels, is used to cover a trochanteric ulcer (after [31])

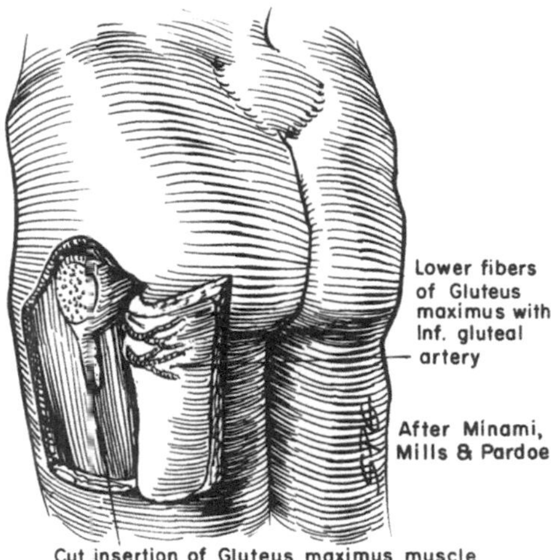

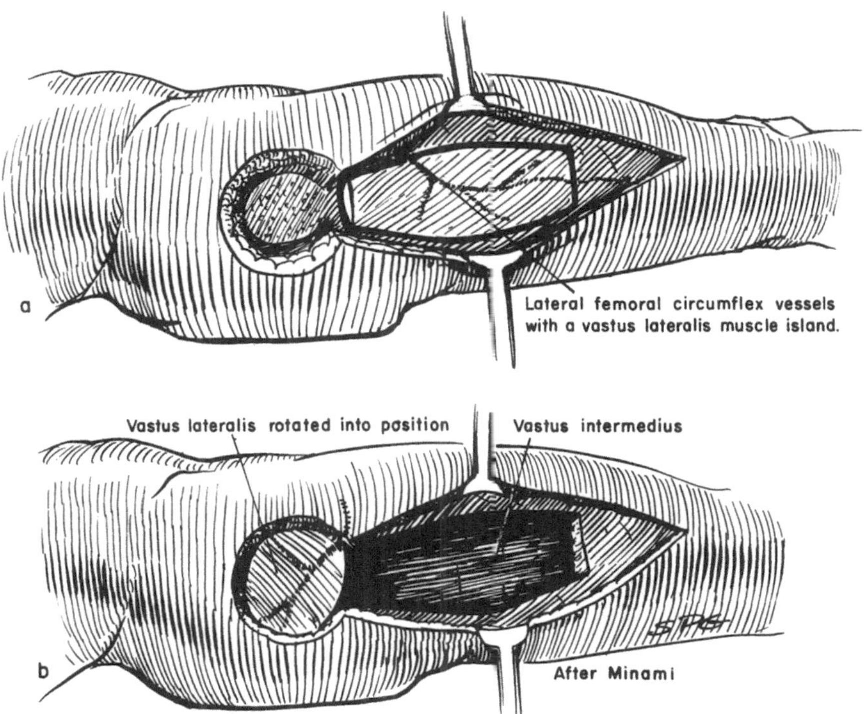

Fig. 15a,b. A vastus lateralis island muscle flap is rotated upward to cover a trochanteric decubitus ulcer (after [26])

Tensor Fasciae Latae Skin–Muscle Flap. This flap is probably the most useful flap in the management of trochanteric ulcers [30] (Fig. 11). Its location and ease of dissection greatly simplify the repair. A skin graft is needed on the donor area.

Massive Ulcerations

Fortunately, massive ulcerations, called "end-stage" decubitus ulcers, with contiguous cavities and sinus tracts, occur infrequently since they present a formidable challenge to the patient and physician. Every attempt should be made to devise a treatment approach short of amputation and total thigh flap because of the attendant blood loss (7–20 units), risk to the patient, postoperative difficulties with balance, and effects on body image. In selected patients, no reasonable alternative exists, however, and the procedure may be life saving by ridding the patient of a chronic source of sepsis, fluid loss, and a metabolic sink. Indications for this procedure can be drawn from an extensive experience by Royer et al. [37]:

1. Multiple or recurrent ulcers with insufficient adjacent tissue
2. Large trochanteric ulcers complicated by pyarthrosis and/or osteomyelitis of the femur
3. Multiple ulcers associated with ankylosed hip and knee joints
4. Single ulcers too large to be covered by rotation flaps
5. Ulcers with associated pelvic osteomyelitis

Several operative approaches have been used by different authors (Figs. 16–18). The procedure essentially consists of circumscription of the ulcer, infected and involved tissues, and subperiosteal filleting of the thigh (to include the leg below the knee if necessary) through a posterolateral or posterior thigh incision. The femoral vessels are protected. In Weeks and Brower's [36] operation, the femoral vessels are mobilized through Hunter's canal to gain 8–10 cm of pedicle length to permit passage through the posterior thigh muscles (Fig. 18) for inset of the flap. When the dissection is continued into the lower leg to gain additional cover, the incisions are brought forward anteriorly to protect the vasculature.

The risk of postoperative complications is significant – 34 complications in 41 flaps performed – with a recurrence rate of 60% [37]. Furthermore, rehabilitation is not always facilitated, particularly in bilateral cases since the center of gravity is changed.

Fig. 16. Coverage of massive ulceration by total thigh flap. A posterolateral approach is used. The femur is dissected subperiosteally to protect the femoral vessels (after [32])

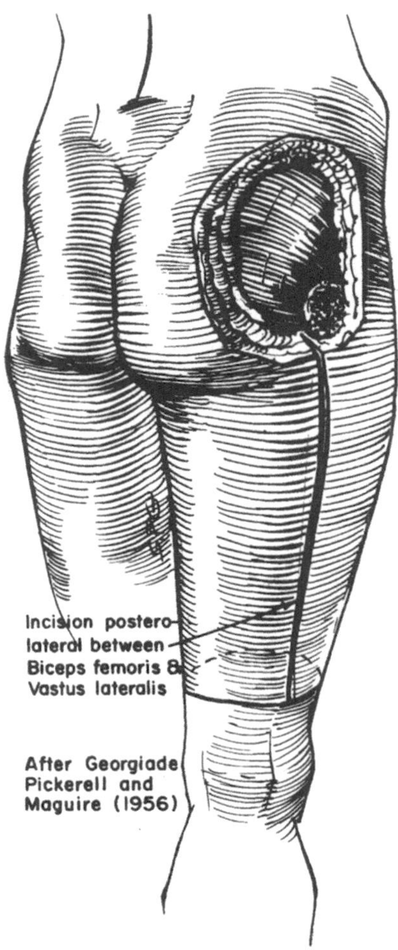

Coverage of Miscellaneous Ulcerations

Occiput and Chin

These usually occur secondary to pressure from devices such as a four-poster collar and usually resolve spontaneously with removal of the offending device. Local skin flaps or skin grafts may hasten recovery.

Shoulder, Scapula, Spinous Processes of the Vertebrae, Iliac Crests

Ulcerations in these locations occur most frequently in emaciated patients and are usually superficial and easily cared for. Protection and local wound care will usually suffice. Occasionally, excision and skin grafting will be necessary.

Fig. 17. The dissection is carried into the lower leg to create a total leg skin–muscle flap for coverage of massive ulceration (after [66])

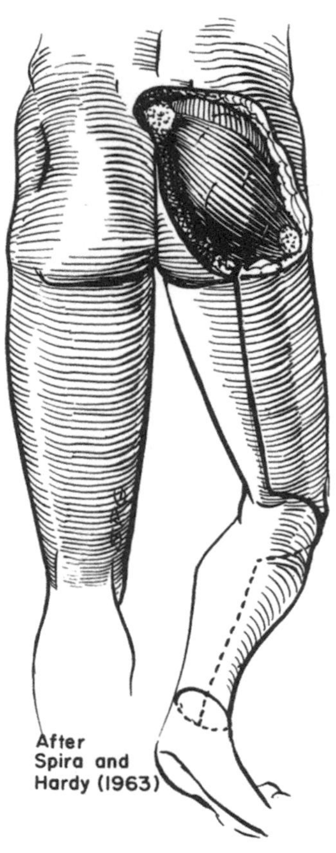

Elbows

Most ulcerations are superficial, but occasionally a deep would will be encountered in these rare ulcers. Excision, bone debridement, and flap coverage may be necessary. A posteriorly based chest flap or anteriorly based abdominal flap can be used (Fig. 19). Both are essentially "random pattern" flaps, and the usual 1–1.5:1 dimensions should be respected. Division can be accomplished 2 weeks following the primary procedure.

Ankles and Heels

Most ulcerations over the malleoli will respond to local care. Skin grafts will often hasten closure. Heel ulcerations may be resistant to permanent closure. In this case, local muscle flaps (abductor hallucis, abductor digiti minimi, and flexor digitorum brevis) in combination with skin grafts may provide a solution [23, 66] (Fig. 20).

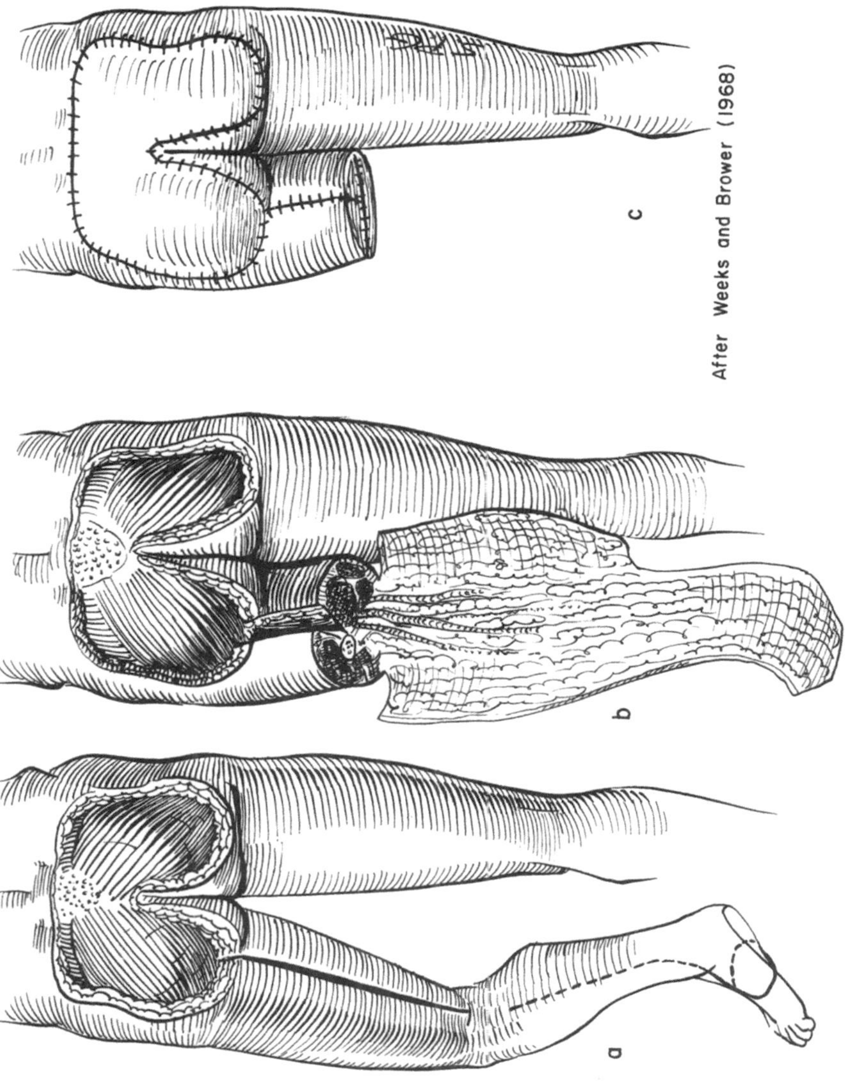

Fig. 18a–c. Coverage of massive ulceration by Weeks and Brower's modification preserves upper thigh by delivering the femoral vascular pedicle through Hunter's canal (after [36])

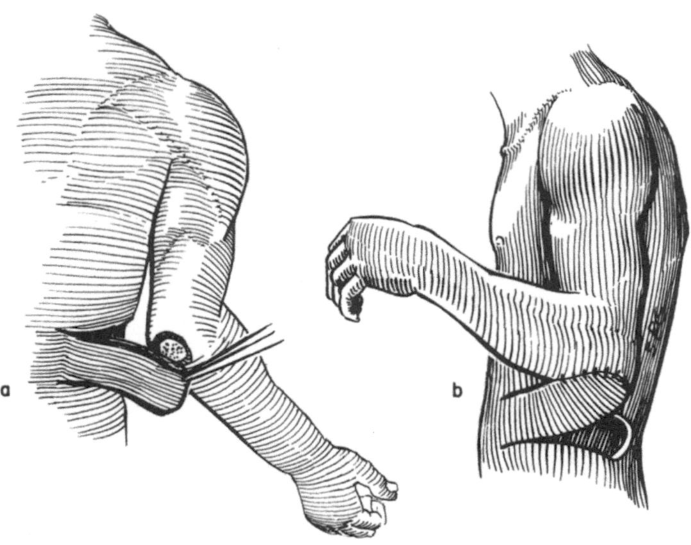

Fig. 19a,b. Elbow pressure sore can be covered by random pattern anteriorly based abdominal flap or posteriorly based chest flap

Fig. 20. The abductor digiti minimi, flexor digitorum brevis, and abductor hallucis muscles alone or in combination can be used to cover heel pressure sores. Final coverage is with a skin graft over the muscle flap (after [68])

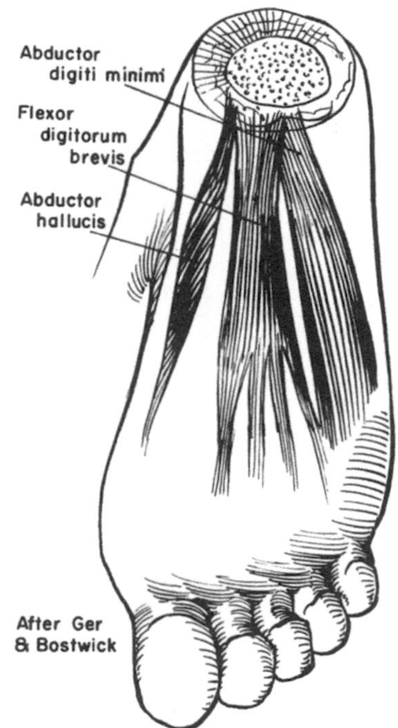

Surgical Complications

Hematoma and seroma are the most common complications and may beget additional complications. Hematomas should be evacuated as soon as they are recognized since they impair healing of overlying flaps and grafts, prevent obliteration of the plane between flap and ulcer bed, have direct toxic effects on flaps, and serve as a nidus of infection and wound separation.

Flap necrosis and/or wound separation are serious complications since the resultant wound may well be larger than the original decubitus ulcer. Early debridement and nutritional support should be used to return the wound to a state where a secondary closure with skin grafts or readvancement of flaps can be done.

Pulmonary embolus, pneumonia, and urinary tract infections are not infrequent occurrences in these patients where prolonged immobilization is a routine part of their care.

The recurrence rate remains high since the underlying pathology is unchanged in most cases, i.e., lack of sensation. Only through education of patients and continued attentiveness can a significant reduction be made in the recurrence rate.

References

1. Davis JS (1938) Operative treatment of scars following bedsores. Surgery 3:1–7
2. Lamon JG and Alexander EJ (1945) Secondary closure of decubitus ulcers with aid of penicillin. JAMA 127:396
3. Bailey BN (1967) Bedsores. Arnold, London
4. White JC, Hudson HW, Kennard HE (1945) The treatment of bedsores by total excision with plastic closure. US Naval Med Bull 45:445–463
5. Barker DE (1945) The surgical treatment of decubitus ulcers. JAMA 129:160
6. Croce EJ, Schillinger RN, Shearer TP (1946) Operative treatment of decubitus ulcer. Ann Surg 123:53–69
7. Gibbon JH, Freeman LW (1946) The primary closure of decubitus ulcers. Ann Surg 124:1148–1164
8. Barker DE, Elkins C, Poer D (1946) Methods of closure of decubitus ulcers in paralyzed patients. Ann Surg 123:523–533
9. White JC, Hamm WG (1946) Primary closure of bed sores by plastic surgery. Ann Surg 124:1136–1147
10. Croce EJ, Beakes CHC (1947) The operative treatment of decubitus ulcer. N Engl J Med 237:141–149
11. Conway H, Kraissl CJ, Clifford RH et al. (1947) The plastic surgical closure of decubitus ulcers in patients with paraplegia. Surg Gynecol Obstet 85:321–332
12. Kostrubala JC, Greeley PW (1947) The problem of decubitus ulcers in paraplegics. Plast Reconstr Surg 2:403–412
13. Blocksma R, Kostrubala J, Greeley P (1949) The surgical repair of decubitus ulcers in paraplegics. Plast Reconstr Surg 4:123–132
14. Conway H, Stark RB, Weeter JC et al. (1951) Complications of decubitus ulcers in patients with paraplegia. Plast Reconstr Surg 7:117–130
15. Comarr AE, Bors E (1951) Radical ischiectomy in decubitus ischial ulcers in patients with paraplegia. Ann W Med Surg 5:210–213
16. Comarr AE, Bors E (1958) Perineal urethral diverticulum – complication of removal of ischium. JAMA 168:2000–2003

17. Guthrie RH, Conway H (1969) Surgical management of decubitis ulcers in paraplegics. In: Proceedings of the 17th V A spinal cord injury conference. Bronx, NY 29 Sept–1 Oct 1969
18. Gordon S (1947) The surgical treatment of pressure sores. Plast Reconstr Surg 2:557–562
19. Campbell RM, Converse JM (1954) The saddle flap for surgical repair of ischial decubitus ulcers. Plast Reconstr Surg 14:442–443
20. Bors E, Comarr AE (1948) Ischial decubitus ulcer. Surgery 24:680–694
21. Conway H, Griffith BH (1956) Plastic surgery for closure of decubitus ulcers in patients with paraplegia. Am J Surg 91:946–975
22. Ger R (1971) The surgical management of decubitus ulcers by muscle transposition. Surgery 69:106–110
23. Ger R (1975) The surgical management of ulcers of the heel. Surg Gynecol Obstet 140:909–911
24. Stallings JO, Delgado JP, Converse JM (1974) Turn over island flap of gluteus maximus muscle for the repair of sacral decubitus ulcer. Plast Reconstr Surg 54:52–54
25. Ger R, Levine SA (1976) The management of decubitus ulcers by muscle transposition. Plast Reconstr Surg 58:419–428
26. Minami RT, Hentz VR, Vistnes LM (1977) Use of vastus lateralis muscle flap for repair of trochanteric pressure sores. Plast Reconstr Surg 60:364–368
27. Tansini I (1896) Nuovo processo per l'amputazione della mammella per cancro. Reforma Med 1(1):3–5
28. McCraw JB, Massey FM, Shanklin KD et al. (1976) Vaginal reconstruction with gracilis myocutaneous flap. Plast Reconstr Surg 58:176–183
29. McCraw JB, Dibbell DG, Carraway JH (1977) Clinical definition of independent myocutaneous vascular territories. Plast Reconstr Surg 60:341–352
30. Nahai F, Silverton J, Hill HL et al. (1978) The tensor fascia lata musculocutaneous flap. Ann Plast Surg 1:372–379
31. Minami RT, Mills R, Pardoe R (1977) Gluteus maximus myocutaneous flaps for repair of pressure sores. Plast Reconstr Surg 60:242–249 (Commentary by HB Griffith)
32. Georgiade N, Pickrell K, Maguire C (1956) Total thigh flap for extensive decubitus ulcers. Plast Reconstr Surg 17:220–225
33. Chase RA, White WJ (1959) Bilateral amputation in rehabilitation of paraplegics. Plast Reconstr Surg 24:445–455
34. Berkas EM, Chesler MD, Sako Y (1961) Multiple decubitus ulcer treatment by hip disarticulation and soft tissue flaps from the lower limbs. Plast Reconstr Surg 27:618–619
35. Spira M, Hardy SB (1963) Our experience with high thigh amputations in paraplegics. Plast Reconstr Surg 31:344–352
36. Weeks PM, Brower TD (1968) Island flap coverage of extensive decubitus ulcers. Plast Reconstr Surg 42:433–436
37. Royer J, Pickrell K, Georgiade N et al. (1969) Total thigh flaps for extensive decubitus ulcers: a 16-year review of 41 total thigh flaps. Plast Reconstr Surg 44:109–118
38. Burkhardt BR (1972) An alternative to the total-thigh flap for coverage of massive decubitus ulcers. Plast Reconstr Surg 49:433–438
39. Dibbell DG (1974) Use of a long island flap to bring sensation to the sacral area in young paraplegics. Plast Reconstr Surg 54:220–223
40. Daniel RK, Terzia JK, Cunningham DM (1976) Sensory skin flaps for coverage of pressure sores in paraplegic patients. Plast Reconstr Surg 58:317–328
41. Mellesi H (1977) Healing of nerves. Clin Plast Surg 4:459–473
42. Vasconez LO, Schneider WJ, Jurkiewicz MJ (1977) Pressure sores. Curr Probl Surg 14(4):1–62
43. Mulholland JH, CoTui F, Wright AM et al. (1943) Protein metabolism and bedsores. Ann Surg 118:1015–1023
44. Dudrick SJ, Vars HM, Rhoads JE (1967) Growth of puppies receiving all nutritional requirements by vein. Fortschritt der parenteralen Ernährung, West Germany, pp 1–4
45. Yeoman MP, Hardy AG (1954) The pathology and treatment of pressure sores in paraplegics. Br J Plast Surg 7:179–192
46. Dansereau JG, Conway H (1964) Closure of decubiti in paraplegics. Report on 2000 cases. Plast Reconstr Surg 33:474–480

47. McCraw JB, Myers B, Shanklin KD (1977) The value of fluorescein in predicting the viability of arterialized flaps. Plast Reconstr Surg 60:710–719
48. Griffith BH, Schultz RC (1961) The prevention and surgical treatment of recurrent decubitus ulcers in patients with paraplegia. Plast Reconstr Surg 27:248–260
49. Robson MC (1979) Infection in the surgical patient: an imbalance in the normal equilibrium. Clin Plast Surg 6:493–503
50. Lopez EM, Aranha GV (1974) The value of sinography in the management of decubitus ulcers. Plast Reconstr Surg 53:208–213
51. Rocco A, Vandam L (1959) Problems in anesthesia for paraplegics. Anesthesiology 20:348–354
52. Gronert GA, Theye RA (1975) Pathophysiology of hyperkalemia induced by succinylcholine. Anesthesiology 43:89–99
53. Tobey RE (1970) Paraplegia, succinylcholine, and cardiac arrest. Anesthesiology 32:359–364
54. Wesser DRG, Kahn S (1967) The reversed dermis graft in the repair of decubitus ulcers. Plast Reconstr Surg 40:252–254
55. Daniel RK, Williams HB (1973) The free transfer of skin flaps by microvascular anastomoses. An experimental study and a reappraisal. Plast Reconstr Surg 52:16–31
56. McCregor I, Morgan G (1973) Axial and random pattern flaps. Br J Plast Surg 26:202–213
57. Harii K, Ohmori K, Ohmori S (1974) Successful clinical transfers of ten free flaps by microvascular anastomoses. Plast Reconstr Surg 53:259–270
58. Daniel RK, Taylor GI (1973) Distant transfer of an island flap by microvascular anastomoses. Plast Reconstr Surg 52:111–117
59. Landa SJF, Anagnost M, Robson MC (1976) Advances in the surgical treatment of pressure sores. Rev Surg 33:1–4
60. Cunningham EE, Balu V (1979) Cardiac arrest following fluorescein angiography. JAMA 142:2431
61. Stein MR, Parker CW (1971) Reactions following intravenous fluorescein. Am J Ophthalmol 72:861–868
62. Tulenko JF (1967) Surgical treatment of ischial decubitus ulcers with demo-fat flap. Plast Reconstr Surg 40:72–76
63. Orticochea M (1972) The musculocutaneous flap method: an immediate and heroic substitute for the method of delay. Br J Plast Surg 25:106–110
64. Dibbell DG, McCraw JB, Edstrom LE (1979) Providing useful and protective sensibility to the sitting area in patients with meningomyelocele. Plast Reconstr Surg 64:796–799
65. McGregor IA, Jackson I (1972) The groin flap. Br J Plast Surg 25:3–16
66. Bostwick J (1976) Reconstruction of the heel pad by muscle transposition and split skin graft. Surg Gynecol Obstet 143:973–974

12 Rehabilitation Approach

W.E. Staas Jr., H.M. Cioschi, and B. Jacobs

The rehabilitation patients of this decade and of the future are taking on a very distinct profile for being at risk for decubitus ulcer development. Patients admitted to an acute, comprehensive rehabilitation program are typically only a few days to a few weeks post onset of their disability, trauma, or surgical intervention. It is not uncommon for the needs of these patients to be complex, as well as for them to be medically unstable. Even more common is the rehabilitation patient who has not been fully mobilized and requires high technological intervention, including ventilator management, total parenteral nutrition, and multiple parenteral chemotherapeutic regimens, coupled with other intensive therapies throughout their comprehensive rehabilitation program. This new profile of the rehabilitation patient aggravates their "at risk" status for the development of decubitus ulcers.

Decubitus ulcers continue to be a major societal health problem throughout the entire term of care. They are a primary or secondary cause for admission and readmission to acute, subacute, and rehabilitation programs.

The magnitude of the costs of this significant health problem is reflected in the study by Miller and Delanzier [1], of elderly post-traumatic hip surgery patients. Treatment and physician costs of 34 000 in-patients with this primary diagnosis was estimated at $836 million for the acute care setting, $355 million in nursing home facilities and $60 million in home care settings. Another at risk group is persons with spinal cord injuries. Approximately 23 %–30 % will develop decubitus ulcers within the first 2 years after injury [2, 3]. Young and Burns [2] reported that at least 5 %–7 % of these patients will require readmission to a hospital for the management of severe pressure ulcers during their follow-up years. In addition, the complications of decubitus ulcers are multiple and life threatening and account for 7 %–8 % of deaths of spinal cord injury (SCI) patients [4].

Despite more than 40 years of research on decubitus ulcers, "preventable" decubitus ulcers continue to be a major cause of hospital admission, temporary interruption of life style, activities of daily living, and lost vocational and educational time.

Although the health care statistics are staggering, the costs to patients and their care takers in lost income, productivity, progress towards vocational goals, independence, and self-esteem are also significant [5]. Decubitus ulcer prevention and ongoing treatment is a constant reminder of the person's "at risk" status [6]. Patients with SCI and others who are motor or sensory compromised need to learn and apply preventive skills, develop a new repertoire of health maintenance behaviors, and know when and how to intervene if signs of skin breakdown are identified.

Many patients with traumatic injury, progressive disability, or chronic illness need education regarding skin management. This includes detecting skin changes early, exploring possible causes, seeking help early, and taking actions to prevent further skin trauma and comorbidity. There are, however, situations where basic resources in health care, professional intervention, or individual (patient) detection may not be available, timely and/or aggressive enough to prevent tissue destruction resulting in a decubitus ulcer.

Interventions directed at decubitus ulcers can be divided into categories that include preventive (medical, both local and systemic), functional (including rehabilitation issues and the use of special equipment), and behavioral or educational. Preventive interventions include proper positioning and posturing, frequent weight shifts and other pressure relief interventions, the elimination of shear force and friction, the proper use of equipment, frequent skin inspections, and early intervention. These techniques direct care providers and patients toward the goal of maintaining intact skin and preventing extensive tissue destruction. Preventive interventions are directed at educating patients to prevent or reduce the development of decubitus ulcers by avoiding or minimizing the major contributing risk factors of pressure, friction, shear, moisture, and other trauma.

Other preventive interventions include the use of overlays, specialty mattresses and "high-tech" beds, and wheelchair cushions. The critical issue of pressure distribution and its effect on decubitus ulcer development has been identified [7, 8], as well as "time at pressure", and the intensity and duration of pressure in contributing to decubitus ulcer formation. In Kosiak's [7] study, no changes were noted in tissues subjected to constant pressures of 35 mmHg for as long as 4 h or to varying intermittent pressures of as much as 190 mmHg for 1 h. However, the constant application of a pressure of 70 mmHg produced irreversible cellular changes after 2 h. This points to the need to frequently reduce tissue surface interface pressure. Based on these early studies, most "surface" interventions were directed toward keeping surface pressures below capillary pressures (15 mmHg venous to 32 mmHg arteriolar) to reduce the external compression of capillary blood flow and thus prevent ischemia and necrosis. Most overlay and cushion products attempt to acheive readings below capillary pressure.

During the past 30 years, a variety of overlays, mattresses and cushions, including foam, sheepskin, gel, and air products, have become available. For the most part, these devices provide relief by partially reducing pressure in a supine, side-lying, or sitting position. They also may decrease pain. Studies involving normal, healthy subjects using mattress overlays have shown that mean trochanteric and sacral interface pressures at slightly below closing capillary pressure were achieved in a supine and side-lying static position. One study [9] compared the sacral, trochanteric, and heel pressures among hospital mattresses, 5-cm foam, a flotation foam pad, and an air cell overlay. The air cell overlay reduced pressures for sacral and trochanteric areas. As would be expected, the highest pressures for all mattress overlays were in the heels.

In selecting a product, caution should be exercised about generalizing these results to compromised patients or to patients at high risk for decubitus ulcer development. The latest generation of these products is the high-technology bed, which is typically a hospital bed that is modified to provide pressure relief through fluidized air systems or a pulsating, alternating, and possibly oscillating air system. These beds suspend the patient on the support surface, providing flotation and, therefore, pressure relief. Air-fluidized therapy is effective for the prevention and management of decubitus ulcers in postsurgical patients with sacral, trochanteric, or ischial rotation flaps; it assists with positioning of patients who have severe contractures and spasticity; and it provides a comfortable support surface for cancer and burn patients who typically experience pain from frequent repositioning or constant pressure.

The limitations of high-technology beds include patient temperature control, potential dehydration, limited mobility from bed to chair or other surfaces, thereby limiting patient independence and increasing care giver dependence, patient adjustment to flotation, bed design, cost, and limited applicability to the home setting.

The water mattress, or water-filled overlay, has been shown to provide significant pressure reduction below capillary closing pressures. In a flotation device, the patient's weight is distributed over a greater surface area, thus decreasing the pressures over bony prominences. Some water mattresses, when properly inflated, will float the patient over the surface with documented mean capillary pressure of 11 mmHg CM^2 body surface in the supine position [10]. Since all water mattresses will not accomplish pressure reduction and some mattresses will not have enough structural capacity to float the patient properly, care should be taken in prescribing the proper mattress. In addition, special caution must be taken in the set up and maintenance of the water mattress to assure adequate flotation.

Although more cost effective, water mattresses, similarly to air-fluidized therapy, cause added mobility difficulties with transfers, may worsen spasticity, and may cause motion sickness. Despite these limitations, water mattresses may be used effectively in hospitals and in the home. In addition, some patients can remain in a supine position for a prolonged period (as long as 8 h) without showing any signs of compromise to the skin. However, caution and individualization of the patient's tolerance must be utilized when considering this extended positioning schedule. Careful pre- and post-positioning skin assessments should be completed with any lengthening of a turning/positioning schedule. Hospitals and home care equipment costs are minimized when water mattresses are utilized in that high-technology beds require significant expenditure, use of electrical systems, and electrical backup to maintain mattress effectiveness during blackouts. It is critical to restate that, regardless of the type of mattress overlay, mattress, or specialty bed, great consideration must be given to the initiation, progression, and assessment of a patient's turning regimen and bed positioning. Patients and care givers should not develop a false sense of security through the use of any device, as no device is fail-safe. Before a device is selected, the risk–benefit ratio should be determined by assessing patient tolerance, acceptability, functionality, comfort, costs, care delivery, and patient goals.

In addition to selecting a pressure relief surface, the following basic guidelines must be adhered to for prevention of ulcer development:

1. Repositioning at least every 2 h if consistent with overall patient and treatment goals. This will include a written plan for implementation. (Some limitations to this might include alterations in cardiopulmonary status which limits patient tolerance of turning or prone positioning.)
2. Utilization of supportive surfaces, including foam wedges, heel protection, and pillows to reduce shear and pressure on and between bony prominences.
3. Positioning to reduce or minimize direct pressure on bony prominences.
4. Positioning to reduce shear forces including appropriate head elevation (not greater than 30°) (except during feeding) and appropriate transfer techniques with appropriate use of transfer aids.
5. Incorporating pressure relief measures at least every 30 min for 30 s, including forward pressure relief, reclining positions, and lateral shifts to decrease pressure over ischial, sacral, and trochanteric sites while sitting in a wheelchair or geriatric chair.

Functional and medical interventions must also be taken into consideration to prevent decubitus ulcer development. These are outlined in the Appendix [10]. Numerous wheelchair cushion products are also available, including foam, air, and gel products. With wheelchair cushions, it is not possible to achieve pressure relief adequate enough to reduce capillary compression. Therefore, cushion selection is based on achieving the lowest possible pressure, with a surface that manages heat and moisture build up while facilitating wheelchair posture, mobility, and transfers.

Henderson et al. [11] have identified patients who are unable to perform or adequately achieve total pressure relief as a result of preexisting conditions, insufficient upper extremity strength and endurance, and who require staff and care takers to be particularly aware of their role in the prevention of decubitus ulcers. This study examined pressure relief measures and their effectiveness. Three pressure relief interventions, including the 65° backward tip, the 35° sideway tip, and forward lean chest to thigh were studied. The forward lean consistently reduced pressures on the ischial tuberosites to near or below 32 mmHg [11]. Power and manual chair products that are currently available attempt to achieve effective pressure relief at incremental stages through tilt and recline mechanisms. Safety, stability, postural maintenance, and minimal shearing can be achieved through the proper selection and use of these advanced wheelchair systems.

Concern regarding pressure relief management is also identified with the use of special equipment such as the shower–commode chair. Many sensory and motor-impaired patients require a bowel and bladder program. At a minimum, many bowel programs are regulated on an every other day or third day routine. Frequent transfers to the commode chair, as well as overuse of the commode, particularly with ineffective bowel routines, may lead to sacral, ischial, or trochanteric decubitus ulcers. This occurs because of prolonged sitting, shearing of unprotected skin while transferring, and ineffective or no pressure relief during the routine. A study [12] compared three types of shower chairs measuring interface pressure at risk sites during commode chair use. All three shower chairs posed significant risk as each exceeded maximum acceptable pressures for these sites. In addition [13], SCI patients, unlike the able-bodied individual, is more at risk for ischemia at moderate pressures at all bony sites. Therefore, prolonged sitting, whether in a wheelchair or on a padded commode chair, may place the patient at risk if pressure relief interventions are not incorporated into the activity.

These studies, although limited in design, also verify the need to assess all components of an individual's rehabilitation program and careful management of all aspects of care which may contribute to decubitus ulcer development.

The challenges of decubitus ulcer treatment selection and surgical management are addressed elsewhere in this text (Chaps. 10, 11). A brief discussion of the approaches in a rehabilitation program identifies the ever-changing approaches to decubitus ulcer prevention and treatment.

Managing preexisting medical conditions is essential for the optimal healing of wounds and for the prevention of decubitus ulcers. In the rehabilitation population, certain medical problems that contribute to the development of decubitus ulcers include altered cognition; altered sensation and mobility; hemodynamic changes; anemia; edema; musculoskeletal problems; contractures, heterotopic ossification, and spasticity; infection; malnutrition; undernourishment or overnourishment; incontinence; and iatrogenic causes. Aging patients, trauma patients, and neurologically impaired patients typically experience many of these problems throughout their hospital stays as well as in the community. The early recognition of these medical problems at any point in the continuum of care will help to reduce the risk and severity of decubitus ulcers. Given the medically compromised rehabilitation patient of the 1990s, the primary concern of physicians and rehabilitation staff is to restore health and manage or eliminate complications which place the patient at risk for decubitus ulcer development.

Treatment options for managing pressure ulcers are rapidly growing and changing. Controversy continues over the use of cleansing agents, wet to dry dressings, and certain topical agents for the management of wounds. Although various articles identify the potential cytotoxicity of these agents, many practitioners continue to use solutions to cleanse the ulcer and to provide bacteriostatic control. According to Baxter and Rodeheaver [14], "Antiseptic solutions and washing agents, such as free iodine, alcohol, merbromin, chlorhexidine, soaps/detergents, and hydrogen peroxide, while suitable for healthy, unbroken skin surrounding the wound, are too caustic for the wound itself." In addition, the authors say the actual volume and force of irrigation are more important than the solution itself for cleansing the wound of debris, necrotic tissue, and bacteria. They also question the use of topical antibiotics in wound management and recommend that, due to their unestablished efficacy and the risk of developing resistant organisms or sensitization, they should be used cautiously and for a limited time. When a clinical infection is suspected, parenteral antibiotics should be employed.

Decubitus ulcer cleansing and debridement are usually provided through mechanical, enzymatic, osmotic, or autolytic means. In our view, mechanical debridement often includes surgical debridement, irrigation with a saline solution and other agents, wet to dry dressings, or whirlpool. Enzyme preparations that break down fibrin clots and exudate provide an optimal wound environment for new tissue growth. These agents must be used cautiously and monitored because they may be nonselective and could impair new tissue growth. To work most effectively, these agents require a moist wound bed. Osmotic debridement includes the use of products such as dextranomers, granular absorbers, and gels that absorb exudate and create this moist wound environment.

Other newer topical products include calcium alginate, a product made from seaweed, which provides a high absorptive capacity and conformability to wounds and growth factors [15, 16].

Behavioral, Educational Management of Decubitus Ulcers in a Rehabilitation Setting

There is a dearth of information regarding the behavioral, educational, and psychosocial factors that contribute to decubitus ulcer development. Probably the most cited study, Anderson and Andberg [17], attempted to determine factors other than physiologic and mechanical that relate to the development of decubitus ulcers in quadriplegic and paraplegic persons. The study showed a strong association between decubitus ulcer incidence and psychosocial variables, as well as a relationship between the level of injury and the presence or absence of help with skin care. The most important factor noted in this study was the influence of self-esteem and life satisfaction on a person's feelings about practices and responsibility in skin care. These psychosocial factors were related to the occurrence, recurrence, and persistance of decubitus ulcers in persons with paraplegia.

Through our experience as a rehabilitation provider of the regional spinal cord injury program, we identified the need to develop a comprehensive educational/behavioral program for the management of decubitus ulcers. In the early 1980s, a subgroup of our SPI population had an 80 % recurrence of decubitus ulcers within 3 months of successful treatment of the decubitus ulcer as an in-patient or out-patient in our spinal cord follow-up program. This prompted an interdisciplinary team to develop a decubitus ulcer readmission program. The goals of this program include learning specific information and behaviors related to skin care and disability management, and to define and attain goals related to psychosocial and vocational outcomes which would build healthy behaviors. The team recognized that the incidence of recurrent decubitus ulcers was related not only to biomechanical, biochemical, medical, and functional issues but also to psychosocial and vocational ones. The ability to initiate, perform, or direct care, the availability of a health care professional, and the knowledge to seek help seemed to have a substantial effect on a person's ability to maintain intact skin and good health, and this was reflected in our patient subgroup.

The program is based on the premise that multifaceted approach to educating patients will help alter behaviors and reduce the incidence of recurrent decubitus ulcers [18].

Through the assistance of a coach, a decubitus ulcer program team, and patients already in the program, a patient learns new skills in avoiding decubitus ulcer "at risk" activities. The role of the coach is to assist the patient with program participation and completion, to enhance learning and compliance, and to facilitate optimal patient outcomes including decubitus ulcer healing. The coach meets weekly with the patient, reviews individual and program goals, administers "knowledge" tests before and after program completion and reviews the results, assists with resolving program agreement violations, and monitors the patient's progress and readiness for progression or discharge from the program.

Before entering the program, the patient formally agrees to the goals mutually established by signing a written agreement. The agreement outlines staff responsibilites for assuring patient success and the patient's responsibilities for participating in the program. Patients are also informed of hospital policies and procedures, including those related to the use of substances not prescribed by the attending physician. Screening for substance abuse is done periodically, and a positive urine or serum screen results in discharge from the in-patient program with ongoing monitoring provided on an as-needed basis in the out-patient follow-up system, as well as referral to a substance abuse program.

The program has evolved into three phases. Phase I (core) is for patients admitted for the first time with a primary diagnosis of decubitus ulcer (grade II or greater). It is also for persons who previously participated in the program but required readmission to the acute hospital. Phase II is designed for persons who successfully complete the program but who are readmitted with another skin problem. Successful completion is defined as a 70 % or higher score in the postprogram tests or if a patient shows an adequate knowledge of proper skin care and healed skin. Phase II classes, titled "Challenge and Enrichment," focus on community and other psychosocial issues as well as on medical-functional and equipment issues. Phase III is a specialized program for patients admitted with a primary diagnosis other than skin breakdown and with decubitus ulcers as a secondary diagnosis.

The decubitus ulcer program begins at the point of referral from another hospital or anywhere within our hospital programs, the out-patient system of care, or the community. Preprogram screening is completed by the physiatrist, nurse clinician, and/or social worker. Controlling spasticity, treating infection, improving respiratory and nutritional status, evaluating the patient's possible response to decubitus ulcer treatments and interventions, maintaining or improving bowel and bladder status, and addressing functional and home-maker activities are a part of this evaluation process. If surgical debridement is indicated, consultation is provided by the program's plastic surgeon. Pre-operative education regarding the surgical procedure, postoperative care, and rehabilitation management is provided before hospital admission. Functional and equipment issues are coordinated by a nurse clinician in consultation with a physical or occupational therapist.

The surgical phase (7–10 days) involves admission to an acute care hospital. During this admission, the patient is monitored by the readmission team which includes an acute care physiatrist, the SCI project coordinator, and the follow-up nurse clinician to assure that the acute care team adheres to disability-specific issues, such as bowel, bladder, or spasticity management; responds to patient's individual needs; and facilitates a timely admission to the rehabilitation phase of the program.

The patient actively participates in an individually designed program comprising classes based on program placement, successful testing, or both. The program has expanded to more than 40 possible educational sessions on topics such as skin management, functional equipment issues, assertiveness classes, and vocational and community survival issues. During this phase, the patient is expected to attend a "community" meeting, patient and team meetings, and a coping group. Also during this phase, the goals are to facilitate wound healing, educate, reinforce behavioral skills, and maintain skin integrity. Finally, integrated throughout the program are community skills groups which focus on avoidance and identification of at-risk behavior and/or situations that the patient will encounter after discharge which may place him or her further at risk for decubitus ulcer development.

The program has also been modified to include a day treatment program, incorporating many components of the comprehensive in-patient program so that patients with reimbursement limitation can benefit from this intense educational and behavioral approach to treatment and future prevention of decubitus ulcers.

For evaluation and outcome purposes, patient performance and success in maintaining skin integrity is measured through intact skin. Conversely, failure is measured through the development of or a nonhealing of the decubitus ulcer. It is critical, however, to view nonhealing not as failure but as a result of repeated trauma from sustained pressure, shear, moisture, compromised health, psychosocial status, or all of these factors.

As a significantly complex health problem, it is essential for all health care and rehabilitation professionals to assist the patient and each other in understanding success and failure for maintaining skin integrity. Success may be measured through the patient's ability to independently and consistently perform and direct others to perform the skin care program. This includes the ability to direct or demonstrate skin care techniques, including the use of inspection mirrors, appropriate pressure relief techniques, appropriate use of equipment and knowledge to solve equipment problems, the ability to detect skin problems early and intervene immediately and seek appropriate attention from the health care system. One could also utilize the same expectations to measure the effectiveness of the care provided by the health care professionals throughout the health care continuum.

Questions to evaluate outcomes or effectiveness in maintaining skin integrity include:

1. Have we prevented decubitus ulcers and over what length of time post onset of disability trauma has skin integrity been maintained?
2. Have we been timely and consistent in our prevention measures and early interventions?
3. Have we properly instructed staff, care providers, and patients in maintaining skin integrity?
4. Have we selected the appropriate equipment that will minimize decubitus ulcer occurrence and persistance?
5. Have we thoroughly explored the needs of the patient and his or her care provider in adhering to a realistic skin care program?
6. Do we provide ongoing support and accesss for problem solving, early intervention, and program modification?

Success in maintaining skin integrity is based on "professional" and "individual" vigilance, and a realistic and consistent approach to preventing and managing decubitus ulcers. As identified by Petro [19], responsibility for illness and injury (decubitus ulcers) lies with the health care givers in institutions as well as with patients themselves.

It our responsibility as rehabilitation professionals to provide these prevention and treatment interventions and to assist the patient in achieving independence with this crucial aspect of care.

Appendix

Functional and Medical Interventions

Forces and activities contributing to pressure development	Interventions to relieve and avoid pressure
Scapula	
Direct Pressure	
Supine position: Insufficient pressure relief	Inspect skin every shift if wearing immobilizer

	Bed: relieve pressure in supine position
	  Use turning schedules
	  Use water mattress if indicated

Sitting position
  Semi-reclined position with sufficient
  pressure relief by weight shifting
	Wheelchair: relieve pressure in semi-reclining position
	  Perform 15–30 min weight shifts (independently by patient or assisted by staff)
	  Use tilt/recline wheelchair systems

Shearing forces	

Sitting position
  Sliding down in bed while head of bed
  is raised
	Bed: prevent shearing over scapula; avoid elevating head of bed more than 30°
	  Use footboards, pillows, bolsters between patients' feet and board of bed to prevent sliding when sitting up in bed

Forces and activities contributing to pressure development	Interventions to relieve and avoid pressure
Other contributing factors Plastic body jackets; cervical spine immobilized with body jackets	Use water mattress or other effective pressure-reducing overlay when patients are in body casts and body jackets

Elbows
Direct Pressure

Prone position Insufficient pressure relief when leaning on elbows for support	Bed prone carts: prevent pressure/trauma when elbows are used for leaning and support; use elbow protectors Instruct patients in proper positioning and trauma prevention Provide patient with bolsters and wedges so that elbows are not used to support upper trunk and head
Other contributing factors Trauma Elbows are used for leverage and changing position	

Sacrum
Direct pressure

In the supine position Pressure unrelieved by turning; insufficient time off back In sitting position Slumping in a wheel chair	Bed: relieve pressure Use turning schedule at least every 2 h Use appropriate foam wedges for support Wheelchair: correct slumping Correct poor wheelchair seat (seat "hammocks"); replace with new seat or use a seat board under wheelchair cushion Evaluate posture and lower extremity positioning and support

Shearing forces

In sitting position Sliding down in bed when the head of bed is raised; sliding forward on the wheelchair seat	Bed: prevent sliding Do not elevate head of bed more than 30° Use footboards, wedges, pillows between lower extremities Wheel chair: prevent forward sliding Select appropriate chair back support Use seat belts, lapboards Correct wheelchair seat height – seat must be low enough for hemiplegic, incomplete quadriplegic, to propel Should not need to pull self forward in wheelchair to propel with foot
In supine position Inappropriate turning techniques	Bed: prevent shearing Use correct turning techniques; do not slide or pull body across sheets Roll and lift hips, ankles and shoulders across bed Medical management of spasticity Reclining wheelchair: prevent shearing; select reduced shear power chair; use a wheelchair cushion that gives with movement, i.e., Roho air cushion

Forces and activities contributing to pressure development	Interventions to relieve and avoid pressure
Other contributing factors Body casts, plastic body jackets, other immobilizing devices	Bed and wheelchair: prevent pressure from plaster casts, body jackets Increase frequency of turning use water mattress, trim casts over bony prominences if possible insure proper fit of body jacket, vests

Trochanters

Direct pressure Side lying position Prolonged pressure unrelieved by turning; insufficient time between turns	Relieve pressure Position in a 30° oblique position to sacrum, trochanter ischium Relieve pressure Use turning schedule
Sitting position Poor wheelchair fit – too narrow	Wheelchair: relieve pressure Check for adequate room for hips in wheelchair seat Hips should not touch either armrests or wheels Assess for weight gain, edema, development of heterotopic ossification
Shearing forces Side lying position Lower extremity spasticity draws hips across bed sheets	Bed: prevent shearing Adjust position to insure legs do not rest on one another Use pillows to bolster position when side lying; this action will deter the sliding that occurs with spasticity Arrange turning schedule to avoid side involved with heterotopic bone or shorten period of time on that trochanter Medically manage spasticity
Other contributing factors Heteroptic bone	

Ischeal Tuberosites

Direct pressure Sitting position Prolonged pressure unrelieved by adequate weight shifting; improper position of leg and footrest of wheelchair; poor condition of wheelchair seat – the "hammock" effect	Wheelchair: relieve pressure Perform weight shifts in wheelchair every 15–30 min (independently by patient or assisted by staff) Use lateral, posterior, or forward shift techniques Correct improper footrest positioning; if footrests are positioned too high, weight is born directly over ischium – adjust so that body weight is distributed evenly over thighs and buttock Increase depth of wheelchair cushion, this will cause weight to fall forward on thighs Use seat board under cushion to correct "hammock" effect of wheelchair seat

Forces and activities contributing to pressure development	Interventions to relieve and avoid pressure
Shearing forces	
Sitting position	Wheelchair: prevent shearing
Poor technique when transferring from one surface to another; sliding the skin over a board used to assist the transfer	Avoid sliding buttocks across transfer board (if necessary, buttocks should be lifted over board in a series of short pushups)
	Avoid hitting brakes and wheel rims during transfers
	Commode chair: do not use over prolonged period
	Perform pressure relief measures
	Select tilt/recliner wheelchair with minimal shearing
Other contributing factors	Bed and wheelchair: prevent shearing over compromised skin/tissue
Previous skin breakdown with scarring heterotopic bone	Increase frequency of turns in bed
	Avoid turning onto side of involvement
	Lift when turning; do not pull or slide across bed or wheelchair seat
	Use wheelchair cushion that "gives" with movement, i.e., Roho air cushion
	Medically manage spasticity
Knees	
Direct pressure	
Prone position	Bed: prevent pressure in prone position
Insufficient pressure relief	Use correct positioning techniques; bolster pillows to bridge bony prominences when on regular mattress
	Use water mattress if indicated
Side lying position	Bed: prevent pressure on lateral knees (side lying position)
Insufficient pressure relief	Use turning schedule
	Use water mattress if indicated
Shearing forces	
Side lying position	Bed: prevent shearing on lateral knees (side lying position)
Lower extremity spasticity drawing knees across bedsheets	Proper positioning with pillows or wedges avoiding contact between knees
	Medically manage spasticity
Ankles	
Direct pressure	
Side lying position	Bed and wheelchair: prevent pressure on lateral ankle
Insufficient pressure relief	Use turning schedule
	Use water mattress if indicated
	Use foot/ankle protectors that completely support ankle off of bed
Sitting position	Position foot correctly on footplate; foot should rest squarely on footplate and not rest against pins or heel loops
In wheelchair – poor position of foot on footplate of wheelchair, trauma during transfers	

Forces and activities contributing to pressure development	Interventions to relieve and avoid pressure

Other contributing factors
  Ankle edema, poor shoe fit
	Bed and wheelchair: relieve edema
	  Elevate feet
	  Use elastic stockings
	  Correct shoe fit (advise larger shoe size if edema is a chronic problem)

Toes

Direct pressure
Sitting position
  Trauma during transfers, wheelchair maneuvering
	Wheelchair: prevent trauma
	  Instruct patient's staff in proper transfer techniques
	  Proper size footplate to support and protect foot and toes
	  Instruct patient to wear shoes when up in wheelchair
	  Wear correct size footwear
	  Avoid shear with application of footwear

Prone position
  Poor positioning and insufficient relief
	Bed: relieve pressure in prone position
	  Use correct positioning; toes should not touch mattress
	  Position feet over end of mattress or use pillows or bolster

Other contributing factors Ingrown, infected toenails; tight elastic stockings, poor fitting shoes	

Heels

Direct pressure
Supine position
  Prolonged pressure on heels unrelieved by proper relief or elimination of pressure
Side lying position
  Prolonged pressure on malleoli unrelieved by proper relief or elimination of pressure
Foot positioning in wheelchair
  Improper leg rest length and improper foot plate positioning increases heel pressure
	Decrease lower extremity swelling through use of elevating leg rests
	Wear properly fitting shoes to avoid shearing on heel with application and removal and to accommodate dependent pedal edema
	
	Elevate heels off mattress through the use of pillows or bolsters under lower extremity – egg crate under Achilles tendon

Shearing forces	Avoid trauma to feet and lower extremities with transfers Inspect heels and feet for abrasions, blisters, induration in morning, prior to activity, and at night with evening routine
Supine and side lying position Increased by improper semi-Fowler's/ position and improper positioning (sliding) instead of lifting up in bed with repositioning	Assess for contractures, lower extremity spasticity and treat appropriately to minimize shear and pressure forces

Other contributing factors
  Lower extremity swelling
  Pedal edema
  Clonus
  Lower extremity spasticity
  Foot deformities
	Apply transparent film or extra-thin occlusive dressing over bony prominences if reddened to decrease friction and shear
	
	Position heels and lateral medial malleoli so that all surface pressure is eliminated with bolsters, pillows, heel boots

Other Factors Contributing to Pressure Ulcer Development

Change in support systems
Change in care takers
Changes in bowel and bladder routines resulting in incontinence
Accessibility – stair and "surface"/curb management; repetitive
trauma from aggressive mobility activities
Malfunctioning equipment and failure to identify and intervene
(e.g., punctured cushions, power recliner chair failure, mattress
overlay malfunction)
Change in financial resources which affect regimen and care
delivery
Health habits (smoking, ethyl alcohol and substance abuse, weight
management, over or under nourished)
Change in activity schedule without incorporating appropriate
pressure relief measures (return to work, school, travel)

References

1. Miller H, Delozier J (1994) Cost implications of the pressure ulcer treatment guideline. Columbia, MD: center for health policy studies, 1994. Sponsored by Agency for Health Care Policy and Research. Contract no 282-91-0070
2. Young J, Burns P (1981) Pressure sores and the spinal cord injured. Model Syst SCI Dig 3(PTI):9–18
3. Whiteneck G, Carter R, Charlifue S et al. (1985) A collaborative study of high quadriplegia. (Rocky Mountain Regional Spinal Cord Injury System, Northern California Regional Spinal Injury System and Texas Regional Spinal Cord Injury System). Craig Hospital, Englewood CO
4. Cooney T, Reuler J (1984) Pressure sores: topics in primary care medicine. West J Med 140:622–624
5. LaMantia J, Hirschwald J, Goodman et al. (1987) A program design to reduce chronic readmission for pressure sores. Rehabil Nurs 12:22–25
6. Woodbury B, Redd C (1987) Psychosocial issues and approaches. In: Buchanan L, Nawoczenski (eds) Spinal cord injury: concepts and management approaches. Williams and Wilkins, Baltimore, pp 185–218
7. Kosiak M (1961) Etiology and pathology of ischemic ulcers. Arch Phys Med Rehabil 42:19–29
8. Lindan O (1961) Etiology of decubitus ulcers: an experimental study. Decubitus ulcer. Arch Phys Med Rehabil 774–783 ·
9. Maklebust J, Mondoux L, Sieggreen M (1986) Pressure relief characteristics of various support surfaces used in prevention and treatment of pressure ulcers. J Enterostom Ther 85–89
10. Staas W, LaMantia J (1983) Rehabilitation approach. In: Parish L, Witkowski J, Crissey J (eds) The decubitus ulcer, Chap 9. Masson, New York, pp 83–90
11. Henderson J, Price S, Brandstater M, Mandac B (1994) Efficacy of three measures to relieve pressure in seated persons with spinal cord injury. Arch Phys Med Rehabil 75:535–539
12. Nelson A, Malassigne P, Murray J (1994) Comparison of seat pressures on three bowel care/shower chairs in spinal cord injury. SCI Nurs 11:105–107
13. Patterson R, Cranmer H, Fisher SV, Engel R (1993) The impaired response of spinal cord injured individuals to repeated surface pressure loads. Arch Phys Med Rehabil 74:947–953

14. Baxter C, Rodheaver G (1990) Interventions: hemostasis, cleansing, topical antibiotics, debridement, and closure. In: Wound care manual. Convatec: a Squibb Company, Princeton, pp 71–82
15. Chapius A, Dolfus P (1990) The use of a calcium alginate dressing the management of decubitus ulcers in patients with spinal cord lesions. Paraplegia 28:269–271
16. Frylling C (1989) Comprehensive wound management with topical growth factors. Ostomy/Wound Care Management, 36:42–51
17. Anderson T, Andberg M (1979) Psychosocial factors associated with pressure sores. Arch Phys Med Rehabil 60:341–346
18. Staas W, Cioschi H (1991) Rehabilitation medicine – adding life to years. Pressure sores – a multifaceted approach to prevention and treatment. West J Med 154:539–544
19. Petro J (1990) Ethical dilemmas of pressure sores. Decubitus 3(2):28–31

Therapy – Specific

13 Occlusive Dressings

L.L. Bolton and L. van Rijswijk

More than 40 years have passed since Gilje [1], a dermatologist, discovered that leg ulcers covered with tape healed faster than those covered with gauze. His observations not only stimulated wound healing research in general, but also inspired researchers and clinicians to evaluate the effect of topical agents on the healing process. As a result, we now know that almost every aspect of the healing process can be affected by what we put on, or in, a wound [2]. With the realization that dehydration is detrimental to wounds came the development of would care products that "provide a moist environment" and their use in the management of chronic wounds such as decubitus or pressure ulcers. Specifically, clinicians can now choose from more than 70 dressings, wound filler products, gels, and creams designed to be "occlusive, to promote moist wound healing, to prevent unnecessary loss of body fluids or to provide a moist environment" [3]. Unfortunately, neither the definitions of these terms, nor their clinical relevance have been clearly defined.

Therefore, before discussing the clinical use of these dressings, it is important to establish an operational definition of moisture-retentive dressings based on objective criteria.

Defining Moisture-Retentive Dressings

Literally, to occlude means to "shut or stop up so as to prevent anything from passing in, out, or through" [4]. Thus, occlussive dressings can include dressings that provide a barrier to all combinations or mixtures of chemical elements (solids, liquids, gases), as well as microorganisms. Some products are defined as occlusive because they exclude topical oxygen from the wound surface; hence, they may facilitate angiogenesis [5]. Others are called "semi-occlusive," usually defined as "permeable to oxygen but relatively impermeable to moisture vapor transmission." Indeed, when compared to gauze-type dressings, these semi-occlusive dressings will facilitate the growth of new blood vessels. However, angiogenesis is significantly more pronounced in wounds dressed with occlusive as compared to semi-occlusive dressings [6]. The definition of semi-occlusive may also have been introduced to help clinicians overcome their fear of infection under occlusion, which has proven to be unfounded [7]. Specifically, wounds dressed with moisture-retentive dressings are less likely to become infected than those dressed with conventional dressings. This may, in part, be related to the fact that fluid from wounds dressed with moisture-retentive dressings has been found to contain viable polymorphonuclear leucocytes, macrophages, lymphocytes, and monocytes [8]. The reluctance to use occlusive dressings and fear of infection was most often based on observing folliculitis and maceration following the use of occlusive plastic film, such as Saran wrap, to treat dermatologic conditions. Of course, these plastic films are not only completely occlusive to moisture vapor, but are also unable to absorb any fluid.

In today's practice, the term "occlusive dressing" is most often used to describe a product that retains moisture at the wound site. Since most occlusive and semi-occlusive dressings are designed to prevent dessication of the wound bed, which has been shown to benefit the healing process, the most practical and objective operational definition of occlusion should be based on a dressing's ability to retain moisture. In addition, dressing moisture vapor transmission rates (MVTR) can be measured objectively and are clinically relevant since research has shown that greater dressing moisture retention (i.e., lower dressing MVTR) is correlated with faster wound healing. For exuding partial-thickness wounds, MVTR values of < 35 g/m^2 per hour are sufficient to facilitate moist wound healing [9, 10]. Theoretically, MVTR levels higher than 35 g/m^2 per hour may provide moist healing if wounds are deeper and more exudative, or when the dressing or wound filler is covered with a moisture-retentive dressing. For example, in vivo research has shown that calcium alginate dressings may dry the wound when covered with gauze, but that they maintain a moist wound bed when covered with a hydrocolloid dressing [11]. Similarly, in vitro studies have shown that the MVTR of wound dressings decreases when additional bandages are used [12].

Unfortunately, research in this area remains very limited. Most importantly, few dressings have been clinically tested to substantiate common product descriptions such as "provides a moist wound-healing environment." This may be important because, in addition to the effect of secondary dressings discussed, variations among "similar" dressing types do exist. For example, in one study of superficial wounds in humans, MVTR for film-type dressings was found to range from 14.6 to 34.1 g/cm^2 per hour [9]. Similarly, we have found differences in MVTR and corresponding reepithelialization rates for different hydrocolloid dressings (Fig.1). To be clinically relevant, MVTR values should apply to the complete dressing (all layers) as measured on a real or simulated exuding wound at body temperature and away from sources of moving air or moisture such as air vents or vaporizers.

Using Moisture-Retentive Dressings on Decubitus Ulcers

Decubitus ulcers present the clinician and researcher with unique challenges, including limited research upon which to base treatment decisions. With respect to the existing literature, study design methods and data analysis methods often do not control for the effect of covariates that have been found to influence the healing rate of these ulcers, e.g., ulcer depth, patient nutritional

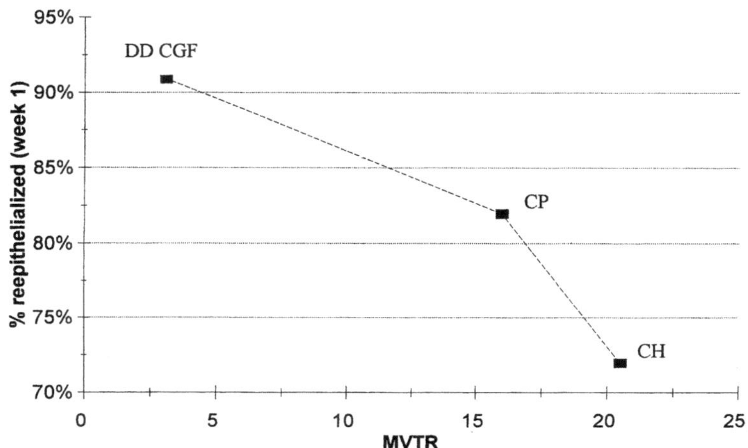

Fig. 1. Percentage return of cutaneous barrier function after 7 days of dressing five to eight dorsal swine donor sites as a function of the MVTR of three different hydrocolloid dressings. *DD CGF*, DuoDERM Control Gel Formula dressings; CP, Comfeel Plus ulcer dressing; *CH*, Cutinova Hydro

status, use of pressure-relieving devices, incontinence, mobility, and patient age [13]. However, once the challenge of managing the underlying etiology has been met, there appears to be little difference between the acute and chronic wounds. Compared to wounds dressed with conventional dry or impregnated gauze dressings, chronic wounds covered with a moisture-retentive dressing heal more expediently and are less painful [14–16].

Use of Moisture-Retentive Dressings in Patients with Erythema

Nonblanchable erythema is commonly referred to as a stage I decubitus ulcer or "the heralding lesion of skin ulceration" [17]. Even though decubitus ulcer prevalence survey data indicate that stage I ulcers are more common than stage II or III ulcers, information about their treatment is very limited [18]. Also, because there is no apparent break in the skin, measures that may prevent this from occurring are often not reimbursed [19]. If the presence of erythema is discovered shortly after its occurrence and the cause of the erythema (pressure, shear, friction, exposure to feces or urine) addressed, skin breakdown may be prevented.

General measures designed to reduce pressure such as frequent repositioning, specialty beds, mattresses, and chair pads can be augmented by protecting the skin from shear, friction, and/or the deleterious effects of exposure to feces and urine [20]. Proper (re)positioning techniques as well as the

Table 1. Selecting a moisture-retentive dressing for decubitus ulcers

Dressing type	Dressing characteristics			Indications						Comments
	Moisture retentive	Facilitate autolysis	Secondary dressing needed	Erythema	Partial-thickness wounds	Deep wounds	Dry wounds	Light/ moderately exudative wounds	Highly exudative wounds	
Film dressings	Yes	Yes	No	Yes	Yes	Not generally recommended	Yes	Yes	Not generally recommended	Use with caution in patients with fragile skin
Thin hydrocolloid dressings	Yes	Yes	No	Yes	Yes	Wound filler may be needed	Yes	Yes	Absorption dressing is needed	Adheres to slightly moist skin; remove with caution in patients with fragile skin; some provide microbial barrier
Hydrocolloid dressings	Yes	Yes	No	Yes	Yes	Wound filler may be needed	Yes	Yes	Absorption dressing may be needed[a]	Will adhere to slightly moist skin; some provide microbial barrier

Foam dressings	Yes for some	Not all do	Yes if non-adherent	No	Yes	Wound filler may be needed	No	Yes	Absorption dressing may be needed	Dressing characteristics and adhesive properties vary; discontinue use if removal causes tissue damage
Alginate dressings	Yes[b]	Yes[b]	Yes	No	Yes	Yes	No	No	Yes	Available in sheets and ropes; discontinue use if removal causes tissue damage
Hydrophylic beads, powders, paste, and dressings	Yes[b]	Not all do	Yes	No	Yes	Yes	No	No	Product dependent	May be difficult to remove from deep sinus tracts if not in sheet/dressing form
Hydrogel dressings	Yes for some	Yes	Yes, if non-adherent	No	Yes	No	Yes	Yes	No	Bacterial barrier/adhesive properties vary
Amorphous hydrogel dressings	Yes[b]	Yes[b]	Yes	No	Yes	Yes	Yes	Yes[c]	No	Often used for autolytic debridement

[a]Depending on amount of exudate and type of hydrocolloid dressing used.
[b]If covered with moisture-retentive dressing.
[c]Some hydrogel paste products have the capacity to release as well as absorb moisture.

use of lubricants or protective dressings, particularly those with a smooth top layer, will reduce shear and friction [21]. In incontinent patients, moisture-retentive dressings with a smooth top layer (e.g., polyurethane film or thin hydrocolloid dressings) are particularly helpful because they will not only reduce shear and friction but will also protect the skin against contamination and prevent dehydration. These dressings, providing they are adhering properly and the skin remains intact, should remain in place for 5–7 days. Frequent removal is neither necessary (skin breakdown can be assessed through the dressing) nor recommended because the longer they remain in place, the easier it is to remove them.

Choosing a Moisture-Retentive Dressing to Manage Partial-Thickness and Full-Thickness Ulcers

The general principles of wound care, cleanse, debride, protect, and provide a moist wound environment, apply to superficial, partial-thickness as well as full-thickness decubitus ulcers. The type of moisture-retentive dressing to use depends on the condition of the wound bed, wound margins, the amount of wound exudate as well as the depth of the ulcer (Tables 1, 2).

Moisture-retentive dressings, used alone, retain moisture as described above. Their low MVTR prevents dessication and facilitates healing (e.g., hydrocolloid or film dressings). Additional primary dressings may be needed to fill wound dead space or quickly absorb copious amounts of exudate (e.g., alginate and Hydrofiber dressings). Very dry, necrotic, wounds may need additional moisture to permit endogenous enzymes to digest the devitalized tissue. Moisture-releasing (supplemental) primary dressings can provide this additional moisture to dry wounds (e.g., DuoDERM Gel dressing, IntraSite gel). A moisture-retentive dressing used as a secondary dressing over absorption or moisture-releasing dressings will protect the wound against contamination while preventing leakage of exudate or drying of the wound bed. These additional dressings are not designed to be used during the entire wound healing process. When the wound is no longer highly exudative or dry, their use should be discontinued.

The most commonly used moisture-retentive dressings, e.g., hydrocolloid and film dressings, are designed to remain in place for up to 7 days. In clinical practice, they are usually changed once every 2–5 days. The frequency of dressing changes depends on the method of application, the type of dressing used, the location of the wound, the presence/absence of incontinence, and the amount of wound exudate. Dressing wounds in the sacral area, particularly in incontinent patients, can be very challenging. Indeed, the same factors that may have contributed to the formation of the ulcer in the first place (shear and friction) may dislodge the dressing. Proper positioning/re-positioning techniques may help prevent this problem. In addition, selecting the right dressing and applying it carefully will help increase dressing wear time. For example, in one study of sacral decubitus ulcers, it was found that triangle-shaped hydrocolloid dressings (DuoDERM Control Gel Formula border dressing) re-

Table 2. Examples of moisture-retentive dressings and manufacturers[a] in the United States

Dressing type[b]	Examples	Manufacturer
Film dressings	Bioclusive	Johnson & Johnson Med.
	Biofilm	Sherwood Medical
	Flexfilm	Dow B. Hickham, Inc.
	OpSite	Smith & Nephew United
	Pro-Clude	ConvaTec
Thin hydrocolloid	Comfeel transp. HCD	Coloplast Inc.
dressings (HCD)	DuoDERM CGF Extra Thin	ConvaTec
	Restore Extra Thin	Hollister Inc.
Hydrocolloid	CombiDERM ACD dressing	ConvaTec
dressings (HCD)	DuoDERM/DuoDERM CGF	ConvaTec
	Restore/Restore CX	Hollister Inc.
	Tegasorb	3M Health Care
	Ultec	Sherwood Medical
Foam dressings	Allevyn	Smith & Nephew United
	Lyofoam	Acme United Corp.
	Mitraflex	ConvaTec
	PolyMem	Ferris Manuf.
Alginate dressings	Algosteril	Johnson & Johnson Med.
	Kaltostat	ConvaTec
	Sorbsan	Dow B. Hickham, Inc.
Hydrophylic beads,	Aquacel Hydrofiber	ConvaTec
powders, paste, and	Bard absorption dressing	C.R. Bard Inc.
Hydrofiber dressings	Debrisan Hydrofiber	Johnson & Johnson Med.
	Multidex hydrophilic powder	DeRoyal Wound Care
Hydrogel dressings	Aquasorb	DeRoyal Industr. Inc
	Elasto-Gel	Southwest Technologies
	Nu-gel	Johnson & Johnson Med.
	Vigilon	C.R. Bard Inc.
Amorphous hydrogel	Carrasyn gel	Carrington Laboratories
dressings	DuoDERM Hydroactive gel	ConvaTec
	IntraSite gel/SoloSite gel	Smith & Nephew United

[a]This table does not provide a complete listing of all products available. Inclusion does not constitute endorsement. All products are copyrighted or registered trademarks.
[b]See Table 1 for dressing characteristics, ability to retain moisture, and indications.

mained in place longer when applied with the point down in the anal fold as compared to the oval (Tegasorb) or triangle-shaped dressings applied with the point up [22]. In general, using a hydrocolloid dressing that is large enough (covering 3.8–5.1 cm of the surrounding skin) as well as holding the dressing in place for a few seconds following application may increase dressing wear time [23].

Film dressings may be difficult to apply on curved areas and their acrylic adhesive can injure intact or new skin [21]. If the right dressing has been carefully applied but the dressing still needs to be changed every 24–48 h, or the surrounding skin is macerated (not to be confused with newly formed epithelium), an exudate-absorbing dressing may be applied underneath the moisture-retentive dressing.

Dressings for Highly Exudative Wounds

In the past, highly exudative wounds were packed with gauze. The capillary action of gauze "wicks" excess exudate (as well as endogenous enzymes, growth factors, and white blood cells) away from the wound bed. In addition to removing all cells needed for protection and repair, a dressing that is left to dry may cause re-injury of the wound bed upon removal. Finally, bacteria travel rapidly through layers of damp conventional gauze-type dressings [24]. Generally speaking, the newer exudate-absorption dressings are designed to retain exudate without dehydrating the wound bed or adhering to the granulation tissue. For example, alginate dressings (e.g., Algosteril, Kaltostat, Sorbsan) will absorb fluid while forming a gel from the alginate fibers, whereas a Hydrofiber dressing (Aquacel) will absorb fluid into the fibers while forming a gel sheet. Hydrophilic paste, powder, or beads (e.g., Comfeel or DuoDERM Paste, Bard absorption dressing) will fill wound cavities, while absorption of the exudate converts them to a gelatinous mass. Debrisan beads are designed to cleanse (not debride!) wounds and absorb exudate. Studies of acute wounds using alginate dressings have shown that they are safe and easy to use. In addition, compared to conventional gauze dressings, alginates are less painful to remove [25]. Studies using other wound exudate-absorbing products to manage decubitus ulcers also seem to indicate that they will facilitate healing, providing they are used appropriately. As mentioned earlier, these dressings will not retain moisture unless they are covered by a moisture-retentive dressing. The product package insert should be read to determine which secondary dressings can (and should) be used to cover them, and whether the product is indicated for use in deep cavity wounds. Not all dressings are indicated for use in sinus tracts because it may be difficult to remove them. In the course of treatment, as soon as the exudate-absorbing dressings are not liquefied upon removal, or if they adhere to the wound bed, their use should be discontinued.

Dressings for Dry/Necrotic Wounds

Dry ulcers often contain a significant amount of dead black/brown or fibrinous (yellow) tissue. Moisture-retentive dressings facilitate autolytic debridement of dead tissue. Specifically, studies have shown that proteinases can be found in the fluid from wounds dressed with a polyurethane film (OpSite) or a hydrocolloid (DuoDERM Hydroactive) dressing [26, 27]. In addition, dissolution of fibrin has been shown to be enhanced with the use of this hydrocolloid dressing [6]. Prompt removal of necrotic tissue is particularly important in patients who are at risk of developing infection. In these instances, sharp/surgical debridement may be the treatment of choice, providing the wound contains black/brown necrotic tissue and the patient can tolerate the procedure. Removing fibrinous slough using a sharp instrument is virtually impossible without damaging healthy tissue; thus, even though different debridement methods are often discussed separately, many can be effectively used in combination. For example, clinicians can choose sharp debridement to remove black necrotic tissue followed by autolytic debridement using a moisture-retentive dressing to help dissolve any remaining devitalized tissue or fibrinous slough [28].

If the ulcer is dry, a gel dressing can be used to provide moisture or hydrate devitalized tissues. The water-based hydrogels are available as sheets (dressings) or as amorphous gels in sachets, tubes, etc. The latter can be used to fill deep wounds and always require a secondary dressing (Table 1). Hydrogel dressing sheets do not always require tape or bandages to secure them. They should be used cautiously in exudating wounds because maceration of the surrounding skin can occur. In addition, some are very poor barriers to bacteria [29]. Amorphous hydrogels need to be covered with a moisture-retentive, e.g., hydrocolloid or film, dressing. Apply the gel sparingly, do not fill the entire wound so as to prevent maceration of the surrounding skin. Particularly if the wound contains devitalized tissue, application of a moisture-retentive dressing will facilitate autolysis and, as a result, the amount of wound exudate will increase. Most amorphous gel dressings (e.g., Carrasyn, SoloSite) will donate fluid to the wound, whereas one amorphous gel (DuoDERM Hydroactive Gel) will donate fluid when the environment is dry but absorb exudate if the environment is moist [30]. To prevent maceration of the surrounding skin and frequent dressing changes, it is important to discontinue the use of hydrogel dressings (particularly the fluid-donating-only types) as soon as the wound becomes moist/lightly exudative.

Common Concerns

Infection

As mentioned earlier, most moisture-retentive dressings need to be changed once every 2–5 days. Clinicians not familiar with their use may be uncomfortable leaving a dressing on for more than 24 h as it violates the long-held tradition of looking at wounds every day. This tradition, possibly adopted from the practice of looking at surgical incisions, is based on the assumption that we can see an infection in chronic wounds. Unfortunately, it is not easy to diagnose infected decubitus ulcers or, most importantly, osteomyelitis. For example, a recent clinical study involving 36 patients with decubitus ulcers found that clinical judgement of osteomyelitis was correct in only 20 of 36 patients. Only one of the six patients with osteomyelitis had purulent drainage from the wound (compared to 20% of patients who did not have osteomyelitis), three (50%) had bone exposure and none had a fever or leukocytosis [31]. All wounds, particularly those that have existed for some time, are colonized by a variety of bacteria but most do not become infected. Thus, even though clinicians should know the classic signs and symptoms of wound infections (fever, erythema, pain, induration, swelling), they should also remember that these signs may be absent in patients with infected decubitus ulcers. If they do exist, they can be assessed without looking at the wound itself; cellulitis, induration, and swelling are readily observed by assessing the surrounding skin. Conversely, culturing a wound without the classic clinical signs of infection can be misleading because all chronic wounds are contaminated with noninvading bacteria. As mentioned earlier, studies have shown that wounds dressed with moisture-retentive dressings are less likely to become infected than those covered with conventional gauze-type dressings [7] (Fig. 2). There are several explanations for these findings, including the ability of some of these dressings to retain viable polymorphonuclear leucocytes, macrophages, lymphocytes, and monocytes [8]. At least one hydrocolloid dressing (DuoDERM CGF) has also been found to exhibit in vivo bacterial and in vitro viral barrier properties [29, 32]. Compared to conventional gauze-type dressings, cross-contamination of wounds may also be greatly reduced when using these hydrocolloid dressings [33]. These findings may have significant infection control implications, particularly in patients with methicillin-resistant *Staphylococcus aureus* (MRSA), aminoglycoside-resistant enterococci (R-ENT), and ceftriaxone- and/ or gentamicin-resistant Gram-negative bacilli (R-GNB) which has been found to occur in 10%–20% of patients in long-term care facilities [34]. Indeed, Dunn and Wilson [35] have used these hydrocolloid dressings to prevent the spread of MRSA in colonized chronic venous ulcers in hospitalized patients.

Because wound odor has long been associated with the presence of infection, it is important to realize that all wounds will emit an odor when a dressing is removed after a few days. Fresh, clean wounds tend to have a "sweet" odor that resembles fresh blood, whereas necrotic wounds tend to have a more "repulsive" odor. Wounds infected with anaerobic bacteria tend to produce a distinct acrid or putrid smell [36]. A descriptive odor assessment can provide important information about the wound because it may be indicative of a

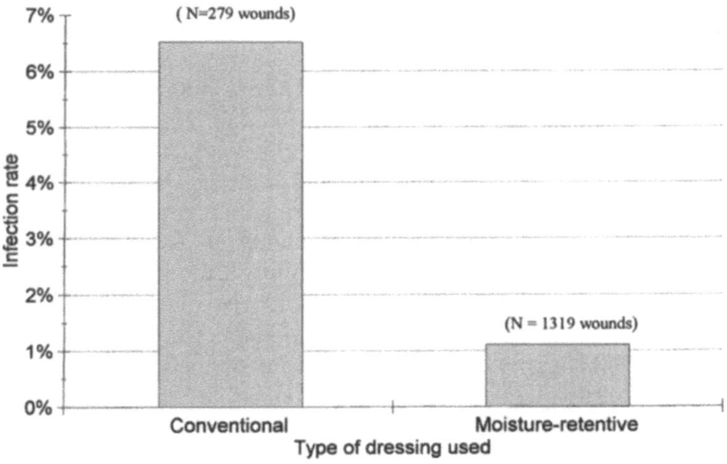

Fig. 2. Infection rates of Chronic wounds (leg and decubitus ulcers) based on 40 studies (1598 chronic wounds). The majority of wounds studied were dressed with impregnated or non-impregnated gauze-type dressings (conventional; n = 279 wounds) or with hydrocolloid or film dressings (moisture retentive; n = 1319 wounds) adapted from [7]

change in the wound status. Standardizing the terms to describe wound odor, e.g., "like fresh blood, putrid, sweet" may be very helpful [37]. Decubitus ulcers often contain a yellowish coating. It is important to realize that this is not pus, rather, it is fibrin which will dissolve when a moisture-retentive dressing is used, producing fribrin fragments which play a role in angiogenesis [6]. Similarly, the dissolved components of (yellow) hydrocolloid dressings may be mistaken for pus. However, cleansing of the ulcer usually reveal a healthy granulating wound bed.

The presence of erythema in decubitus ulcers, another clinical sign of infection, should not be confused with erythema caused by chronic inflammation as a result of, for example, unrelieved pressure or inappropriate topical treatment modalities. Erythema can also be caused by the careless removal of adhesive dressings or allergic reactions to the dressings themselves [38]. In this context, it is important to realize that, in addition to the varying MVTR among similar "classes" of products, variations in product components, and the incidence of allergic reactions do exist. For example, in one controlled study involving 103 decubitus ulcers, the incidence of treatment-related adverse experiences (e.g., erythema, pain) was 0% for one type of hydrocolloid (DuoDERM CGF) compared to 10% for another type of hydrocolloid dressing (Tegasorb) [22]. The "classic" definitions of wound infection may indeed be too narrow for granulating wounds such as decubitus ulcers, and other assessment criteria that should be considered include: delayed healing, discoloration, friable granulation tissue, and wound breakdown [36].

Cost

The price of a moisture-retentive dressing is always higher than the price of a 10×10 cm piece of gauze. However, ascertaining the price of any treatment modality using the "per unit product cost" only does not address the true cost of care. Cost of care also includes the number of dressing changes per day, cost of ancillary supplies used, as well as the cost of care giver time. Depending on the patient care setting, other cost factors may include: disposal of materials, travel time by care giver or patient, and treatment efficacy (e.g., time to healing, complications) [39]. For example, it has been shown that using a film or hydrocolloid dressing to manage decubitus ulcers is less expensive than using moist saline gauze dressings because the cost of care giver time is significantly reduced. Because this can permit care of more patients in the same time, it is recommended that care giver time be taken into consideration when selecting a moisture-retentive dressing [40].

Using Moisture-Retentive Dressings: What to Expect

An apparent increase in wound exudate can be expected as soon as a moisture-retentive dressing is applied to an existing decubitus ulcer, particularly if it contains devitalized tissue. In addition, as with other debridement methods, autolytic removal of devitalized tissue may cause a slight increase in wound size. During this time, the dressings may have to be changed once every 24 or 48 h. Once the wound bed is clean and granulating, the amount of exudate will decrease and the dressings usually remain in place for longer periods of time. Controlled clinical studies have shown that, not unlike acute wounds, many partial-thickness decubitus ulcers can be expected to heal after 1–3 weeks if a moisture-retentive dressing is used [14, 15]. Full-thickness decubitus ulcers, on the other hand, may take 8–12 weeks to heal [41]. In addition to systemic conditions associated with wound healing, the percentage reduction in ulcer area after 2–4 weeks of treatment is a signficant predictor of treatment outcome. In general, it is recommended that patients whose deep wounds do not exhibit a considerable reduction in ulcer area (20%–30%) after 2–4 weeks of treatment be reevaluated [40, 41].

Conclusions

Dressings do not heal decubitus ulcers but they can have a profound impact on the body's ability to heal. With proper usage, moisture-retentive dressings have been found to affect the rate of decubitus ulcer healing as well as the incidence of wound infection. However, as with any treatment modality, careful selection of products and using dressings that have been shown to be safe and effective for the intended indication is crucial. In addition, consistent and regular wound assessments will help clinicians decide whether or not the selected treatment modalities are safe and achieving the desired effect for each patient.

Acknowledgement. Lou Pirone, Karyn Monte, and Arlene Hancock provided data and analysis for this chapter.

References

1. Gilje O (1948) On taping (adhesive tape treatment) of leg ulcers. Acta Derm Venereol (Stockh) 28:454–467
2. Field CK, Kerstein MD (1994) Overview of wound healing in a moist environment. Am J Surg 167(IA):2S–6S
3. Thomas Hess C (1995) Nurse's clinical guide: wound care. Springhouse, Springhouse
4. Oxford English dictionary, 26th edn. (1987) Oxford University Press, Oxford
5. Knighton DR, Silver IA, Hunt TK (1981) Regulation of wound healing angiogenesis – effect of oxygen gradients and inspired oxygen concentration. Surgery 90:262–270
6. Lydon MJ, Hutchinson JJ, Rippon M et al. (1989) Dissolution of wound coagulum and promotion of granulation tissue under DuoDERM. Wounds 1(2):95–106
7. Hutchinson JJ, McGuckin M (1990) Occlusive dressings: a microbiologic and clinical review. Am J Infect Control 18:257–268
8. Witkowski JA, Parish LC (1986) Cutaneous ulcer therapy. Int J Dermatol 25:420–426
9. Bolton LL, van Rijswijk L(1991) Wound dressings: meeting clinical and biological needs. Dermatol Nurs 3:146–161
10. Shelanski MV, Nicholson JE, Shelanski JB, Constantine BE (1989) The influence of moisture vapor transmission rates of polymer dressings on the rate of wound healing and bacterial proliferation on wound surfaces. Wounds 1(2):115–121

11. Pirone LA, Bolton LL, Monte KA, Shannon RJ (1992) Effect of calcium alginate dressings on partial-thickness wounds in swine. J Invest Surg 5:149–153
12. Wu P, Fisher AC, Foo PP et al. (1995) In vitro assessment of water vapor transmission of synthetic wound dressings. Biomaterials 16:171–175
13. Polanksy M, van Rijswijk L (1994) Utilizing survival analysis techniques in chronic wound healing studies. Wounds 6:150–158
14. Gorse GJ, Messner RL (1987) Improved pressure sore healing with hydrocolloid dressings. Arch Dermatol 123:766–771
15. Xakellis GC, Chrischilles EA (1992) Hydrocolloid versus saline gauze dressings in treating pressure ulcers: a cost-effectiveness analysis. Arch Phys Med Rehabil 73:463–469
16. Sebern MD (1986) Pressure ulcer management in home health care: efficacy and cost effectiveness of moisture vapor permeable dressing. Arch Phys Med Rehabil 67:726–729
17. National Pressure Ulcer Advisory Panel (1989) Pressure ulcers: incidence, economics, risk assessment. Consensus development conference statement. Decubitus 2:24–28
18. Meehan M (1994) National pressure ulcer prevalence survey. Decubitus 7:27–38
19. Turnbull G (1995) Weaving reimbursement of surgical dressings into the plan of treatment. Ostomy Wound Man 41(7A):103S–110S
20. Panel for the Prediction and Prevention of Pressure Ulcers in Adults (1992) Pressure ulcers in adults: prediction and prevention. Clinical practice guideline no 3. AHCPR Publ no 92-0047. Agency for Health Care Policy and Research, Public Health Service, US Department of Health and Human Services, Rockville
21. Maklebust JA, Sieggreen M (1995) Pressure ulcers; guidelines for prevention and nursing management, 2nd edn. Springhouse, Springhouse
22. Day A, Dombranski S, Farkas C et al. (1995) Managing sacral pressure ulcers with hydrocolloid dressings: results of a controlled, clinical study. Ostomy Wound Man 41:52–64
23. Erwin-Toth P (1995) Cost-effective pressure ulcer management in extended care. Ostomy Wound Man 41(7A):64S–68S
24. Lawrence JC (1994) Dressings and wound infection. Am J Surg 167(1A):21S–24S
25. Dawson C, Armstrong MWJ, Fulford SCV et al. (1987) Use of calcium alginate to pack abscess cavities: a controlled clinical trial. J R Coll Surg 37:177–179
26. Chen WY, Rogers AS, Lydon MJ (1992) Characterization of biologic properties of wound fluid collected during early stages of wound healing. J Invest Dermatol 99:559–561
27. Grinnell F, Ho CH, Wysocki A (1992) Degradation of fibronectin and vitronectin in chronic wound fluid: analysis by cell blotting, immunoblotting, and cell adhesion assays. J Invest Dermatol 98:410–416
28. Fowler E, van Rijswijk L (1995) Using wound debridement to help achieve the goals of care. Ostomy Wound Man 41:23S–35S
29. Mertz PM, Marshall DA, Eaglstein WH (1985) Occlusive wound dressings to prevent bacterial invasion and wound infection. J Am Acad Dermatol 12:662–668
30. Thomas S, Hay P (1995) Fluid handling properties of hydrogel dressings. Ostomy Wound Man 41:54–59
31. Darouiche RO, Landon GC, Klima M et al. (1994) Osteomyelitis associated with pressure sores. Ann Intern Med 154:753–758
32. Bowler PG, Delargy H, Prince D, Fondberg L (1993) The viral barrier properties of some occlusive dressings and their role in infection control. Wounds 5:1–8
33. Lawrence JC, Lilly HA, Kidson A (1992) Wound dressings and the airborne dispersal of bacteria. Lancet 339:807
34. Terpenning MS, Bradley SF, Wan JY et al. (1994) Colonization and infection with antibiotic-resistant bacteria in a long-term care facility. J Am Geriatr Soc 42:1062–1069
35. Dunn LJ, Wilson P (1990) Evaluating the permeability of hydrocolloid dressings to multiresistant Staphylococcus aureus. Pharm J 248:50
36. Cutting KF, Harding KG (1994) Criteria for identifying wound infection. J Wound Care 3:198–201
37. van Rijswijk L (1996) Wound assessment and documentation. In: Krasner D (ed) Chronic wound care; a clinical source book for health care professionals, 2nd edn. Health Management, Wayne

38. Nielsen PG, Madsen SM, Stromberg L (1990) Treatment of chronic leg ulcers with a hydrocolloid dressing. Acta Dermato Venereol (Stockh) 152[Suppl]:2–12
39. International Committee on Wound Management (ICWM) (1995) An overview of economic model of cost-effective wound care. Adv Wound Care 8:46
40. Bergstrom N, Bennett MA, Carlson CE et al. (1994) Treatment of pressure ulcers. Clinical practice guideline, no 15. US Department of Health and Human Services, Public Health Service, Agency for Health Care Policy and Research, Rockville. AHCPR Publ no 95-0652
41. van Rijswijk L, Polansky M (1994) Predictors of time to healing deep pressure ulcers. Wounds 6(5):159–165

14 Support Systems

T.P. Stewart

Support surfaces are as integral a part of the clinical management of decubitus ulcers as medical intervention and nursing care. So important is this concept that any protocol on the prevention and treatment of decubitus ulcers that either omits or is confined solely to a discussion of the use of support surfaces is incomplete.

In the past, the task of matching a support surface to a particular patient was difficult. Hundreds of different support surfaces were available, no standardized methods had been developed to evaluate them, and there were few prospective, randomized clinical trials. Although these issues have not been entirely resolved, it should no longer be difficult to determine a patient's need for a support surface and to select the most appropriate option.

It is now understood that support surfaces can be evaluated accurately on the basis of their performance [1], that the individual support surface needs of patients also can be assessed accurately, and that it is better to use a well-informed, educated approach, rather than case-by-case emergencies to determine whether a facility has a sufficient selection of support surface equipment. Although no standards yet exist for evaluation of support surfaces, some consensus has been reached on performance-based criteria for evaluation [1, 2]. Based on this, the most efficient approach for facility operators and care givers at present is to stock the minimal array of support surfaces that are required to cover all recognized patient needs.

The best way to evaluate support surfaces is through randomized, prospective, controlled clinical trials; however, few such trials exist [3, 4], and it is unlikely that more will occur because of their cost and the large number of surfaces that must be evaluated. Another approach to evaluating the ability of support surfaces to reduce or relieve pressure is through the use of interface pressure measurements. This is the best tool available for a relatively straightforward evaluation of support surfaces [1, 5]. An important concept to understand, as it relates to support surfaces and interface pressure measurements, is the distinction between the therapeutic effects of pressure reduction and pressure relief. *Pressure reducing devices* are defined as those which reduce tissue interface pressure (measured at the trochanter) as compared to a conventional hospital mattress, but are unable to consistently maintain tissue interface pressure below capillary closure pressure. *Pressure relieving devices* are defined as those which consistently maintain tissue interface pressure below capillary closure pressure (i.e., 32 mmHg).

Because hundreds of different support surfaces are available for the recumbent patient, the issue of support surface selection becomes unnecessarily complicated [1, 3, 6–14]. While there is no perfect support surface [1, 14], continuing to search for one misses a basic point and may cause a caregiver to dwell too much on individual surfaces rather than on creating a unified approach to prevention and treatment. There can be no perfect support surface because these surfaces alone are not the perfect method of preventing and treating decubitus ulcers. A methodologic approach to selecting support surfaces will achieve its maximum value only if it is used as an integral part of an effective overall program. The types and numbers of specific support products that one institution or care site needs to achieve optimum overall success may be quite different from those required by another.

A plan for the prevention and treatment of decubitus ulcers in an individual must also acknowledge that the decubitus ulcer patient is a subclass of the immobilized patient. The immobilized patient has many needs. Prolonged immobilization of the body, whether because of illness, injury, or other cause, has extensive harmful physiologic and biochemical consequences for practically every major organ system of the body. Decubitus ulcers are only one of these consequences.

Factors in the Cause of Decubitus Ulcers

If an important cause of decubitus ulcers is accepted as point pressure in excess of capillary closure (i.e., 32 mmHg) for a prolonged time, then this can be considered the cause of a deformation of the surrounding tissue which then causes a collapse or occlusion of the capillaries and ischemia to the area supplied by the affected vessels (Fig. 1). Prolonged ischemia leads to cell death and tissue necrosis [15–19].

Shear is another mechanical force which may contribute to the development of decubitus ulcers and is a matter of concern as related to support surfaces. Shear is defined as a force parallel to the plane of interest [20]. In order for shear force to act on the human body, there must be friction. Friction causes the body to remain adherent to the support surface, while the underlying tissues move. This can happen at both shallow and deep tissue depths. Shear forces can cause the occlusion of capillaries, causing ischemia which can lead to the development of decubitus ulcers [20–22]. In the clinical setting, shear often occurs simultaneously with pressure. When the head of the hospital bed is elevated above 30°, it causes shear in the area of the patient's sacrum [2, 5, 21] (Fig. 2).

The seated individual is also at risk for the development of decubitus ulcers. The seated individual represents special considerations when it comes to identifying the etiology or cause of decubitus ulcers and also choosing appropriate support surfaces. Disabled individuals who spend most of their time in the seated position are clinically different from the "typical" geriatric decubitus ulcer patients who spend most of their time (both developing decubitus ulcers and suffering from them) in bed in recumbent positions. There are age

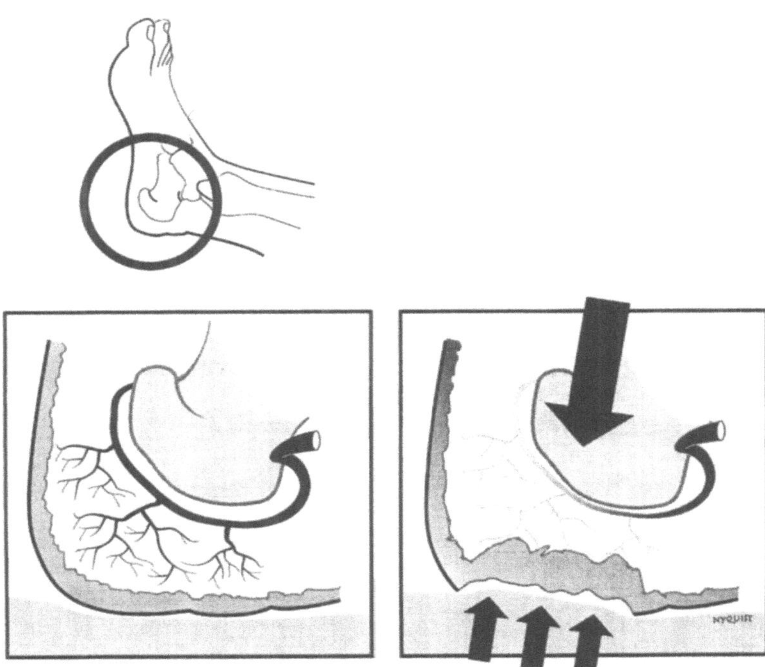

Fig. 1. Capillaries supplying tissues between a bony prominence and the surface: pressure less than 32 mmHg (*left*) with blood flow in capillaries and pressure greater than 32 mmHg (*right*) causing tissue deformation and occlusion of capillaries

differences, muscle and nervous system differences, and hemodynamic differences based on position.

Rationale for Support Surfaces

All human beings are subjected to pressures and shearing forces which could cause decubitus ulcers; however, in the healthy nondisabled individual, there are built-in protective mechanisms that provide feedback preventing us from remaining at a damaging pressure for too long a time. The healthy individual will make conscious or unconscious postural shifts or movements in order to relieve pressure. These movements are all that is required to provide protection from developing decubitus ulcers. These protective mechanisms may be inhibited or absent in many patients due to their underlying medical problem. Postural moves may cause such severe pain in some patients that they will choose not to move even if it means the development of decubitus ulcers. These patients do not or cannot move often enough or in a fashion that is consistent with the prevention of decubitus ulcers.

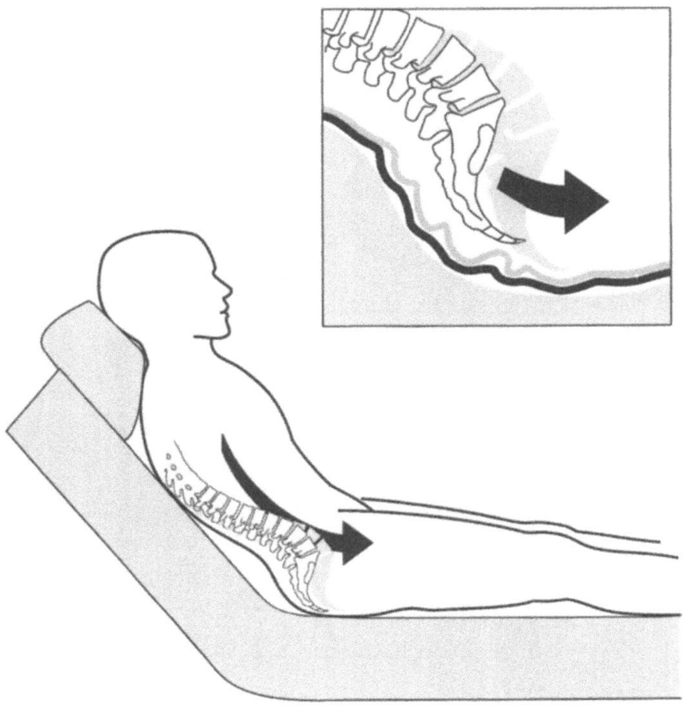

Fig. 2. Raising the head of the bed beyond 30° causes shear in the sacral area. (*inset*) The patient's skin adheres to the bed surface, but the bony skeleton moves in the direction of the *arrow* causing tissue deformation and capillary occlusion

One strategy to prevent or treat decubitus ulcers if patients cannot move or turn themselves is to provide help from someone else. This is the basis for the 2 h turning schedule that is widely used in institutions. The 2 h turning schedule probably evolved from the observation of Guttman and his turning and lifting team at the Stoke Mandeville Spinal Cord Centre in England in the late 1940s. They determined empirically that patients turned every 2 h did not develop decubitus ulcers.

Theoretically, there would be no need for special support surfaces if patients could be moved often enough. In practice, however, many patients are not turned every 2 h (as if the 120-min interval had some magic quality to it), or have existing conditions that make it impossible for them to be moved at all. Therefore, special support surfaces are employed which can relieve the pressure and shear on the body so that, even in the absence of movement, the patient will be less likely to develop a decubitus ulcer. When a patient develops a decubitus ulcer, then the pressure and shear must be eliminated, or the ulcer will not heal.

One of the early concepts/techniques for the relief of pressure was the plaster of Paris bed [23] (Fig. 3) which permitted an individually contoured

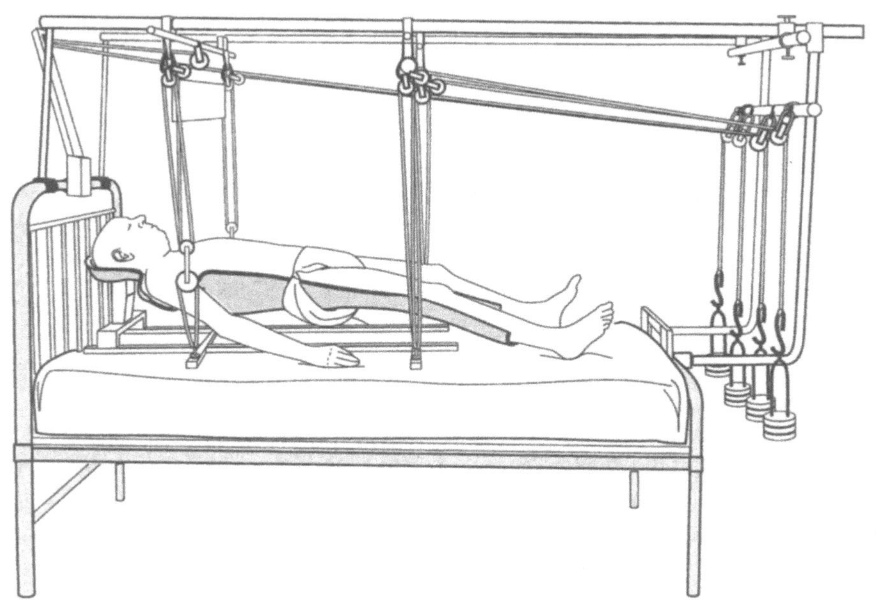

Fig. 3. Plaster of Paris support

device to provide low interface pressures. Unfortunately, this device immobilized the patient and was not suitable in most cases.

In 1948 Gardner [24, 25] described the alternating pressure mattress which
consisted of two distinct sets of cells that alternately inflated and deflated. Its
purpose was to move the pressure points around the body so that pressure at
any one point would not be permitted for too long. As the mattress inflates, it
lifts the body up off the bed, supporting it first on one set of cells and then on
another. No part of the body remains in contact with the mattress for a long
period of time.

In 1961 Scales [26] described the use of temperature-controlled air to support the patient so that the patient was levitated. He developed the High Air
Loss Patient Support system which supported the patient (levitated) on a
cushion of air [27–29]; the body was suspended without touching any surface.
This permitted a very even distribution of pressure on the body. Scales et al.
[30] then described a Low Air Loss Bed system which consisted of a series of
vapor-permeable air sacs arranged on a bed. The air sacs provided support to
the patient. Because the sacs contoured to the patient, even distribution of
pressure over the entire body could be achieved.

In 1963 Hargest [31, 32] conceived the idea of patient support by air fluidization. In this system the patient floats on 100-μm ceramic beads that have
been fluidized by air flowing through the beads. The beads are separated from
the patient by a porous covering that constrains the beads but permits the
passage of air.

Keane [33] first described the minimum physiologic mobility requirement (MPMR) for human support on a soft surface in 1978. Keane's description was based upon observations and studies of normal healthy subjects and their average spontaneous movement during sleep [34–36]. The frequency for movement for healthy individuals during sleep was found to be, on the average, one movement every 11.6 min. He referred to this as the MPMR [33].

There is evidence that frequency of movement declines with age. For the mobility-impaired individual, Keane suggested that kinetic nursing would be defined "as the automatic and continuous turning of a patient equally from side to side in a given posture, through a maximum excursion of 124° at a minimum rate of 124° in 4.5 minutes." The maximum excursion provided by the kinetic treatment bed is 160°.

Subsequent studies have demonstrated the effectiveness of kinetic nursing for various medical problems including, but not limited to, decubitus ulcers, atelectasis, multiple trauma, respiratory distress, pneumonia, and spinal cord injury [5, 37–41]. The Roto Rest (Ethos Medical Ltd., Athlone, Republic of Ireland) bed was developed in response to Keane's work [42, 43].

Since the 1970s, hundreds of different support surfaces have been developed to assist in the management of decubitus ulcers.

Types of Support Surfaces: Physical Construction, Features, Advantages, and Disadvantages

When compared to a standard hospital bed, support surfaces used for the management of decubitus ulcers take three basic physical or mechanical forms: mattress overlays, mattress replacements, or full-framed special beds. Each of these forms is able to accommodate many different means/functions to achieve either pressure reduction or pressure relief [44]. These means or functions can be grouped as either static, alternating, flotation, or rotation. The combinations of form and function are illustrated in Table 1.

Table 1. Form versus function shows the various possibilities for performance and indicates that just knowing the form or function will not predict the ability of a support surface to relieve pressure

	Overlay	Mattress	Bed
Static	ABCD	ABCD	ABCD
Alternating/pulsating	ABC	ABC	ABCD
Low air loss	ABCD	ABCD	ABCD
Immersion			
Air fluidized			ACD
Water	AB	AB	ACD
Gel	AB	ABC	
Turning/rotating/ oscillating	BCD	ABCD	ABCD

A, comfort; *B*, pressure reduction; *C*, pressure relief; *D*, pressure relief plus

Mattress Overlays

An overlay is a general term to describe a support surface placed on top of a standard hospital mattress. The most common overlays are foam, static air, alternating air, gel, water, or low air loss. Some overlays are constructed of a combination of these components.

Foam overlays (Fig. 4) have been used extensively in the management of decubitus ulcers. The height, density, and other physical parameters of foam will affect its pressure-reducing performance [45–48]. Five-centimeter convoluted foam overlays do not reduce pressure when compared to a standard mattress and should only be used for comfort [2]; 7.5-and 10-cm foam may offer some pressure reduction, but foam performance varies according to the manufacturer. Interface pressure studies should be used to evaluate the relative performance of a specific foam [49].

Static air overlays (Fig. 5) are made of a series of interconnected cells that can be inflated with a powered blower. Some air-filled overlays are pressure reducing while others are pressure relieving. One overlay has been extensively studied and has been demonstrated to provide pressure relief similar to an air-fluidized bed [50] with improved clinical outcomes [51]. Static air-filled overlays can be used for either short- or long-term use.

Alternating air overlays (Fig. 6) are connected to a pump. The alternating overlay functions by a cyclical inflation and deflation of the overlay's air cells. The alternation of the cells shifts the patient's support from one body area to another and thus relieves the pressure on any one body part for prolonged periods of time. In addition to relieving pressure, it has been suggested that such overlays also increase perfusion; however, one study of an alternating overlay failed to demonstrate an increase in skin perfusion [52].

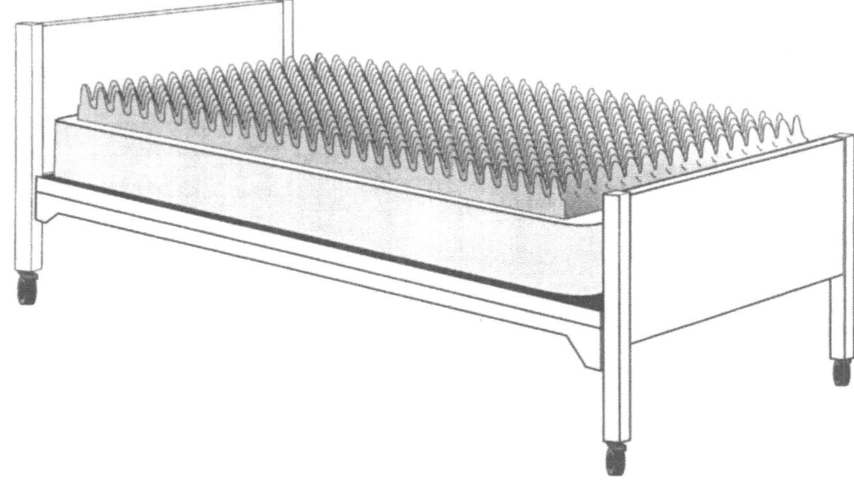

Fig. 4. Convoluted foam overlay

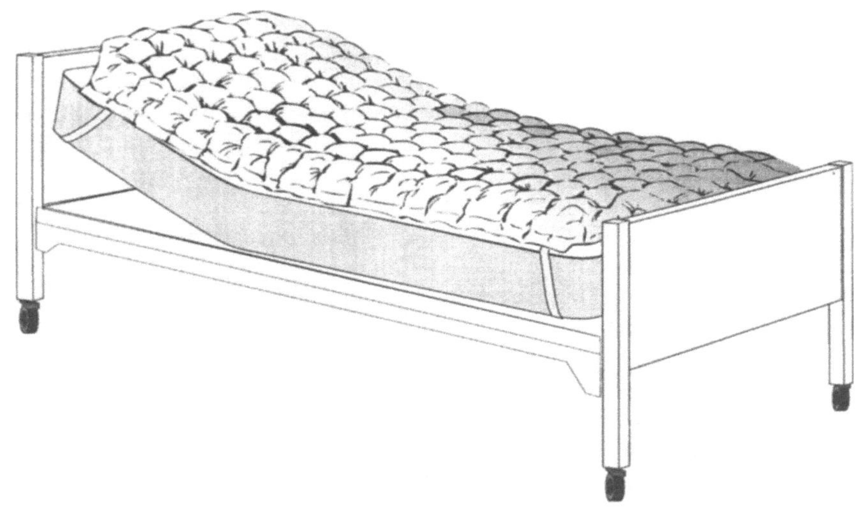

Fig. 5. Example of a pressure relieving static air overlay

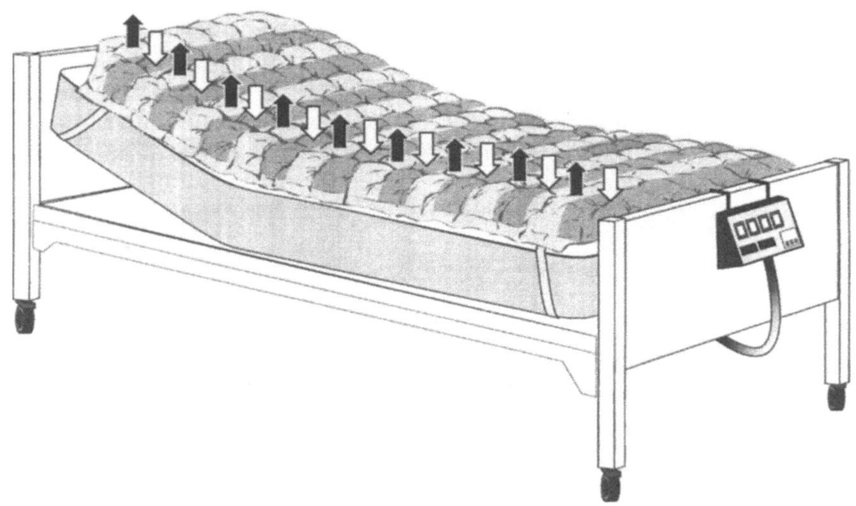

Fig. 6. Alternating air overlay. Adjacent rows of cells (*black and white arrows*) are alternately inflated and deflated to relieve pressure

Gel-filled overlays may consist of either a rigid or a compliant gel. The rigid gels do not appear to provide pressure relief or reduction. They do generally provide some shear force relief. The more compliant or conforming gels may reduce pressure as well as shear.

Water-filled overlays are an attempt to provide the patient with the benefits of immersion. Because the water depth is not great, true immersion cannot be achieved [53]. Therefore, these types of overlays generally provide pressure reduction rather than true pressure relief.

Low air loss overlays are generally similar to static air overlays except that they are connected to a pump or blower which maintains the pressure in the overlay while allowing air to escape through the surface of the overlay to help manage heat and moisture on the patient's skin (Fig. 7).

Bottoming or Bottoming Out. Some overlays may become fully compressed under the weight of the body. If the overlay is fully compressed, then the patient will be resting on the underlying mattress and defeating the purpose of the overlay. When this occurs, the phenomenon is called bottoming or bottoming out. One way to test for bottoming is to perform a "hand check". To perform a hand check, the care giver inserts a hand between the overlay and the underlying mattress. The hand must be flat, palm up with fingers outstretched. If the patient's body can be felt resting directly on the care giver's hand, then the overlay is not providing adequate support (Fig. 8).

Mattress Replacements

Replacement mattresses are, as the name implies, intended to replace the standard hospital mattress (Fig. 9). They have been designed to reduce pressure to below those seen on a conventional hospital mattress. The mattress

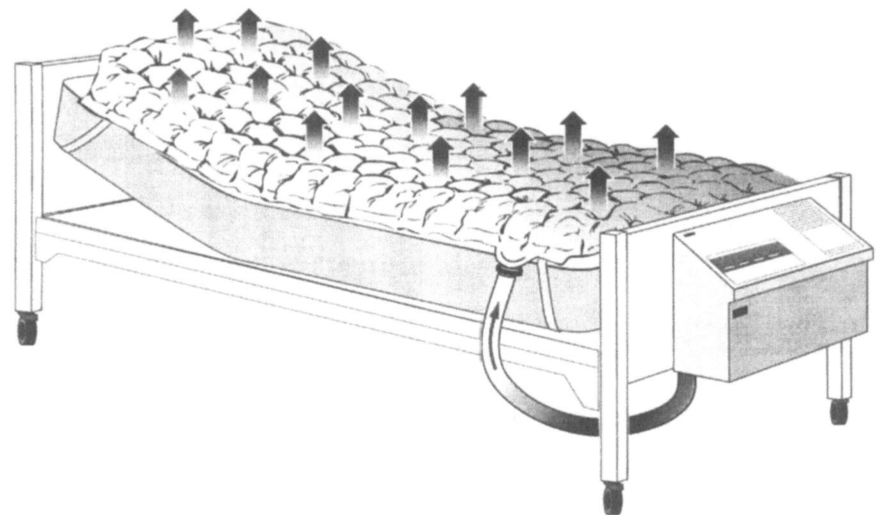

Fig. 7. Example of a low air loss overlay. Air escapes from the surface of the overlay (*arrows*) to help manage moisture as it relieves pressure

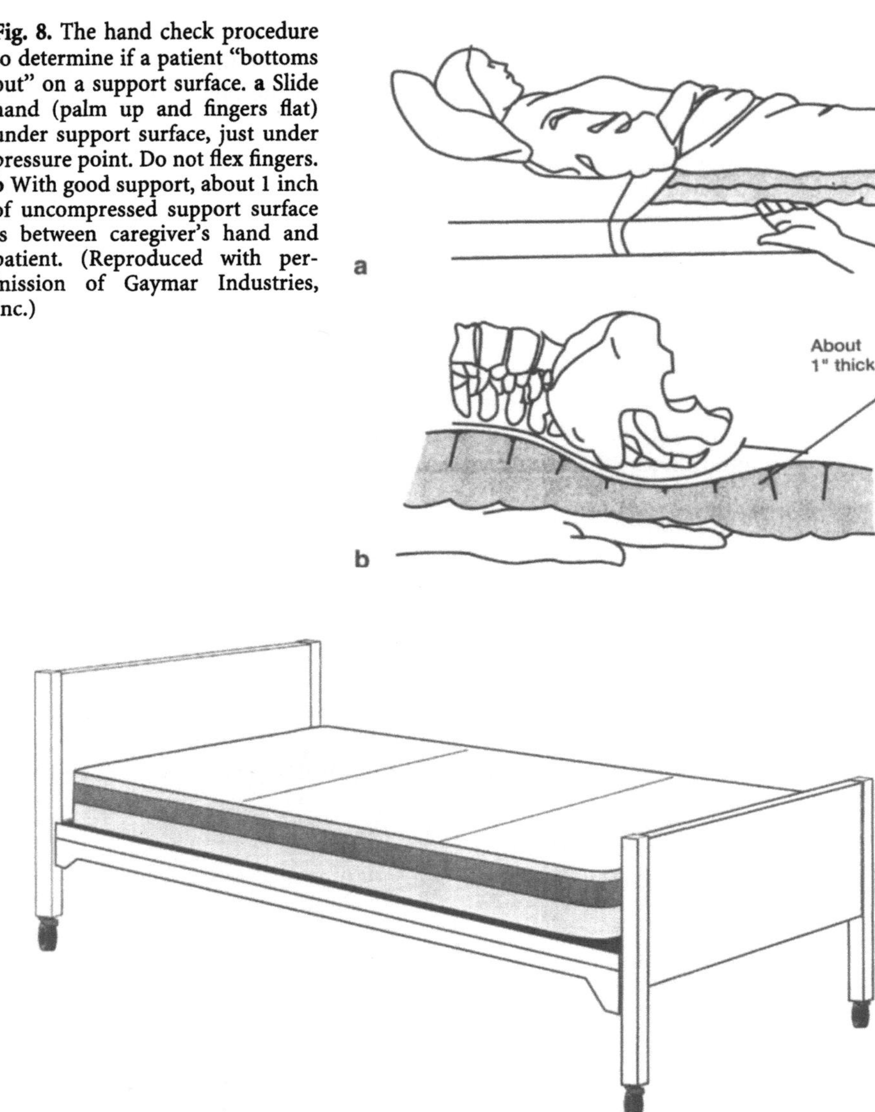

Fig. 8. The hand check procedure to determine if a patient "bottoms out" on a support surface. **a** Slide hand (palm up and fingers flat) under support surface, just under pressure point. Do not flex fingers. **b** With good support, about 1 inch of uncompressed support surface is between caregiver's hand and patient. (Reproduced with permission of Gaymar Industries, Inc.)

Fig. 9. Nonpowered replacement mattress. May be one piece or divided into different sections. Composition of the sections may vary

replacement can be either nonpowered or powered by a blower (or pump) (Fig. 10). Like overlays, they are often constructed of static air, foam, alternating air, water, or gel, or they provide low air loss. The first mattress replacements were not powered and were constructed of foam or a combination of foam and gel. These mattresses have been found to be pressure-reducing devices [54]. Although not pressure relieving, these types of mattresses can

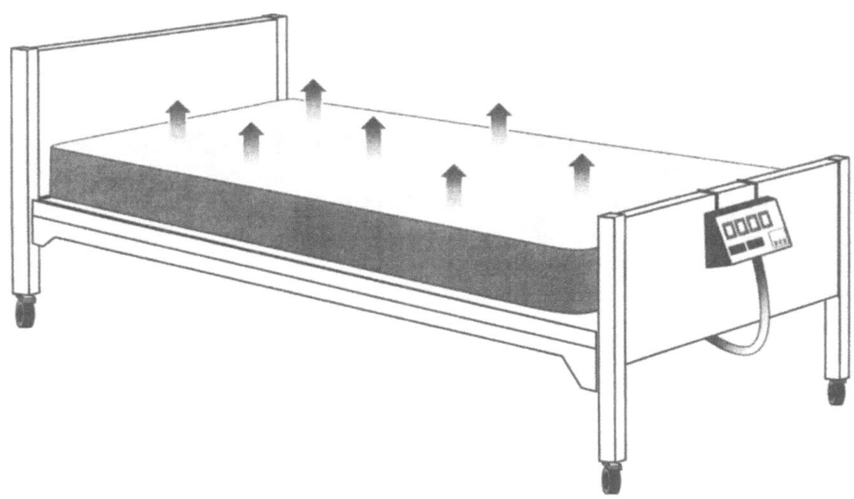

Fig. 10. Example of a powered mattress replacement. The *arrows* indicate that this mattress provides low air loss through the top surface

help prevent decubitus ulcers for some patients. The mattresses are very similar in performance to their respective overlays (i.e., foam and gel). Because they are designed to have the same thickness as conventional hospital mattresses, they are much less susceptible to bottoming out [55]. The additional depth provided by the mattress enables some gel and water mattresses to provide pressure relief because the patient can actually be immersed in the fluid.

Powered mattress replacements can also be placed directly on a bed frame. These mattresses can be either pressure reducing or pressure relieving. They can be used in any setting because they are generally easy to transport and set up. The most popular powered mattresses are either alternating powered mattresses or low air loss-powered mattresses. They are generally greater than 12.5 cm in height, are attached to a blower or motor, and their surfaces or cover have been designed to reduce friction and shear. Some powered mattresses also provide turning or rotational capabilities.

Full-Framed Special Beds

These are usually the most technically complex and expensive support surfaces. The pressure-relieving support surface is integrated into a bed frame such that the entire conventional hospital bed is replaced with the special bed. These full-framed beds are usually low air loss beds, air-fluidized beds, water immersion beds, rotational beds, or a combination of the low air loss and rotational bed.

Low Air Loss Beds. The surface of a low air loss bed generally comprises a number of cushions (Fig. 11). The pressure in these cushions may or may not be individually adjustable or adjustable by zone. Some air escapes through the surface of the bed. This low air flow is intended to enhance patient comfort and assist in moisture/heat control. It has been suggested that, in order for a surface to be considered low air loss, it should, as a minimum, be able to remove moisture at a rate that is equivalent to the rate of insensible water loss (1.2 mg/cm^2 per hour) [56] although, at present, no universally accepted standard exists. Low air loss beds provide the same therapeutic benefit as low air loss overlays and mattresses [57]. The beds, however, provide for a low air loss surface with the controls integrated with the bed frame and usually some additional features or options. Low air loss beds have been shown to significantly improve the healing rates of decubitus ulcers when compared to foam overlays [58]. Some low air loss beds have alternating or pulsating cushions incorporated into the bed to provide additional therapy to the patient. The benefit of such therapy remains to be proven [52].

Water Immersion Bed. Another type of full-framed bed is the water immersion bed (Fig. 12). It consists of a frame and vessel that contains water or other fluid [59, 60]. The water is heated to provide warmth and comfort to the patient. The patient is separated from the immersion fluid by a waterproof sheet. On demand, the patient can be raised out of the water through the use of a built-in airlift surface. The airlift can be used during transfers, repositioning, and various nursing treatments. This type of bed provides pressure relief and a very

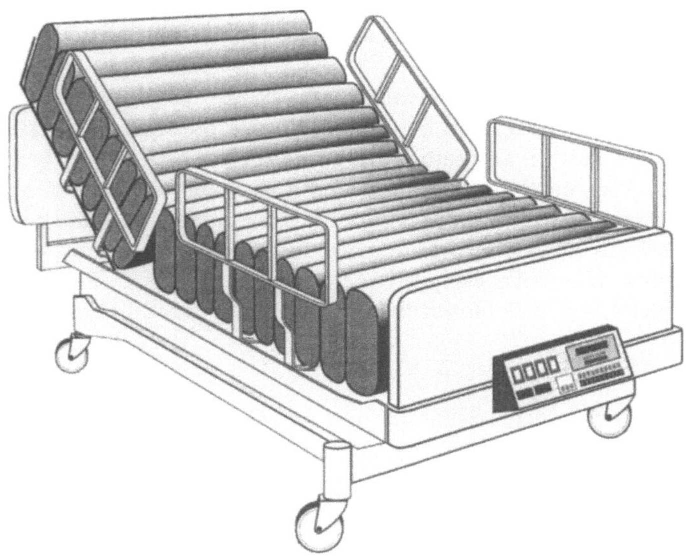

Fig. 11. Low air loss bed. Controls are integrated into the bed frame and may permit different zones to be adjusted independently

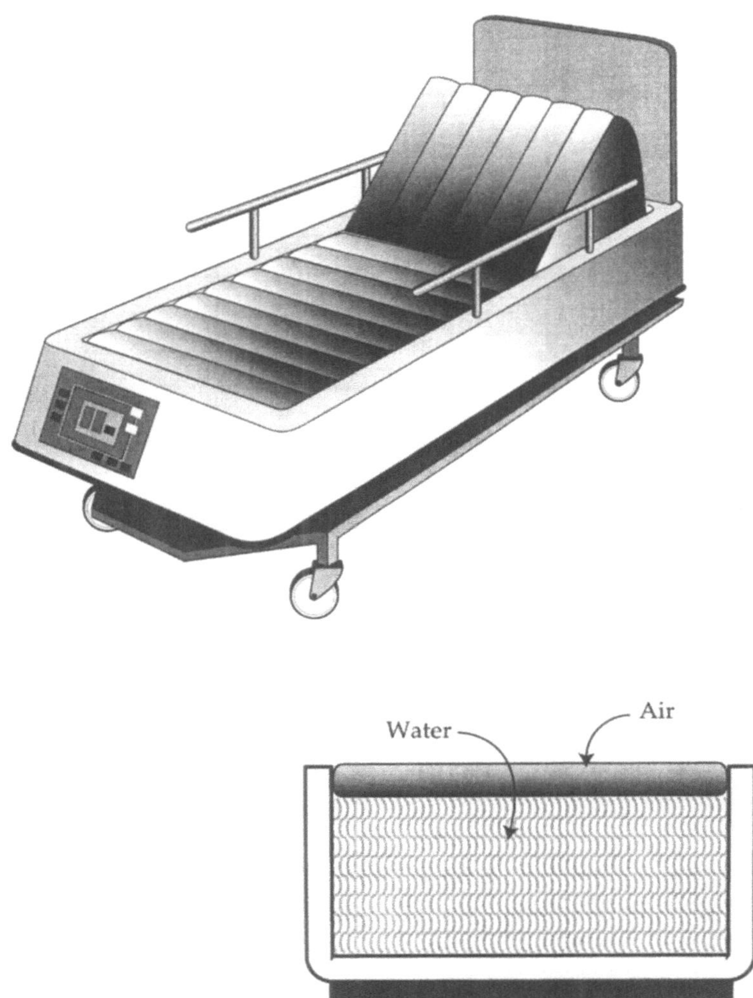

Fig. 12. Fluid immersion bed. Provides pressure relief through immersion in a temperature controlled fluid (*inset*). The air chamber is used to move the patient in or out of the fluid

low shear surface. One uncontrolled clinical trial has reported the ability of the water immersion bed to heal stage III and IV decubitus ulcers [59].

Rotational Beds. The original rotational bed was the Roto Rest bed (Fig. 13). It consisted of a frame and padded support surface that held patients as they were rotated from side to side. Newer designs of rotational beds usually incorporate a turning/rotational feature in a low air loss bed (Fig. 14). Although rotational therapy does provide pressure reduction or relief, the primary indication for rotational therapy is for pulmonary therapy for the critically ill, immobilized

Fig. 13. Diagram of the Roto Rest bed

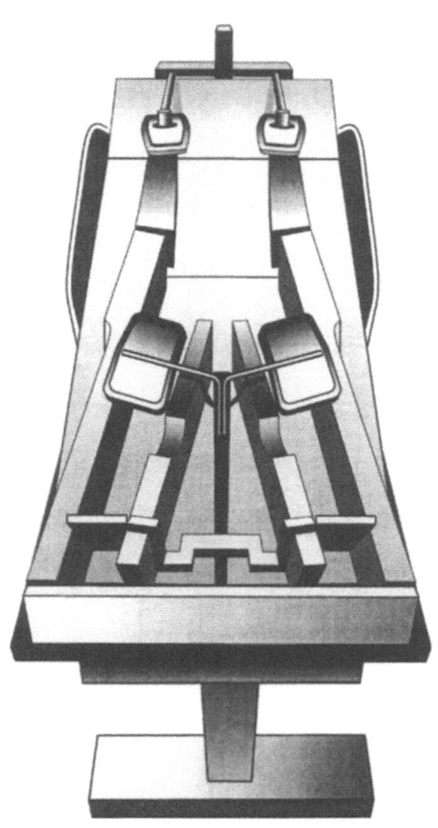

patient [37–40]. Numerous studies have demonstrated the benefits of rotational therapy for these patients [39].

Air-Fluidized Bed. An air-fluidized bed consists of a vessel attached to a frame. The vessel contains very fine ceramic beads and a pump or blower. The beads are fluidized by pumping air through them (Fig. 15). This fluidization causes the beads to behave like a liquid (fluid) [31, 61, 62]. The temperature of the air is controlled to keep the patient warm and comfortable. The patient is separated from the beads by a permeable filter sheet that permits a high rate of upward flow of air to the patient. The filter sheet also permits the downward flow of body fluids into the beads. When contacted with fluid, the beads clump and fall to the bottom of the vessel for removal. Numerous studies have been conducted to demonstrate the pressure-relieving capabilities and clinical outcome of patients treated on air-fluidized beds [3, 31]. Air-fluidized beds have become, and remain, the "gold standard" for pressure-relieving support surfaces. They also provide a surface with very low shear forces; however, air-fluidized beds have been known to cause dehydration and electrolyte imbalance due to the high air flow that reaches the patients' skin and the resulting

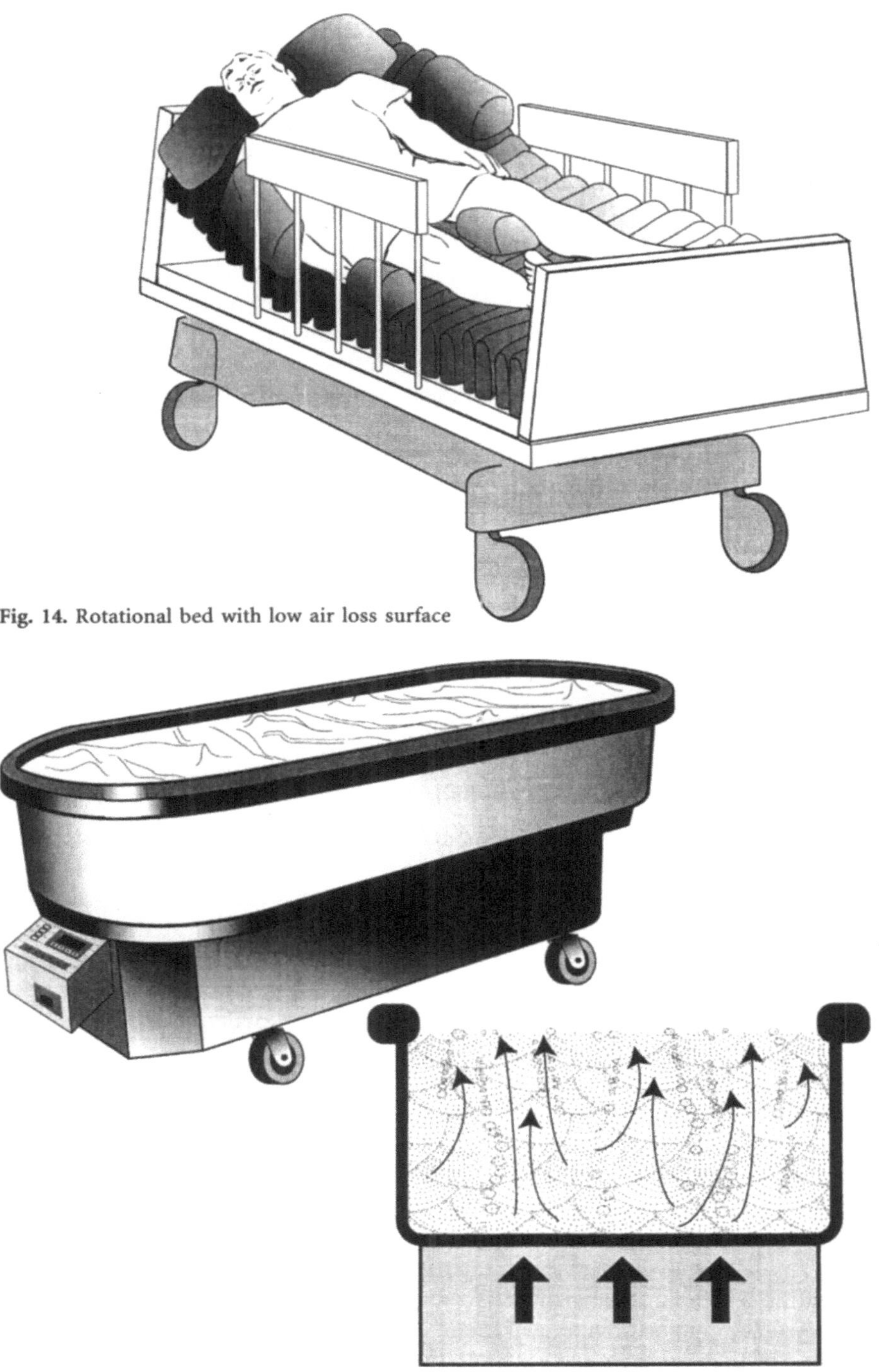

Fig. 14. Rotational bed with low air loss surface

Fig. 15. Air fluidized bed (*inset*). Blower beneath vessels supplies air at high velocity and fluidizes the ceramic beads in the vessel

high rate of evaporative fluid loss [63, 64]. Such beds are currently used for only the most severely compromised patients.

Adverse Events. In addition to the advantages and disadvantages listed (Table 2), there have been isolated reports of adverse events for support surfaces. There is one report for the air-fluidized bed where iatrogenic occiput and heel decubitus ulcers occurred [65]. Air-fluidized beds may cause dehydration and electrolyte imbalances in the healthy and the severely ill [63, 64]. An accidental extubation of a patient occurred when placed on a rotating low air loss system [66]. Most of the support surfaces used to prevent and treat decubitus ulcers are contraindicated for the unstable spine following acute injury or surgery. This is of particular concern because these types of patients are at high risk for decubitus ulcer development.

Support surfaces can be categorized by their mechanical form (overlay vs. mattress vs. bed) or mechanical features (static, alternating, flotation, etc.). These methods of categorization do not indicate the clinical effectiveness of the support surface. For instance, an overlay can be either a comfort device, a pressure-reducing device or a pressure-relieving device. It is not enough to only know the mechanical structure or features. These characteristics are not a measure of the clinical effectiveness of a support surface. As can be seen from Table 1, the performance of a particular mechanical category can vary widely.

Clinical Application

Clinical Goals. The decision of choosing the support surface appropriate for a specific patient should be made within the context of the patient care plan and the clinical goals of that plan. While many decubitus ulcers can be prevented [2, 5, 67], most of those that do occur can be successfully treated and healed. Considering the end stages of life for some patients, the development of decubitus ulcers may be inevitable and irreversible [68]. A number of papers have been written concerning the clinical goals and ethics involving the prevention and treatment of decubitus ulcers [69–71].

Many methodologic approaches have been devised to match the patient needs to the appropriate support surface [6, 14]. These approaches usually include two important elements: patient·assessment and a support surface assessment. The combination of these two elements permits for a single, straightforward method for the proper utilization of support surfaces [72, 73]. The first step in the process is to decide into what category a support surface falls. The next step is to assess the patient and, from the patient assessment, determine which support surface is required. One such method for matching patient and support surface involves an assessment of the patient based on the number of uninvolved sleep surfaces the patient has available. Based on this type of patient assessment, a support surface recommendation can be arrived at via a flow diagram (Fig.16) [74–77].This method can also be visualized in tabular form (Table 3). Another method involves the use of the Norton, Bra-

Table 2. Advantages and disadvantages for various support surfaces

Advantages	Disadvantages
Foam overlays	
One time charge, no set-up fee	May increase perspiration
Lightweight	Difficult to reposition patient
Needle or metal traction cannot damage	Added height to bed, difficulty getting patient out of bed
No maintenance required	Washing removes flame-retardant coating
	Limited life
	Plastic protective sheet promotes maceration of skin
Static air overlays	
Easy to clean	Sharp objects can damage
Low maintenance	Regular monitoring required to determine proper inflation
Durable	May cause increase of perspiration
More effective than foam for heavier patients	Added height to bed, difficulty getting patient out of bed
Alternating air overlays	
Easy to clean	Inflation and deflation of mattress may give patient sensation of motion
Quick deflation for emergencies	Electricity required
Gel-filled overlays	
Low maintenance	Heavy
Easy to clean	Expensive
Reusable	Limited research on effectiveness
Water-filled overlays	
Baffle system controls motion effects	Water heater required to maintain comfortable water temperature
Easy to clean	Fluid motion makes procedures difficult
	Patient transfers may be difficult
	Inadvertent needle puncture may cause leaks, creating safety hazard
	Maintenance needed to prevent microorganism growth
	Heavy
	Over-or under-filling possible
Low air loss overlays	
Easy assembly	Large pump at foot of bed
Easy to clean	Motor noise
Level of pressure reduction	Electricity required
Maintained automatically	
Reusable pump	
Quick deflation for emergencies	
Replacement mattress	
Reduces need for overlay mattress	Initial high cost
Level of pressure reduction automatically controlled	Removable sections may be misplaced
	No therapeutic benefit when used with overlays

Table 2 (*Cont.*)

Advantages	Disadvantages

Reusable
Easy to clean
Hospital linens may be used
Low maintenance

Powered replacement mattress

Advantages	Disadvantages
Easy to clean	Sharp objects can damage
Constant inflation maintained	Motor noise
Deflation facilitates transfers and procedures	
Company sets up	
Moisture controlled	

Full-framed low air loss bed

Advantages	Disadvantages
Head and foot of bed can be elevated and lowered	Heavy portable motor
Transfers easily accomplished	Slippery surface: patient may slide down or out of bed during transfer
Portable motor maintains inflation during transfers	Must use incontinence pad recommended by manufacturer
Pressure relief in any position	Difficult to transfer patient in and out of bed
Set-up, monitoring, on-call services provided	
Most have built-in scale	
Shear friction fabric surfaces	

Full-framed air-fluidized bed

Advantages	Disadvantages
Improves patient comfort	Continuous circulation of warm, dry air may dehydrate patient
Quickly becomes firm for cardiopulmonary resuscitation	
Shear and friction reduced at site	Bed generates heat to patient and elevates room temperature
Wound drainage or incontinence managed	Additional care measures to prevent wound dissication.
Set-up, monitoring and on-call services provided	Leakage of beads – irritates eyes and respiratory track, and makes floor slippery
	Width – (narrow) may preclude care to obese patients with contractures
	Difficult to transfer patient
	Height of bed makes some nursing difficult; step is needed to facilitate care
	Dependent drainage of catheters may be compromised due to low position of patient immersed in bed, and the catheter tubing must be elevated over the rigid bedside to the catheter bag
	Head of bed cannot be raised: semi-Fowler's position is achieved by using foam wedges
	Heavy

Oscillating low air loss bed

Advantages	Disadvantages
Pressure relief and low friction surface with gentle repositioning	
Most models have built-in scales	

Advantages	Disadvantages
Rotational bed	
Pressure reduction may be provided Frequent turning of patient with unstable spine possible	
Water immersion bed	

Improves patient comfort
Shear, friction reduced at site
Set-up, monitoring and on-call services
  provided
No dehydrating effects
	Dependent drainage of catheters may be
	  compromised due to low position of patient
	  immersed in bed, and the catheter tubing
	  must be elevated over the rigid bedside to the
	  catheter bag
	Head of bed cannot be raised: semi-Fowler's
	  position is achieved by using foam wedges

Table 3. A method for matching a patient's assessment to the appropriate support surface

Patient assessment	Outcome criteria	Appropriate support surface function
Turning surface (AHCPR)		Static Alternating
At high risk for development of decubitus ulcers	Pressure reduction	Flotation Rotation
Existing decubitus ulcer on one turning surface	Pressure reduction	Static Alternating Flotation Rotation
Existing decubitus ulcer on two or three turning surfaces	Pressure relief	Static Alternating Flotation Air fluidized Rotation

Existing pressure ulcer on
  one or more turning
  surfaces plus incontinence
  or large-volume drainage
	Pressure relief plus	Static
		Alternating
		Flotation
		Air fluidized
		Rotation

Post-operative repair procedure	Pressure relief plus	Static Alternating Flotation Air fluidized Rotation

If additional conditions are present – immobility, burns, pain, anasarca – consider specialty beds with needed features.
AHCPR, Agency for Health Care Policy and Research, US Department of Health and Human Services, Rockville, MD (Publication Number 95-0652).

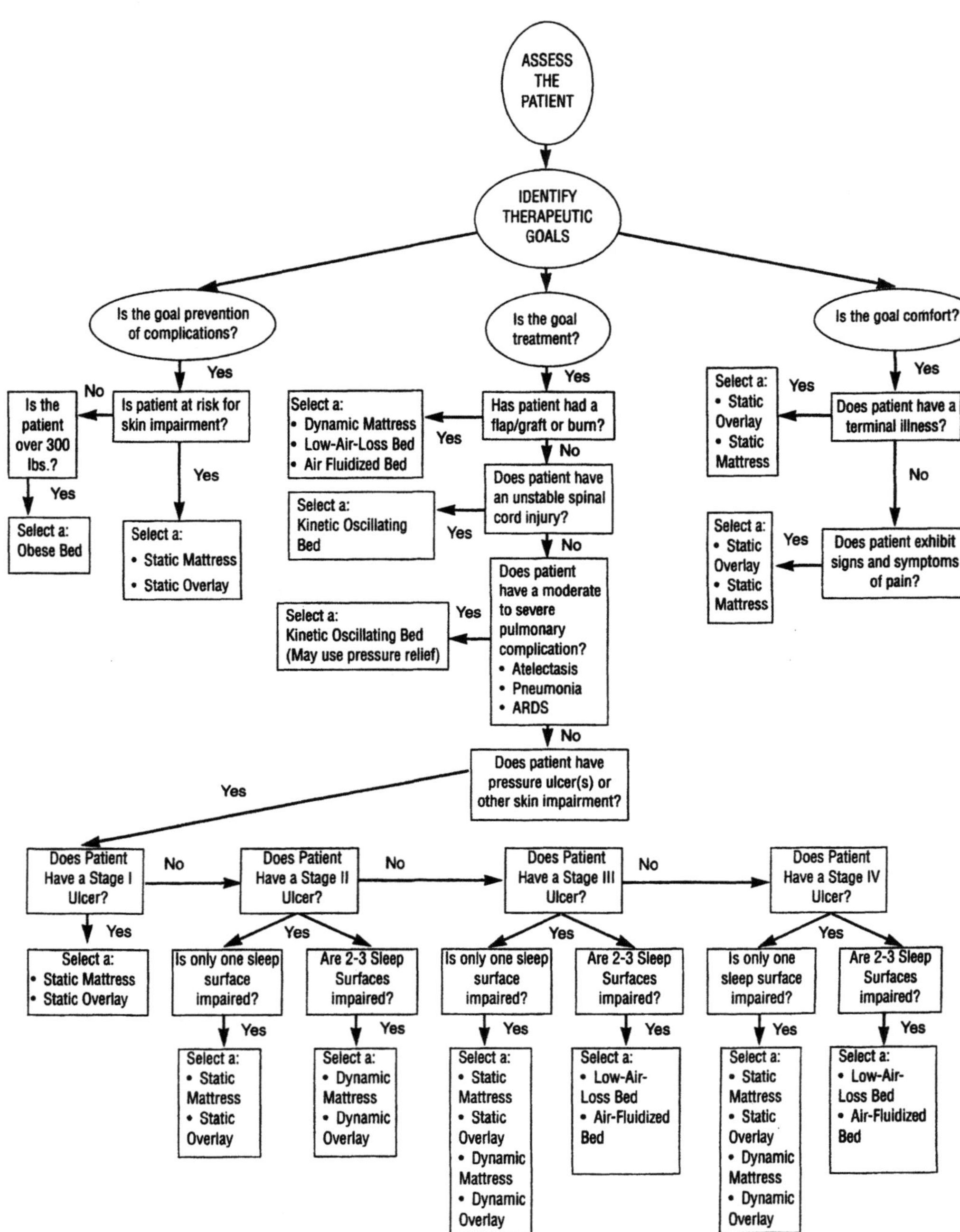

Note: If only one sleep surface is impaired, it is assumed the patient will not be turned on the affected site. A device with *pressure relief* is indicated if two-to-three sleep surfaces are impaired.

Fig. 16. Support surface algorithm (reprinted with permission from the November 1993 issue of *Decubitus*, Copyright 1993, Springhouse Corporation)

den, or similar type patient assessment and uses only the scores of the appropriate risk factors (mobility, activity, sensory perception) to help determine the patients need for a support surface (Fig. 17). These methods are universal in their approach for they will work with any risk assessment method and for any formulary of support surfaces [78].

The Operating Room and Emergency Room. Decubitus ulcers continue to develop in the operating room [79] because of the high pressures [79, 80] and shear stresses experienced by the immobile patient on the conductive operating room pad [81]. Often these lesions are mistakenly identified as burns even when there is insufficient or little evidence to draw such a conclusion [80]. The proper use of pressure-reducing and -relieving support surfaces during surgery could dramatically reduce the incidence of decubitus ulcers occurring during surgical procedures, but relieving pressure often interferes with the surgical procedure itself. The emergency room is another area where patients may lie immobilized on a hard, high-pressure surface for many hours before treatment and admission. Adequate pressure-reducing or -relieving support surfaces should be used with all partially or fully immobilized patients.

Facility and User Consideration for Support Surfaces. The clinical effectiveness of a support surface and matching a patient's needs are the most important criteria for selection of support surfaces but there are other criteria such as cost, ease of use, and service and support supplied by the manufacturer which should be evaluated [1, 14].

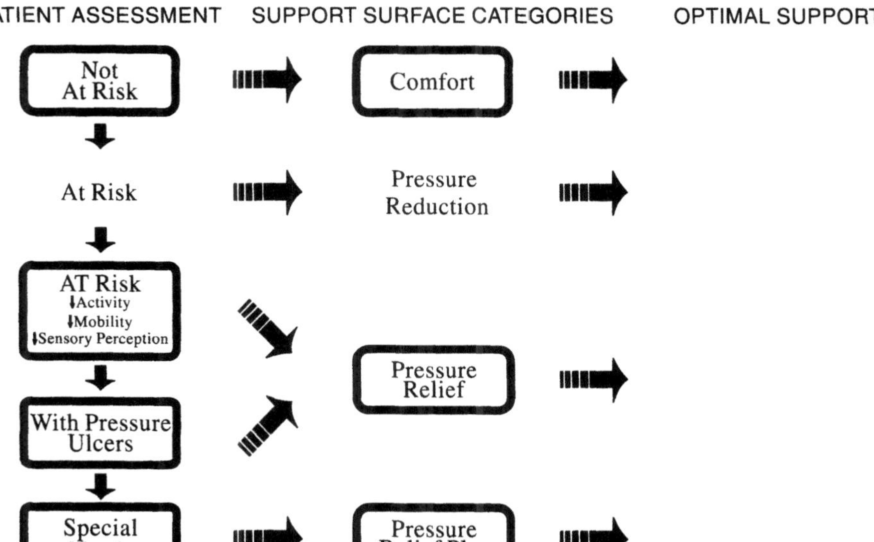

Fig. 17. A methodological approach to the selection of support surfaces (S.T.O.P.S.)

Conclusions

Support surface use and selection was once a mysterious art that confounded the care giver. By understanding the mechanical forces which cause decubitus ulcers and the form and function of various support surfaces, a methodologic approach can be achieved. Such an approach requires the use of patient assessment and support surface assessment and leads to a matching of the patient's needs to the capabilities of a support surface. A methodologic approach assures that patients receive the appropriate support surfaces in a cost-effective fashion.

References

1. Krouskop T, van Rijswijk L (1995) Standardizing performance-based criteria for support surfaces. Ostomy/Wound Management 41:34–45
2. Bergstrom N, Allman RM et al. (1994) AHCPR guidelines: treatment of pressure ulcers. AHCPR 1:1–154
3. Allman RW, Walker JM, Hart MK et al. (1987) Air-fluidized beds or conventional therapy for pressure sores: a randomized trial. Ann Intern Med 107:641–648
4. Inman KJ, Sibbald WJ, Rutledge FS, Clark BJ (1993) Clinical utility and cost-effectiveness of an air suspension bed in the prevention of pressure ulcers. JAMA 269:1139–1143
5. Bergstrom N, Allman R, Carlson C et al. (1992) Pressure ulcers in adults: prediction and prevention. Quick reference guide for clinicians. Decubitus 5(3):26–30
6. Sylvia CJ (1993) Determining the right mix of support surfaces to minimize hospital acquired pressure ulcers. Ostomy/Wound Management 39:12–16
7. Krasner D (1991) Patient support surfaces. Ostomy/Wound Management 33:57–60
8. Thomas C (1989) Specialty beds: decision making made easy. Ostomy/Wound Management 31:51–59
9. Stewart TP (1987) Materials management and decubitus care purchasing for prevention. J Healthcare Materiel Management 5:32–34
10. Stewart TP, Adamczyk L (1988) Decubitus care and prevention: manufacturers respond to growing concerns. J Healthcare Materiel Management 6:50–55
11. Anderson KE, Jensen O, Kvorning SA, Bach E (1982) Decubitus prophylaxis: a prospective trial of the efficiency of alternating pressure air mattresses and water mattresses. Acta Derm Venereol (Stockh) 63:227–230
12. Cuzzell JZ, Willey T (1987) Pressure relief perennials. Am J Nurs 87:1157–1160
13. Braun JL, Silvetti AN, Xakellis GC (1988) Decubitus ulcers: what really works? Patient Care 22:22–34
14. Doughty D, Fairchild P, Stogis S (1990) Your patient: which therapy. J Enterostmal Ther 17:154–159
15. Romanus M (1977) Microcirculatory reactions to local pressure induced ischemia. Thesis, University of Goteborg, Goteborg, Sweden, pp 1–30 [Abstract]
16. Maklebust J (1987) Pressure ulcers: etiology and prevention. Nurs Clin North Am 359–377
17. Kosiak M (1961) Etiology of decubitus ulcers. Arch Phys Med Rehab 19–29
18. Stewart TP, Grove McKay M, Magnano S (1990) Pressure relief characteristics of an alternating pressure system. Decubitus 3(4):26–29
19. Romm S, Lynch D, Tebbetts J, White R (1982) Pressure sores: state of the art. Texas Med 78:52–60
20. Bennett L, Lee BY (1985) Pressure versus shear in pressure sore causation. In: Lee BY (ed) Chronic ulcers of the skin, 1st edn. McGraw-Hill, New York, pp 39–56
21. Reichel SM (1955) Shearing force as a factor in decubitus ulcers in paraplegics. JAMA 166:762–763

22. Bennett L, Kavner D, Lee BK, Trainor FA (1979) Shear vs. pressure as causative factors in skin blood flow occlusion. Arch Phys Med Rehab 60:309–314
23. Roaf R (1976) The causation and prevention of bed sores. In: Kenedi RM, Cowden JM, Scales JT(eds.) Bedsore biomechanics, 1st edn. University Park Press, Baltimore, MD, pp 5–9
24. Gardner WJ, Anderson RM (1948) Alternating pressure alleviates bedsores. Mod Hosp 71:72–73
25. Gardner WJ (1948) Prevention and treatment of bedsores. JAMA 138:583
26. Scales JT (1961) Levitation. Lancet II:1181
27. Scales JT, Hopkins LA, Muir IFK (1968) Levitation – a means of treating burns. Pharmacol Treat Burns, pp 333–342
28. Scales JT, Hopkins LA, Bloch M et al. (1967) Levitation in the treatment of large area burns. Lancet I:1235–1240
29. Scales JT, Winter GD, Bloch M (1966) Levitation, a possible means of treating burns. Res Burns, p 266
30. Scales JT, Lunn HF, Jeneid PA et al. (1974) The prevention and treatment of pressure sores using air support systems. Paraplegia 12(2):118–131
31. Hargest TS, Artz CP (1969) A new concept in patient care: the air-fluidized bed. AORN 10:50–53
32. Artz CP, Hargest TS (1971) Air-fluidized bed clinical and research symposium, 1st edn. Medical University of South Carolina, Charleston, pp 1–92
33. Keane FX (1978) The minimum physiological mobility requirement for man supported on a soft surface. Paraplegia 16:383–389
34. Hartmann E et al. (1971) Sleep need. How much sleep and what kind? Am J Psych 127:41–48
35. Johnson M et al. (1930) In what position do healthy people sleep? JAMA 94:2058–2062
36. Laird DA (1935) Did you sleep well? Rev Rev 91:23, 86, 321
37. Nelson LD, Anderson HB (1989) Physiologic effects of steep positioning in the surgical intensive care unit. Arch Surg 124:352–355
38. Summer WR, Curry P, Haponik EF et al. (1989) Continuous mechanical turning of intensive care unit patients shortens length of stay in some diagnostic-related groups. J Crit Care 4:45–53
39. Whiteman K, Nachtmann L, Kramer D et al. (1995) Effects of continuous lateral rotation therapy on pulmonary complications in liver transplant patients. Am J Crit Care 4:133–139
40. Choi S, Nelson L (1992) Kinetic therapy in critically ill patients: combined results based on meta-analysis. J Crit Care 7:57–62
41. Fink MP, Helsmoortel CM, Stein KL et al. (1988) Lower respiratory tract infection in critically ill victims of non-penetrating trauma: effect of continuous postural oscillation. Depts of Surgery and Anesthesiology, University of Massachusetts Medical Center (Abstract)
42. Exton-Smith AN, Sherwin RW (1961) The prevention of pressure sores: significance of spontaneous bodily movements. Lancet II:1124–1126
43. Keane FX (1967) Roto-rest. B M J I:731–733
44. Hess CT (1995) Nurse's clinical guide to wound care, 1st edn. Springhouse, Springhouse, PA, pp 1–294
45. Krouskop TA, Garber S (1987) The role of technology in the prevention of pressure sores. Ostomy/Wound Management 29:44–54
46. Noble PC, Goode B, Krouskop TA, Crisp B (1984) The influence of environmental aging upon the loadbearing properties of polyurethane foams. J Rehab Res 21:31–38
47. Krouskop TA, Noble P, Brown J, Marburger R (1986) Factors affecting the pressure-distributing properties of foam mattress overlays. J Rehab Res Dev 23:33–39
48. Kemp MG, Krouskop TA (1994) Pressure ulcers: reducing incidence and severity by managing pressure. J Geronitol Nurs 20:27–34
49. Maklebust J, Mondoux L, Sieggreen M (1986) Pressure relief characteristics of various support surfaces used in prevention and treatment of pressure ulcers. J Enterost Ther 13:85–89
50. Maklebust J, Sieggreen M, Mondoux L (1988) Pressure relief capabilities of the Sof Care bed and the Clinitron bed. Ostomy/Wound Management 30:32–44

51. Maklebust J, Brunckhorst L, Cracchiolo-Caraway A et al. (1988) Pressure ulcer incidence in high risk patients managed on a special three-layered air cushion. Decubitus 1(4):30–40
52. Mayrovitz HN et al. (1993) Effects of rhythmically alternating and static pressure support surfaces on skin microvascular perfusion. Wounds 5(1):47–55
53. Jay R (1995) Pressure and shear: their effects on support surface choice. Ostomy/Wound Management 37:36–45
54. Johnson G, Daily C, Franciscus V (1991) A clinical study of hospital replacement mattresses. J Enterost Ther 18:153–157
55. Fletcher J, Billingham G (1993) Mattress replacements: assessment and evaluation. J Tiss Viabil 3(4):123–126
56. Flam E (1990) Skin maintenance in the bed-ridden patient. Ostomy/Wound Management 32:49–54
57. Caley L (1994) Randomized prospective trial of two types of low air loss therapy. Ostomy/ Wound Management 36:138
58. Mulder GD, Taro N, Seeley JE, Andrews K (1994) A study of pressure ulcer response to low air loss beds vs. conventional treatment. J Geriatr Dermatol 2:87–91
59. Murphy PK, Fenske NA (1994) Assessment of a new dynamic pressure relief air fluid bed for management of stage III-IV decubitus ulcers in geriatric patients. J Geriatr Dermatol 2:72–79
60. Berjian RA, Douglas HO, Holyoke ED et al. (1983) Skin pressure measurements on various mattress surfaces in cancer patients. Am J Phys Med 62:217–226
61. Thomson CW, Dunkin LJ, Ryan DW, Smith M (1980) Fluidized-bead bed in the intensive-therapy unit. Lancet I:568–570
62. Shore-Myers KM, Mann-Distaso S (1985) Multiple trauma: a case study using an airfluidized support system. Orthopaed Nurs 4:9–10
63. Eusanio PL (1976) Monitoring skin care eliminates decubitus ulcers. Am Health Care Assoc J 2(6):50–51
64. Micheels J, Sorensen B, The physiology of a healthy normal person in the air-fluidized bed. Burns 3:158–168
65. Parish LC, Witkowski JA (1980) Clinitron therapy and the decubitus ulcer: preliminary dermatologic studies. Int J Dermatol 19:517–518
66. Smeele PQ (1988) Accidental extubation and low air loss mattresses. Anaesthesia 43(11):992
67. Stewart TP (1988) Pressure points. Decubitus 1(1):12–14
68. Witkowski J, Parish L (1993) Skin failure and the pressure ulcer. Decubitus 6(5):4
69. Moss R, LaPuma J (1991) The ethics of pressure sore prevention and treatment in the elderly: a practical approach. J Am Geriatr Soc 39:905–908
70. Freedman B, Gilbert J, Kaltsounakis L (1990) Air-support treatment: a case study in the ethics of allocating expensive treatment. J Clin Ethics 1:298–303
71. Blaylock B (1992) Air support therapy: ethical considerations. J Enterost Nurs 19:171–173
72. Gruis ML, Innes B (1976) Assessment essential to prevent pressure sores. Am J Nurs 76(11):1762–1764
73. Swain I (1992) Assessment of support surfaces. Nurs Standard 6:12–14
74. Norton D (1975) Research and the problem of pressure sores. Nurs Mirror 140:65–67
75. Lincoln R, Roberts R, Maddox A et al. (1986) Use of the Norton pressure sore risk assessment scoring system with elderly patients in acute care. J Enterost Ther 13:132–138
76. Gosnell DJ (1987) Assessment and evaluation of pressure sores. Nurs Clin North Am 22:399–417
77. Thomason SS (1988) Pressure ulcers: considerations of intervention strategies. Ostomy/ Wound Management 33:48–54
78. Hasty J, Krasner D, Kennedy KL (1991) A new tool for evaluating patient support surfaces. Ostomy/Wound Management 36:51–58
79. Scott SM, Mayhew PA, Harris EA (1992) Pressure ulcer development in the operating room. AORN J 56:242–250
80. Stewart TP, Magnano S (1988) Burns or pressure ulcers in the surgical patient? Decubitus 1(1):36–40
81. Gendron F (1980) "Burns" occurring during lengthy surgical procedures. J Clin Eng 5(1):19–26

15 Antimicrobial Therapy

J C. Craft

The intact stratum corneum prevents invasion by microbes by acting as a barrier against the many organisms encountered daily. Skin is the first line of defense against infection. In the patient with spinal cord injury, debilitating neurologic disease, and surgical pressure necrosis results in the loss of this barrier. But even the loss of the stratum corneum does not guarantee infection and most patients will be able to defend themselves against the bacteria contaminating the wound; however, this is not true of the elderly patient, the diabetic patient, and patients with other reasons for decreased immunity [1–5].

The skin is constantly populated with microorganisms which reflect the contacts, habits, and general health of the individual. These organisms which are universally present on the skin are mainly the staphylococci, among which *S. epidermidis* outnumber *S. aureus*, aerobic corynebacteria, *Propionibacterium acnes*, mycobacteria, and a few species of usually harmless yeast (Table 1). These organisms are like a double-edged sword in that they protect the patient from infection by preventing colonization of the epidermis with more pathogenic bacteria. On the other hand, they can also cause infection when the condition of the patient skin is compromised by pressure necrosis.

Antimicrobial treatment of infected decubitus ulcers should be easy. The problem is deciding who needs antimicrobial therapy and who does not. The majority of decubitus ulcers are not infected and antimicrobial therapy is contraindicated; however, patients who are infected and who will benefit from antimicrobial therapy may not appear different from those that are not infected. This is particularly true because many of these patients are unable to complain of pain due to their neurologic condition, age, or immunocompromised state with a lack of signs of infection. The decision to treat or not to treat comes with experience and careful evaluation of the patient. Once the diagnosis of infection is made, treatment of infected decubitus ulcers requires a clinical approach that combines antimicrobial therapy and surgical debridement of necrotic/devascularized soft tissue and bone.

Factors Influencing the Choice of Antimicrobial Therapy

Because the antimicrobial therapy for infected decubitus ulcers usually needs to be initiated before microbiology data are available, the initial empiric se-

Table 1. Microorganisms of the skin

Acinetobacter calcoaceticus	*Peptostreptococcus* spp.
Bacillus spp.	*Pityosporum ovale*
Candida albicans	*Propionibacterium acnes*
Corynebacterium spp.	*Sarcina* spp.
Epidermophyton floccosum	*Staphylococcus aureus*
Micrococcus spp.	*Staphylococcus epidermidis*
Mycobacterium spp.	*Trichophyton* spp.
Peptococcus spp.	Viridans *Streptococci*

lection depends on the accurate evaluation and assessment of patient-specific variables (Table 2).

Clinical assessment of the severity of infection is one of the most critical factors in determining appropriate antimicrobial therapy but can be difficult to accomplish. The standard clinical classification of decubitus ulcers does not take into account the presence or absence of infection, only the degree of tissue destruction [3]. Difficulties in assessing infection in these patients is due to the frequent loss of many of the typical signs of infection. These problems may result in underestimation of the severity of the infection. Important clinical features of infection such as fever, rigors, and leukocytosis may be absent. The presence of palpable crepitus is a sign of gas in the soft tissue. This ominous sign of aerobic Gram-negative bacilli and/or anaerobic infection is associated with a high mortality rate. Wet gangrene is also a poor prognostic sign warranting aggressive surgical debridement and antimicrobial therapy.

A clinical classification of the severity of the infected decubitus ulcer infection is shown in Table 3. The empiric choice of antimicrobial therapy depends upon an assessment of the severity of the infection. More directed therapy is based on the results of appropriate culture of the wound and tissue as well as blood culture. Patients with mild infection may or may not need antimicrobial therapy. Frequently they will respond to simple topical decontamination. Oral antimicrobial therapy can be considered since the patient is

Table 2. Factors that influence the choice of antimicrobial therapy for treatment of infected decubitus ulcers

Factors	Characteristics
Severity of infection	Mild – local colonization of ulcer which may be preventing healing
	Moderate – definite infection of the ulcer localized to tissues directly adjacent to ulcer
	Severe – Disseminated infection involving bone and/or bacteremia including sepsis; potentially life threatening
Underlying illness	Age
	Diabetes mellitus
	Neurologic disorders
Microbiology	Frequently polymicrobial
	Nosocomial infection related to other treatment modalities
	Local antimicrobial resistance patterns

Table 3. Classification of decubitus ulcer infections

Severity	Characteristics	Therapy
Mild	Superficial ulceration Nonpurulent discharge Minimal/absent cellulitis Mild necrosis No spread to adjacent tissues	Local debridement Topical decontamination
Moderate	Ulceration to deep tissues Purulent discharge Cellulitis Mild to moderate necrosis Systemic toxicity	Intravenous antimicrobials Surgical debridement
Severe	Ulceration to deep tissues Purulent discharge Cellulitis Necrosis/gangrene Osteomyelitis Systemic toxicity Bacteremia/sepsis	Intravenous antibiotics Surgical debridement Control of other medical conditions

generally in no immediate danger. Moderate infections require broad-spectrum parenteral antibiotics and careful surgical debridement. Severe infections can be life threatening and require urgent medical management of all underlying problems – resection or debridement of the necrotic area, and broad-spectrum parental antibiotics sufficient to cover the more resistant pathogens found in the patients environment.

Underlying Illness

Age. The aging patients develop decubitus ulcers for many reasons related to the progressive organ failure related to aging. These include immobility, age-related skin changes, malnutrition, anemia, immunocompetence, vascular insufficiency, renal impairment, denervation, and cognitive impairment [1, 6]. These factors influence the choice of antimicrobial therapy in several ways. The decreasing immunocompetence of the elderly patient in association with malnutrition and anemia make the decision to treat difficult since many of the signs of infection may be suppressed. It is easy to underestimate the severity of the infection and in such cases the infection is overlooked until the patient is in septic shock. Because of this, one should err on the side of overtreatment when any doubt is present. The patient with vascular impairment may not have sufficient blood flow to achieve adequate concentrations of drug at the site of infection. This can slow the response to antimicrobial therapy and result in the development of resistance. Antimicrobial agents with good tissue penetration are preferred. As the patients age, their renal function also declines and even though they may have normal blood urea nitrogen and creatinine, their renal clearance may be severely impaired. This is important for those drug which are primarily eliminated by the kidney and where toxicity is associated with increased serum concentrations such as aminocyclitols (e.g., gentamycin) which should be avoided unless no suitable alternative exists or serum concentrations can be monitored. Cognitive impairment is of no real concern with the hospitalized patient but would prevent any form of home therapy which requires the patient's assistance.

Diabetes Mellitus. It is associated with neuropathy and vascular insufficiency which can lead to decubitus ulcers [2, 7, 8]. These factors can complicate the treatment of the infected decubitus ulcer in several ways. The neuropathy can prevent the patient from experiencing the pain associated with infection. Because of this, infection may progress much further and be much more severe before it is recognized by either the patient or the physician. The ischemia, particularly of the extremities, in the diabetic patient has the same implications as in the elderly patient. Diabetic osteopathy results in underlying bone changes which interfere with the detection of osteomyelitis. Because of this, regular bone scans may be misleading and technetium-99m bone scans combined with an indium-111 (^{111}In)-labeled white cell scan can be used [8]. The immunocompetence of the diabetic patient is directly related to control of the blood glucose concentrations and is extremely important to the control of infection. Antimicrobial therapy without control of the diabetes is less effective.

Neurologic Disorders. Besides the difficulty in assessing infection in these patients, there is the potential for adverse events with some antimicrobials. Carbapenem, imipenem, and metronidazole are associated with significant central nervous system adverse events such as seizures, myoclonic activity, and confusional states. Pre-existing central nervous system disorders and/or renal disease increase the likelihood of these reactions. These concerns should be weighted carefully before starting these agents.

Microbiology

The technique used to obtain microbiologic cultures from the decubitus ulcer is vital to the accurate identification of pathogens. Because up to 50% of all decubitus ulcer infections are due to a mixture of aerobic and anaerobic organisms, both aerobic and anaerobic cultures should be done [9]. Superficial cultures of the wound and/or purulent exudate usually produce results that over-represent the true pathogenic flora [9, 10]. On the other hand, aspiration specimens generally underestimate the number of isolates found by deep tissue biopsy [9, 10]. Deep tissue biopsy of decubitus ulcers should be considered the standard for isolation of the infecting organism/s. Although surface swab cultures are unreliable indicators of the true cause of infection, they may be useful in monitoring the presence and spread of dangerous multiresistant pathogens such as methicillin-resistant *S. aureus* [11, 12]. Awareness of these problem pathogens, especially among patients transferred between institutions, can allow prompt initiation of required isolation and infection control procedures. In addition, the selection of antimicrobial therapy based on the superficial culture results provide an adequate spectrum of antibacterial activity against pathogens isolated from the more reliable biopsy culture [9]. Thus, antimicrobial therapy chosen solely upon the results of superficial ulcer cultures is likely to be adequate in spectrum, but will be unnecessarily broad in spectrum. Modification of the treatment following the results of deep tissue cultures will provide the optimal coverage generally at the lowest cost.

The spectrum of likely pathogens involved decubitus ulcer infections is shown in Tables 1 and 2 in Chap. 9. In the patient with a single isolate and classic signs of cellulitis *S. aureus* and group A *Streptococcus* are the most common pathogens. Infection with both Gram-negative bacilli and/or anaerobes is frequently seen. Commonly isolated aerobic Gram-negative bacilli include *Proteus* species, *Klebsiella* species, *Escherichia coli*, *Citrobacter* species, and *Pseudomonas* species. Anaerobic infections include *Bacteroides* species, *Peptococcus*, and *Peptostreptococcus*, and *Fusobacterium*. The severely ill patient with bacteremia is most likely to have the following aerobic organisms: *Proteus mirabilis*, *E. coli*, *Klebsiella* species, *Citrobacter* species, *S. aureus*, *Streptococcus pyogenes*, group D *Streptococcus* and/or anaerobes such as: *Bacteriodes fragilis*, *Peptococcus*, *Peptostreptococcus*, and *Fusobacterium* [13]. Gram stains of the material taken from the infected decubitus ulcer may provide useful early information regarding the predominant pathogens, but not necessarily so. Other useful clinical features that may suggest the identity of the pathogen include foul odor for anaerobic infection, subcutaneous gas (palpable crepitus, radiographic gas) with either aerobic Gram-negative bacilli or anaerobic infection, gangrene associated with mixed aerobic Gram-negative bacilli and anaerobes.

Susceptibility patterns vary widely even between hospitals within the same city. Because of this, it is important to do susceptibility testing on all aerobic isolates and on anaerobic isolates if they fail to respond to therapy. If there is any doubt as to susceptibility patterns, consultation with the local microbiologist or infectious disease consultant can usually provide useful information for making an empiric choice of antimicrobial agents.

Antimicrobial Agents

Beta-Lactams

The beta-lactam antimicrobials such as the penicillins, penems, carapenems, monobactams, cephalosporins, oxycephams, and oxa-beta-lactams share many properties. They are among the best tolerated and least toxic of all therapeutic agents, hypersensitivity being the only major contraindication to their use. Because of the spectrum of organisms causing infection in decubitus ulcers, only those with broad-spectrum activity, including anaerobes, should be considered for empiric therapy. The beta-lactam/beta-lactamase combinations such as amoxacillin/clavulanate, ticarcillin/clavulanate, and piperacillin/tazobactam have broad-spectrum activity suitable for the treatment of infected decubitus ulcers. Amoxacillin/clavulanate is the only one which has activity when given orally and the spectrum of activity includes *Staphylococci, Streptococci, Enterococci,* many Gram-negative pathogens (excluding *Pesudomonas* species), and anaerobes. Ticarcillin/clavulanate and piperacillin/tazobactam have better activity against *Pseudomonas* species but lose some of their activity agains *Enterococci.* Imipenem/cilastin has the broad spectrum of activity of any of the beta-lactams, including excellent activity against most pathogens except methicillin-resistant *Staphylococci* and Gram-negative bacilli such as *Pseudomonas cepacia* or *Xanthomonas maltophila.* The major disadvantage to their use is the potential for neurologic complication. The anti-*Pseudomonas* activity of the beta-lactams is not sufficient to insure a good outcome in serious infections because of the rapid development of resistance. The combination of ticarcillin/clavulanate and gentamycin will reduce the development of *Pseudomonas* resistance to both agents.

Cefoxitin, cefotetan, and cefmetazole are the only cephalosporins with anaerobic activity sufficient to be considered for treatment of infected decubitus ulcers. They also maintain good activity against *Staphylococci, Streptococci,* many Gram-negative pathogens (excluding *Pseudomonas* species), but have little activity against *Enterococci.*

Aminocyclitols

The aminocyclitols such amikacin, gentamycin, kanamycin, netilmicin, and tobramycin bind irreversibly to the 30S subunit of the bacterial ribosome. They are active against most aerobic Gram-negative orgainsms (including *P. aeruginosa*), some Gram-positive ones such as *S. aureus.* They have no activity against anaerobic organisms such as, *Pseudomonas cepacia* and *Xanthomonas maltophila,* and resistance to *Enterococcus* is increasing. There is no real difference in the activity of these agents, but it is important to know the local susceptibility patterns to make the decision as to which aminoglycoside to use for empiric therapy. The major draw-back to their use is nephrotoxicity and ototoxicity, both of which can be prevented by careful monitoring of serum concentrations, particularly in the elderly or in patients with impaired renal function.

Glycopeptides

Vancomycin is a glycopeptide which is only active against Gram-positive bacteria. This activity includes Methicillin-resistant *S. aureus* (MRSA), coagulase-negative *Staphylococcus* species, *Enterococcus* species, and anaerobic bacteria. Since vancomycin is the last available antimicrobial for patients with resistant *S. aureus, S. pneumoniae,* and *Enterococci,* it should not be used for empiric therapy except when there is a strong possibility of MRSA or *Enterococci.* The ototoxicity and nephrotoxicity of vancomycin are additive when used in combination with aminocyclitols. Because of this, both vancomycin and aminocyclitols serum concentrations should be followed to minimize toxicity.

Lincosamides

Clindamycin is administered orally and intravenously, and is generally active against nonsporulating, Gram-negative anaerobes including *B. fragilis* and *Staphylococcus* species, but is not optimal against anaerobic cocci and *Clostridium* species. Because of the lack of activity against *Clostrium difficile*, clindamycin can cause pseudomembraneous enterocolitis. Patients should be observed carefully for evidence of diarrhea and clindamycin should be stopped if this becomes apparent.

Nitroimidazoles

Metronidazole is active against anaerobic bacteria including *Bacteroides* species, *Fusobacterium* species, *Clostridium* species, and *Peptococcus* species. It has no activity against aerobic bacteria. Metronidazole is equally bioavailable orally or intravenously, and distribution is essentially to all body tissues. The most common complaint of patients is the metallic taste. Disulfiram-like reactions may occur if patients ingest ethanol and it must be remembered that many elixirs contain ethanol. Seizures and peripheral neuropathy are seen, although rare; they may complicate the care of patients with preexisting neurologic disorders.

Fluoroquinolones

Ciprofloxacin is the most potent of the fluoroquinolones but is poorly absorbed. Ofloxacin has slightly less activity than ciprofloxacin but has better oral bioavailability. They are active against most aerobic Gram-negative bacteria including *Pseudomonas* species, but they are less active against *Staphylococci* species, *Streptococci* species, and anaerobic organisms. Both are available in formulations for oral and intravenous administration and can be used to treat infected decubitis ulcers in combination with other agents. Enoxacin, lomefloxacin, and norfloxacin should not be used because of poor activity and/or toxicity.

Mild Infections

The majority of mild decubitus ulcer infections do not need antimicrobial therapy (Table 4). Local wound care and medical management directed at the cause of the decubitus ulcer should be sufficient. Colonization of the wound with normal flora may sometimes prevent granulation of the wound and prevent healing. In these patients, topical decontamination with chlorhexidine gluconate or polyvinyl pyrrolidone for 1–2 days should decrease the number of organisms and provide the appropriate environment for healing [14]. Prolonged treatment should be avoided because it may interfere with granulation tissue formation [4]. In the rare patient who continues to have heavy coloni-

Table 4. Empirical antimicrobial therapy for infected decubitus ulcers

Severity and modifying circumstances	Usual etiologies	Suggested regimens	
		Primary	Alternative
Mild	Normal skin flora	Topical decontamination with: chlorhexidine gluconate for 1–2 days	Polyvinyl pyrrolidone for 1–2 days
Moderate			
Without sepsis	Aerobic Gram-positive cocci	Clindamycin orally	Amoxicillin/clavulanate orally
	Polymicrobic: groups A,C,D *Streptococci*, anaerobic *Streptococci*, *Enterobacteriacea*, *Bacteroides* spp., *S. aureus*	Cefoxitin	Ticarcillin/clavulanate
Patients without intravenous access		Oral clindamycin and ciprofloxacin	Oral metronidazole and ciprofloxacin
Severe			
With sepsis	Polymicrobic: groups A,C,D *Streptococci*, anaerobic *Streptococci*, *Enterobacteriacea*, *Pseudomonas* spp., *Bacteroides* spp., *S. aureus*	Ticarcillin/clavulanate[a] plus gentamycin[b]	Imipenem plus gentamycin
Possible MRSA		Add vancomycin	Imipenem may have activity against some strains
Osteomyelitis	Polymicrobic: aerobic cocci, bacilli, and anaerobes	Ticarcillin/clavulanate plus gentamycin	Imipenem plus gentamycin

[a]Ticarcillin/clavulanate or pipericillin/tazobactam.
[b]Gentamycin or any other aminoglycoside based on local susceptibility patterns.

zation and is not showing improvement, a short trial of 5–7 days of either oral antimicrobials (amoxicillin/clavulanate or clindamycin) or intravenous cefoxitin can be tried. It must be remembered before trying this that antimicrobial treatment can alter the local flora, resulting in recolonization of the wound with resistant organisms. Superficial culture before and after treatment may help to alert the physician of any adverse changes in the wound flora.

Moderate Infections

Moderate infections can be divided into those due to single pathogens and those that are polymicrobial. Cellulitis surrounding the wound is generally caused by normal skin pathogens such as *S. aureus* and group A *Streptococci*.

Gram stains of the wound will show a predominance of Gram-positive cocci. Treatment with oral clindamycin provides coverage against these aerobic Gram-positive cocci and also has good activity against anaerobic organisms. It does not have activity against Gram-negative aerobic organisms so that treatment is not likely to affect the Gram-negative flora. Amoxicillin/clavulanate is an alternative that can be given orally with similar activity against Gram-positive cocci, less anaerobic activity, and some Gram-negative activity. For the patient with suspected polymicrobial infection intravenous antimicrobials are required. Cefoxitin has sufficient coverage for the patient with a moderately infected decubitus ulcer whose general health is not compromised by any underlying illness. Intravenous ticarcillin/clavulanate is an alternate. In the patient in whom intravenous access is difficult, oral clindamycin plus ciprofloxacin can be used but this is not appropriate for the severe infections or in patient with serious underlying illness. An alternative oral therapy is metronidazole and ciprofloxacin.

Severe Infections

Severe infection is found in the patient with underlying illness such as the elderly and diabetics, and/or in otherwise healthy patient in whom the extent of infection has spread beyond the adjacent tissue. Because of the high mortality associated with sepsis in these patients, empiric therapy should have as broad a spectrum as possible [15]. Combination therapy with ticarcillin/clavulanate plus gentamycin should be effective. If the possibility of MRSA is present in the patient's environment, vancomycin should be added to the regimen. Once sepsis is controlled, and culture and susceptibility data are available, antimicrobial therapy can be optimized.

Osteomyelitis associated with decubitus ulcers will respond to antimicrobial therapy directed at the decubitus ulcer [16, 17]. To insure that the infection is treated adequately and will not return once therapy is stopped, several additional steps must be taken. Cultures must be taken before therapy from the bone and all devitalized bone removed. Therapy can be limited to narrower-spectrum agents once the culture and susceptibility results are available. Therapy must be continued for at least 6 weeks or until there is sufficient healing of the wound to prevent reinfection of the bone. Oral therapy of osteomyelitis is possible but requires initial control of the infection with intravenous therapy. The switch to oral therapy can be started once the causative organism(s) has been isolated and susceptibilities are known.

Conclusions

Infection in decubitus ulcers is a common and potentially life-threatening complication. A clear understanding of the associated issues, principles of antimicrobial therapy, and potential treatment modalities is critical to achieving an optimal outcome.

References

1. Bergstrom N, Braden B (1992) A prospective study: pressure sore risk among institutionalized elderly. J Am Geriatric Soc 40:747–758
2. Jelinek JE (1994) Cutaneous manifestations of diabetes mellitus. Int J Dermatol 33:605–617
3. Leigh IH, Bennett G (1994) Pressure ulcers: prevalence, etiology, and treatment modalities. A review. Am J Surg 167:25S–30S
4. Manley M (1978) Incidence, contributory factors and cost of pressure sores. South Afr Med J 53:217–222
5. Young JB, Dobrzanski S (1992) Pressure sores. Epidemiology and current management concepts. Drugs Aging 2:42–57
6. Perez ED (1993) Pressure ulcers; updated guidelines for treatment and prevention. Geriatrics 48(1):39–44
7. Kertesz D, Chow AW (1992) Infected pressure and diabetic ulcers. Clin Geriatr 8:835–852
8. Laing P (1994) Diabetic foot ulcer. Am J Surg 167[Suppl]:34–36
9. Rudensky B, Lipschits M, Isaacsohn M, Sonnenblick M (1992) Infected pressure sores: comparison of methods for bacterial identification. South Med J 85(9):901–903
10. Sapico FL, Witte JL, Canawati HN, Montgomerie JZ, Bessmann AN (1984) The infected foot of the diabetic patient: quantitative microbiology and analysis of clinical features. Rev Infect Dis 6[Suppl]:171–176
11. Haley RW, Hightower AW, Khabbaz RF et al. (1982) The emergence of methicillin-resistant Staphylococcus aureus infections in United States hospitals: possible role of the house staff–patients transfer circuit. Ann Intern Med 97:297–308
12. Rhinehart E, Shales DM, Keys TF et al. (1987) Nosocomial clonal dissemination of methicillin-resistant Staphylococcus aureus: elucidation by plasmid analysis. Arch Intern Med 147:521–524
13. Galpin JE, Chow AW, Bayer AS, Guze LB (1976) Sepsis associated with decubitus ulcers. Am J Med 61:346–350
14. Rodeheaver G, Ballamy W, Kody M et al. (1982) Bactericidal activity and toxicity of iodine-containing solutions wounds. Arch Surg 117:181–186
15. Bryan CS, Dew CE, Reynolds KL (1983) Bacteremia associated with decubitus ulcers. Arch Intern Med 143:2093–2095
16. Darouiche RO, Landon GC, Klima M, Musher DM, Markowski J (1994) Osteomyelitis associated with pressure sores (see comments). Arch Intern Med 154:753–758
17. Deloach ED, DiBenedetto RJ, Womble L, Gilley JD (1992) The treatment of osteomyelitis underlying pressure ulcers. Decubitus 5(6):32–41

16 Nutritional Perspectives

R. Chernoff

The role of nutrition in wound healing, whether a surgical incision or a decubitus ulcer, is essential to successful treatment, the generation of new tissue, and to lowering of the risk for complications, particularly infection. There are two aspects of nutrition in decubitus ulcers that deserve attention: prevention and treatment.

Nutrition in the prevention of decubitus ulcers requires a knowledge of the nutritional requirements of the long-term care patients, particularly elderly people; a protocol for assessing nutritional status periodically; and a plan for early intervention when nutritional problems are identified.

The guidelines for nutrition in the treatment of decubitus ulcers requires the incorporation of basic principles of applied nutrition, nutrient requirements for healing and tissue regeneration, and the metabolic response to injury [1]. These are very complex processes and the incorporation of nutritional therapy in the treatment plan for decubitus ulcer healing is often challenging.

Nutrition in the Prevention of Decubitus Ulcers

Basic Nutrition for the Long-Term Care Patient

The treatment of chronic diseases sometimes requires more attention to nutrition than is commonly given. In order to avoid weight gain in chair- or bed-bound patients, calories are reduced; however, there is not adequate compensation for the parallel loss of other essential nutrients. Providing all macro- and micronutrients to meet the recommended dietary allowances (RDA) is a reasonable goal for all long-term care patients to contribute to health maintenance and minimize the possibility of concurrent illnesses or other complications.

Protein is the most important of the macronutrients to assure adequate intake [2–4]. Immobilization is a major factor in contributing to negative nitrogen balance; loss of muscle (somatic) protein is a contributing cause for decubitus ulcer development. Protein component loss will also increase the likelihood of an infectious complication. Carbohydrate and fat provide other essential nutrients such as water- and fat-soluble vitamins, but also are the major sources of energy.

Regardless of energy requirements, there is a need for vitamins and minerals; 100% of the RDA per day is a minimal goal. This can be achieved in a diet of nutrient-dense food but for patients who have poor appetites, are on restricted diets due to other chronic conditions, or are anorectic, a complete, daily vitamin supplement that provides the RDA should be considered [1]. Dietary restriction should be considered carefully if there are other ways of managing chronic illness; foods that are low in fat, low in salt, low in protein, or restricted in other nutrients may be unpalatable and may not be appealing to the individual at risk of chronic undernutrition. One of the challenges in long-term care is the identification of nutritional risk and of nutritional status. It is important to establish a plan for nutrition screening and assessment for all long-term care patients.

Nutritional Assessment

Screening and assessment of nutritional status in long-term care and elderly patients can be challenging. Identification of risk factors for malnutrition are the objective of screening protocols, whereas the substantiation of signs and symptoms of nutrient deficits is the objective of nutritional assessment.

Screening risk factors can be cataloged using readily accessible tools (see Table 1), but in long-term care patients these risk factors become less important. Assessing for nutritional deficits is a more reasonable activity. Nutritional assessment should include the following components [5]:

- Anthropometric measurements
- Physical assessment
- Biochemical and laboratory measures
- Dietary assessment
- Social history
- Oral health examination
- Drug profile

Anthropometric Measures. Anthropometric measures are easy to collect; the usual evaluations include height, weight, triceps skinfold, subscapular skinfold, and suprailiac skinfold. Height should be measured as accurately as possible by using erect height, recumbent length, segmental measurements, or knee-to-heel measures. Weight is a relative measure that should be measured at regular intervals. Changes in weight over time are one of the best indicators of

Table 1. Risk factors for malnutrition (adapted from [25])

Inadequate food intake
Institutionalization
Poverty
Chronic conditions with chronic medication use
Dependency/disability/immobilization
Social isolation
Advanced age (over 80 years)

changing nutritional status. In addition to signaling changes in nutritional condition, a relative measure of weight for height will identify individuals who are chronically undernourished or overnourished; one measure used to evaluate weight for height is body mass index [Wt (kg)/Ht (m^2)]. Skinfold measures are best used to track changes in body composition over time by using calipers to pinch a small amount of skin and underlying fat tissue. There have been mathematical formulas derived to estimate the amount of muscle and fat at each site. There are no reference tables that set mean values for older people although it is possible to extrapolate averages from existing data.

Physical Assessment. Physical assessment requires knowing the signs of malnutrition so that they are incorporated into every routine review of systems. These are summarized in Table 2.

Biochemical and Laboratory Measures. Although there are many biochemical and laboratory measures that are often used as part of a nutritional assessment, the most valid one that is associated with nutritional status is serum albumin. Hypoalbuminemia has been associated with the development of decubitus ulcers [6]. Although it is difficult to determine which condition occurs first. It is also sound practice to periodically assess hematocrit and hemoglobin since various anemias may be associated with nutrient deficiencies.

Dietary Assessment. Reviewing the usual dietary pattern of the individual will often offer a good assessment of nutritional intake. A diet that is limited in one or more of the food groups will likely be deficient in one or more essential nutrients. A registered dietitian who can take a thorough dietary history may be able to identify nutritional concerns that may subsequently be confirmed with other diagnostic or laboratory tests. Included in a review of protein, carbohydrate, fat, vitamins, and minerals should be an evaluation of total daily fluid intake. Hydration status is an important component of a nutrition and dietary assessment.

Social History. A social history should provide insight into potential socioeconomic etiologies for nutrition risk. It has been demonstrated that many older people who are living independently are financially dependent, do not have enough money to buy enough food, may require help with shopping or preparing food, may need assistance with feeding, and may be at nutritional risk. Older people who are living on fixed incomes, living alone, who have many chronic conditions, or have risk factors for malnutrition may be eligible for elderly nutrition programs, food stamps, or other assistance. Including a social history in a comprehensive assessment may help identify opportunities for early interventions.

Oral Health Examination. Oral lesions, missing teeth, inflamed or bleeding gums, ill-fitting dentures, abscesses, infections, or bacterial overgrowth may all affect the ability of an individual to eat adequate amounts or variety of foods. Additionally, signs of nutritional deficiency are often first seen in the oral

Table 2. Physical signs of malnutrition

	Clinical sign or Symptom	Nutrient deficiency
Hair	Coiled, keratinized	Vitamin A
	Pluckable, sparse hair	Biotin
Skin	Follicular hyperkeratosis	Vitamin A
	Xerosis	
	Subcutaneous hemorrhage	Vitamin K
	Easy bruisability	
	Nasolabial seborrhea	Niacin
	Angular fissures around eyes and mouth	
	Papillary atrophy	
	Pellagrous dermatitis	
	Nasolabial seborrhea	Riboflavin
	Fissuring around eyes and mouth	
	Magenta tongue	
	Genital dermatosis	
	Nasolabial seborrhea	Vitamin B_6
	Glossitis	
	Glossitis	Folic acid/vitamin B_{12}
	Hyperpigmentation of tongue	
	Pallor	
	Petechia	Vitamin C
	Purpura	
	Swollen, bleeding gums	
	Seborrheic dermatitis	Biotin
	Pallor	
	Pallor	Iron
	Glossitis	
	Spoon nails	
	Pale conjunctiva	
	Seborrheic dermatitis	Zinc
	Poor wound healing	
	Dull, dry "flaky paint" dermatitis	Protein
	Edema	
	Loss of subcutaneous fat	Protein/energy
	Dull, dry, easily pluckable hair	
	Muscle wasting	
	Decubitus ulcers	
Eyes	Bitot's spots	Vitamin A
	Conjunctival and corneal xerosis	
	Keratomalacia	
	Ophthalmoplegia	Thiamine
	Corneal vascularization	Riboflavin
	Photophobia	Zinc
Cardiac	Tachycardia	Thiamine
	Cardiomegaly	
	Congestive heart failure	
Gastrointestinal	Constipation	Thiamine
	Diarrhea	Niacin
		Folic acid
		Vitamin B_{12}

Table 2 (*Cont.*)

	Clinical sign or Symptom	Nutrient deficiency
Hematologic	Anemia	Vitamin E
		Vitamin B_6
		Folic acid
		Vitamin B_{12}
		Biotin
		Iron
Neurologic	Mental confusion	Thiamine
	Irritability	
	Parethesias	
	Mental confusion	Niacin
	Peripheral neuropathy	Vitamin B_6
	Parethesias	
	Depression	Folic acid/biotin
	Ataxia	Vitamin B_{12}
	Optic neuritis	
	Paresthesias	
	Mental disorders	

cavity [7]. An oral examination by a dental health professional or another health professional trained to perform such an examination may provide insight into nutritional problems [8].

Drug Profile. Polypharmacy is a serious problem that is often encountered in older and long-term care patients. There are many potential side effects from the use of multiple medications; drug–drug interactions are well known to many health care professionals. The manifestations of this problem are complex and may take some time to identify but there are other consequences associated with the use of many drugs. There may also be drug–nutrient interactions that contribute to the loss of appetite, the interference with nutrient absorption or metabolism [9]. Each of these conditions may contribute to poor nutritional status. Some examples are provided in Table 3.

Nutritional Requirements

Nutrient requirements for long-term care, elderly, or immobilized patients may change in several ways: (a) they may increase; (b) they may decrease; or (c) they may need to be altered to accommodate metabolic changes associated with acute or chronic disease [10]. Energy needs tend to decrease with age and with immobility. However, adequate energy to protect dietary protein from being burned for calories is important.

Dietary protein requirements (RDA for protein is 0.8 g/kg body weight for adults) appear to increase in older people [11] and negative nitrogen balance is associated with immobility. There is good evidence that protein needs increase to at least 1 g/kg body weight simply to maintain lean body mass and other protein compartments. There also is ample evidence that increased levels of

Table 3. Examples of drugs that interfere with nutrition status

Loss of appetite	Nutrient absorption	Metabolism
Alcohol	Aluminum hydroxide	Cephalosporin
Amphetamines	Cholestyramine resin	Coumarin
Benzodiazepines	Mineral oil	Hydralazine
Captopril	Sodium bicarbonate	Isoniazid
Cisplatin	Sulfonamide	Methotrexate
Hydralazines	Tetracycline	Phenytoin
Minoxidil		Triamterene
Phenothiazines		

dietary protein are well tolerated in elderly and long-term care patients, particularly if they are well hydrated.

Fluid requirements are estimated at 30 ml/kg body weight with a minimum target of 1.5 l per day. Older people are often dehydrated. Thirst sensation decreases with age and people may voluntarily dehydrate to avoid minor incontinence problems [12]. Nursing and dietary personnel should make every effort to encourage adequate daily fluid intake in long-term care patients [12].

Vitamin and mineral requirements do not change significantly with age although there are nutrients for which elderly patients may be at risk of inadequacy [11]. Dietary histories will reveal areas of potential deficiency. Nutrients that may be associated with risk include vitamins B_{12} and B_6, folic acid, vitamin D, and calcium.

Malnutrition as a Factor in Decubitus Ulcer Development

One of the major factors in the development of decubitus ulcers is malnutrition [13]. Malnutrition is associated with weight loss and cachexia, muscle wasting, which occurs with inadequate dietary energy intake when endogenous protein is used for energy; with the use of skeletal protein as a source for essential amino acids; and with atrophy of muscle protein due to immobilization [14].

Malnutrition is also associated with an inadequate dietary intake of all other essential nutrients. Adequate calories from carbohydrate and fat sources serve to protect protein so that it is used to replace or repair muscle or organ tissue or make new protein compounds such as blood cells, platelets, immune bodies, hormones, enzymes, etc. Malnutrition is also frequently associated with dehydration which contributes to lack of skin turgor, lack of tissue elasticity, and blood volume depletion, all of which may contribute to the development of decubitus ulcers.

Nutrition in Decubitus Ulcer Healing

Nutrition has a very important role in the treatment and healing of decubitus ulcers. A great deal of money is invested in special treatments, high-technology devices, surgery, new materials and medicines, but often nutritional intervention is overlooked as an essential part of treatment protocols. Providing a well-balanced, nutritionally adequate diet should be a goal for all individuals in long-term care or who are at risk for decubitus ulcers; however, there are some nutrients that require extra attention.

Protein

Protein has a very important role in decubitus ulcer development and treatment. There appears to be a relationship between serum amino acid profiles, hypoalbuminemia, and the development of decubitus ulcers. Undernutrition, where people are using endogenous protein as a source of energy because energy intake is not adequate to maintain weight and muscle and organ mass, is associated with the development of decubitus ulcers. If the cushion of subcutaneous fat is reduced, the muscle tissue beneath it becomes more vulnerable to the injury associated with pressure, friction, and shearing forces.

The rate-limiting nutritional factor in decubitus ulcer healing is protein. With all the technologic approaches available for the treatment of decubitus ulcers, healing cannot occur unless there is adequate accessible protein to make new tissue. It seems clear that older persons require more than the RDA for adults over the age of 50 years [11]. It is estimated that at least 1 g protein per kilogram body weight is needed simply to achieve nitrogen equilibrium; it is possible that more than 1 g/kg body weight is needed for healthy, active individuals. It has been demonstrated that immobilization leads to skeletal muscle atrophy and negative nitrogen balance even without infection or other conditions that demand a protein substrate. When healing demands become part of the protein requirement, more than 1 g/kg body weight of protein may be needed [12]. There is evidence that a great deal more protein (1–3 g/kg body weight) is required to facilitate decubitus ulcer healing.

There has been apprehension expressed when high levels of dietary protein are prescribed for frail patients who have decubitus ulcers. Some clinicians fear that high dietary protein intake will contribute to the development of renal problems in older patients. There is no evidence that dietary protein will precipitate disease in individuals who do not have pre-existing renal problems [15, 16].

One important factor in enhancing tolerance of high levels of dietary protein is to assure adequate fluid intake and hydration status [12]. Fluid intake should be 1500 ml per day at a minimum. For patients who are tube-feeding dependent, additional liquid should be provided to compensate for the tube formula volume that is actually fluid displaced by solids suspended in the solution (usually 25% of the total formula volume).

Energy

Most physiologic energy is derived from dietary carbohydrate (4 kcal/g) and fat (9 kcal/g). When demands for calories exceed that provided by carbohydrate or fat, protein (4 kcal/g) substrate will be used as an energy source. When this occurs, protein cannot be used to make new tissue. One major goal of nutrition intervention is to protect protein by providing adequate calories to meet energy needs which increase with the demands of healing. Calorie requirements may be as high as 32–35 kcal/kg body weight. Providing enough calories to prevent use of protein for energy is difficult; positive nitrogen balance may help to determine whether adequate calories are being provided.

Vitamins

It is a widely accepted recommendation that individuals at risk of decubitus ulcers take a daily multivitamin supplement [1]. There does not appear to be anything gained by using megadoses or therapeutic doses of vitamins; however, a daily multivitamin that provides 100% of the recommended dietary allowances will assure nutritional adequacy for these essential nutrients.

There is also a widely accepted belief that supplementation with specific vitamins known to be associated with wound healing and infection resistance benefits individuals who have decubitus ulcers. There is much contradictory evidence that this is actually the case. Nevertheless, there are treatment protocols that include high amounts of specific vitamins.

Vitamin C. Vitamin C (ascorbic acid) is one nutrient that is often supplemented at very high levels as part of the treatment for decubitus ulcers. There is no evidence that massive doses of vitamin C enhances wound healing; the limiting factors in wound healing appear to be protein and energy. There is a limit to the amount of vitamin C that can be absorbed and stored in body tissue; anything beyond that will be excreted in urine [17, 18]. It is likely that doses of supplemental vitamin C beyond 1 g per day are wasteful and will not have any positive effect on wound healing; it is also likely that even doses of 1 g per day are more than necessary to synthesize new tissue. The RDA for adults is 60 mg.

Vitamin B Complex. Many of the B complex vitamins are necessary in energy metabolism. To assure the most efficient use of nutrients to maintain homeostasis and to support wound healing, the B complex vitamins must be provided in amounts appropriate to support the physiologic processes associated with these activities [19, 20].

Vitamin A. Vitamin A is an essential nutrient for many physiologic reactions, one of which is the synthesis of new tissue [21]. In order to make new epithelial tissue, vitamin A is needed. For decubitus ulcers to heal, vitamin A is required in at least the RDA amount of 5000 IU. Vitamin A is one of the nutrients that is often deficient in dietary surveys of older people so providing a vitamin supplement that contains not more than the RDA for vitamin A is a valid therapy.

Vitamin D. Although vitamin D is most closely associated with bone metabolism and health, it has an important role in wound healing and immune responses [22]. For individuals who have decubitus ulcers, an adequate supply of vitamin D is needed. Vitamin D is one nutrient for which elderly, institutionalized, and home-bound individuals may be at risk for deficiency. Often, their intake of food sources of vitamin D (i.e., dairy products, oily fish) is deficient. Another source of vitamin D is sunlight exposure; these individuals usually do not have adequate sun exposure to stimulate vitamin D precursors found in skin (7-dehydrocholesterol), and this substance has been reported to decrease with advancing age. There is no need to give large doses of this nutrient, but it is important to meet the RDA of 200 IU or 5 µg.

Minerals

A well-balanced diet that meets all the essential nutrient requirements is a reasonable goal for all individuals who are at risk for or have already developed decubitus ulcers. Perhaps the mineral that has garnered the most attention is zinc. There is great controversy about this element [23, 24]. There are clinicians who believe that amounts of zinc in excess of 50 times the recommended allowance of 15 mg are required. Zinc is necessary to synthesize new tissue, but zinc alone will not lead to effective healing. The amount of protein and energy is what controls the rate of healing so massive doses of zinc are not necessary and may, in fact, have deleterious effects on other essential mineral absorption. Large amounts of any mineral may interfere with the absorption of minerals with similar structure. Provision of elemental zinc at 10–15 times the RDA (150–225 mg) is a maximum dose.

Conclusions

Nutrition is key to the management of decubitus ulcers; without adequate nutritional substrate, all the high technology, wound care materials, surgical interventions, skin care protocols, and nursing techniques will not heal a decubitus ulcer.

Nutritional recommendations include high-protein, high-calorie diets with enough fluid to maintain hydration status, with attention to levels of vitamin C, B complex vitamins, vitamin A, vitamin D, and zinc. A daily multivitamin supplement may contribute to the maintenance of nutritional status in chronically ill patients who do not have appetites sufficient to ingest a nutritionally complete diet.

References

1. Agency for Health Care Policy and Research (1991) Treatment of pressure ulcers: clinical practice guidelines. Public Health Service, USDHHS, Rockville
2. Chernoff R, Milton KY, Lipschitz DA (1990) The effect of a very high-protein liquid formula (Replete) on decubitus ulcer healing in long-term tube-fed institutionalized patients (abstract). J Am Dietet Assoc 90:A130

3. Breslow RA, Hallfrisch J, Guy DG, Crawley B, Goldberg A (1993) The importance of dietary protein in healing pressure ulcers. J Am Geriatr Soc 41:357–362
4. Kaminski MV (1976) Enteral hyperalimentation. Surg Obstet Gynecol 143:12–16
5. Mitchell CO, Chernoff R (1991) Nutritional assessment of the elderly. In: Chernoff R (ed) Geriatric nutrition: the health professional's handbook. Aspen, Gaithersburg, pp 363–395
6. Pinchofsky-Devin GD, Kaminski MV (1986) Correlation of pressure sores and nutritional status. J Am Geriatr Soc 34:435–440
7. Martin WE (1991) Oral health in the elderly. In: Chernoff R (ed) Geriatric nutrition: the health professional's handbook. Aspen, Gaithersburg, pp 107–182
8. Sullivan DH, Martin W, Flaxman N, Hagen JE (1993) Oral health problems and involuntary weight loss in a population of frail elderly. J Am Geriatr Soc 41:725–731
9. Blumberg JB, Suter P (1991) Pharmacology, nutrition, and the elderly: interactions and implications. In: Chernoff R (ed) Geriatric nutrition: the health professional's handbook. Aspen, Gaithersburg, pp 337–362
10. Blumberg JB (1992) Changing nutrient requirements in older adults. Nutr Today 27(5):15–20
11. Gersovitz M, Motil K, Munro HN, Scrimshaw N, Young VR (1982) Human protein requirements: assessment of the adequacy of the current recommended dietary allowance for dietary protein in elderly men and women. Am J Clin Nutr 35:6–14
12. Chernoff R (1994) Thirst and fluid requirements. Nutr Rev 52:S3–S5
13. Guralnick JM, Harris TB, White LR, Cornoni-Huntley JC (1988) Occurrence and predictors of pressure sores in the National Health and Nutrition Examination Survey follow-up. J Am Geriatr Soc 36:807–812
14. Evans WJ (1992) Sarcopenia: the age-related loss in skeletal muscle mass. In: Buckwalter JA, Goldberg VM, Woo SL-Y (eds) Musculoskeletal soft-tissue aging: impact on mobility. American Academy of Orthopedic Surgeons Symposium, Colorado Springs
15. Tobin J, Spector D (1986) Dietary protein has no effect on future creatinine clearance. Gerontologist 26:59A
16. Lindeman RD (1991) The aging renal system. In: Chernoff R (ed) Geriatric nutrition: the health professional's handbook. Aspen, Gaithersburg, pp 253–270
17. Suter PM (1991) Vitamin requirements. In: Chernoff R (ed) Geriatric nutrition: the health professional's handbook. Aspen, Gaithersburg, pp 25–52
18. Moore FD (1983) Surgical care and metabolic management of the postoperative patient. In: Winters RW, Greene HL (eds) Nutritional support of the seriously ill patient. Academic, New York, pp 13–33
19. Russell RM (1992) Micronutrient requirements of the elderly. Nutr Rev 50(12):463–466
20. Alvarez OM, Gilbreath RL (1982) Thiamine influence on collagen during the granulation of skin wounds. J Surg Res 32:24–31
21. Levenson SM, Seifter E (1983) Influence of supplemental arginine and vitamin A on wound healing, the thymus, and resistance to infection following surgery. In: Winters RW, Greene HL (eds) Nutritional support of the seriously ill patient. Academic, New York, pp 53–62
22. Yoder MC, Manolagas SC (1991) Vitamin D and its role in immune function. Clin Appl Nutr 1:35–44
23. Jeejeebhoy KN (1983) Malnutrition and effects of nutritional support in the malnourished patient. In: Winters RW, Greene HL (eds) Nutritional support of the seriously ill patient. Academic, New York, pp 207–221
24. Fosmire GJ (1989) Possible hazards associated with zinc supplementation. Nutr Today 24(3):15–18
25. Nutrition screening manual for professions caring for older Americans (1991) Nutrition Screening Initiative, Washington DC

17 Incontinence Management

B.M. Bates-Jensen

Urinary incontinence affects at least 10 million Americans [1, 2]. It is estimated that that more than half of the 1.5 million residents of nursing homes are incontinent of urine [2, 3]. While data for acute-care settings are few, there are reports of incidence rates of 35% for elderly persons during hospitalization [4]. The incidence and prevalence of urinary incontinence in the non-institutionalized elderly is not well documented, but it has been reported at 15–30% for those persons over the age of 60 years [2]. Fecal incontinence affects an estimated 17%–66% of the hospitalized elderly and 10%–30% of the nursing home population [5]. Expenditures by the federal government on skin care are estimated at $10 billion annually [6]. These costs are conservative estimates and may not include all of the costs associated with complications resulting from incontinence.

One of the major complications resulting from incontinence is skin damage ranging from perineal dermatitis to decubitus ulcers, where incontinence is commonly considered a contributing factor [2]. Nurses choose urinary incontinence as one of the major defining characteristics of patients at risk for decubitus ulcer development [7]. The condition of urinary incontinence, or similar conditions, is included in the major risk assessment tools for predicting risk of decubitus ulcer development [8–11]. This chapter reviews the role of urinary and fecal incontinence as predictors for decubitus ulcer development, describes skin damage associated with moisture, urine, and feces, and presents guidelines for prevention and management of incontinence as it relates to the patient with a decubitus ulcer or at risk for developing the condition.

Incontinence as a Predictor for Decubitus Ulcer Development

The presence of urine, moisture, and feces on the skin would intuitively seem to decrease the tolerance of the tissues to trauma and therefore place the patient at risk for decubitus ulcer development; however, causal relationships have been difficult to define. There are conflicting reports in the literature relating to the exact role of incontinence as a risk factor in the development of decubitus ulcers. Both urinary incontinence and fecal incontinence, along with the associated frequency of incontinence episodes were shown to be a correlate of decubitus ulcer development in 699 nursing homes using the National

Medical Expenditure Survey, although another study was unable to show a relationship between urinary incontinence and decubitus ulcer development in acute hospitalized patients [13]. In contrast, several investigators have identified urinary incontinence as a predictor for decubitus ulcer development in the nursing home population [14–17]. Urinary incontinence may also be a significant risk factor for a community population [18]. The independent contribution of urinary incontinence in predicting decubitus ulcers has not been consistently demonstrated in several studies [19–23]. Urinary incontinence was not found to be a significant predictor in these studies except as a part of the Braden Scale which includes five other subscales (see Chap. 4) [21].

In several studies, fecal incontinence has been studied independently of urinary incontinence. Fecal incontinence was found not significant in cross-sectional and cohort-derived data from nursing homes [20], and conversely found significant in two studies [19, 22]. Fecal incontinence was identified as a significant risk factor along with diabetes mellitus, ambulation difficulty, and difficulty in feeding oneself in nursing homes with a high incidence of decubitus ulcer development [19]. A second study revealed fecal incontinence as a significant risk factor in hospitalized patients with activity limitation (bedridden or chairbound) [22], as did data obtained through five hospital wide audits [23], where the odds of having a decubitus ulcer were 22 times greater for hospitalized patients with fecal incontinence compared to hospitalized patients without fecal incontinence [23]. There are problems with determination of fecal incontinence and with fecal incontinence correlations with other significant risk factor variables, such as immobility, that may limit the ability to assess fecal incontinence as an independent risk factor [24].

Determination of the exact role urinary and fecal incontinence play as predictors for decubitus ulcer development remains unclear. Urinary incontinence, probably in conjunction with fecal incontinence or fecal incontinence alone, may be more appropriate risk factors for decubitus ulcer development than urinary incontinence alone. While the causal relationship between incontinence and decubitus ulceration is muddled, patients with mobility impairment and incontinence seem at higher risk for decubitus ulcer formation and to have delayed healing of existing lesions.

Perineal Dermatitis: Role of Moisture, Urine, and Feces

Pathogenesis of Skin Outcomes

The most common skin damage associated with incontinence is perineal dermatitis. Reviewing the literature demonstrates an obvious void in perineal dermatitis research. Much of our knowledge of the effects of moisture and other irritants on the skin comes from the pediatric literature examining diaper dermatitis. Though the skin of elderly persons with incontinence differs in some significant ways from infants' skin, the information provides a useful base in evaluating skin damage from incontinence. Most of the research that is available focuses on the pathogenesis of the dermatitis [25].

For many years, the popular explanation of diaper dermatitis has been urinary ammonia as a principle etiologic agent. This belief was founded on Cooke's [26] 1921 study which showed an organism that could generate ammonia from urea and demonstrated that the ammonia caused erythema and the subsequent irritation associated with diaper dermatitis. The notion of ammonia as the primary causative factor in the intiation of dermatitis was refuted by the 1970s [27]. Only on skin damaged by scratches sufficient to break the stratum corneum was ammonia able to induce erythema. Ammonia may play a subordinate role in exacerbating already damaged skin, but cannot, alone, induce dermatitis. The possibility of other irritants was raised and research began to focus on other irritant substances in urine and feces.

The combination of urine and the enzymes protease, lipase, and urease in feces increases the pH of the skin making it more alkaline, demonstrated using a hairless mouse animal model [25]. The rise in the pH increases the activity of the fecal proteases and lipases which can damage the skin, promoting irritation and leading to increased microbial growth in the skin. Urine may play a primary role in dermatitis by virtue of contributing water to the diaper environment and continuous exposure to water can have deleterious effects on the skin [28]. Hydration of the skin increases the permeability of the skin and decreases the barrier function of the integumentary system. Most importantly, urine increases both the pH of the skin and the permeability of the skin to irritants [25].

The skin environment least likely to be associated with dermatitis is one in which increases in both the skin wetness and the skin pH are minimized [29]. Increased skin hydration and pH compromises the physical integrity of the epidermis. The epidermis becomes less tolerant of friction, abrasion, chemical and enzymatic irritants, and microbial invasion [28–30].

Skin wetness is proportional to diaper wetness, and increased wetness increases the coefficient of friction, abrasion damage, skin permeability, and microbial growth on the skin [30]. A key factor, then, is the wetness of the skin which initiates the sequence of events responsible for the sequelae of dermatitis [30].

Proteases and lipases in feces have been identified as the primary irritants in feces with bile salts potentiating the damage induced by the action of the fecal enzymes, using the hairless mouse model [31]. The enzymes in feces convert urea into ammonia and increase the skin pH in the perineal area. The rise in pH increases the activity of fecal proteases and lipases which, in turn, irritate the skin directly and make the skin more permeable to other irritants (like bile salts). The entire process is facilitated by the deleterious effect of the water content in urine. These interactions create a skin environment favorable to friction damage, blister formation [30], direct irritation from substances, and microbial colonization. Figure 1 depicts these relationships and the outcomes associated with etiologic factors. While most of the research has been aimed at the pediatric population, perineal dermatitis has been studied in a small sample of gero-pyschiatric in-patients, where results suggest a similar interaction between urine and feces in the incontinent elderly [32].

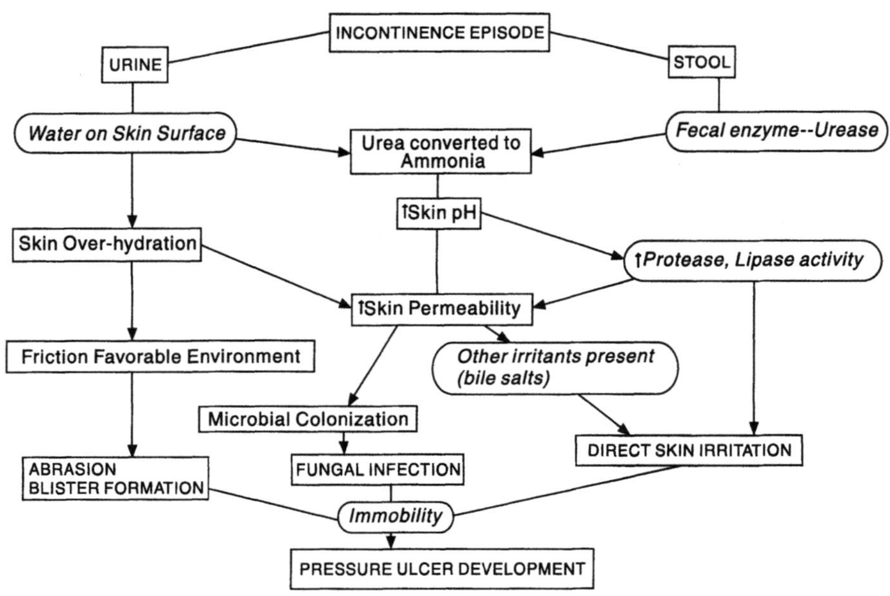

Fig. 1. Model of etiologic factors and outcomes in perineal dermatitis

Perineal Dermatitis: Clinical Presentation

Objective signs, including erythema, swelling, vesiculation, oozing, crusting and scaling, have been used for a conceptual schema for examining perineal dermatitis which includes the concepts of tissue tolerance, perineal environment, and toileting ability [33]. Symptomology includes tingling, itching, burning, and pain. The perineal region is broadly defined as the perineum (area between the vulva or scrotum and anus), buttocks, and perianal, coccyx, and upper/inner thigh regions [34].

The clinical presentation is variable and may be dependent on the frequency of incontinence episode, rapidity and efficacy of post-episode hygiene and duration of incontinence [35].

Skin reactions can be divided into acute reactions and chronic changes. Perineal dermatitis may present with acute episode characteristics or with more long-standing chronic skin changes apparent. In acute eipsodes, the skin characteristics most predominant are erythema, papulovesicular reaction, frank erosions and abrasions and in some cases, evidence of *Candida* infection due to the moist warm environment. In general, a diffuse blanchable erythema is present involving both buttocks, coccyx area, perineum, perianal area, and upper/inner thighs. The extent of the erythema varies and the intensity of the reaction may be muted in immunocompromised and some elderly patients. A papulovesicular eruption is particularly evident in the groin and perineal areas. Secondary skin changes include crusting and scaling, and are usually evident at the fringes of the reaction. Erosions and frank denudation of the skin may be more common with incontinence associated with feces. The distribution of the dermatitis differs between men and women. Typically, the more severe damage in men occurs on the posterior aspect of the penile shaft and the anterior aspect of the scrotum. More damage is seen in the lower perineal regions such as the inner thighs and low buttocks than the higher perineal regions such as the sacral/coccyxgeal area or groin. In women, the skin damage usually involves the vulva and groin areas and spreads distally from those sites.

Chronic skin changes in elderly patients with long-standing incontinence include lichenification where moisture is allowed to maintain skin contact, increased scaling, and the presence of crusting. The thickened appearance resembles the changes seen in peristomal skin of patients with urinary diversions or ileostomy who have pouches with too large an aperture, allowing the urine or fecal effluent to pool around the stoma. This skin is overhydrated and easily abraded with minimal friction. The reaction is notable at the coccyx, scrotum, and vulva. In a cognitively impaired nursing home sample [35], there was also evidence of excoriation from patient's scratching at the affected sites. This provides early clinical validation of the symptom of itching in perineal dermatitis.

In many cases, partial-thickness ulcers are present over the sacral/coccygeal area and medial buttocks region, close to the gluteal fold. Although these lesions may present as typical decubitus ulcers, the underlying etiology may be the effects of incontinence on the skin. There are some characteristics of these partial-thickness ulcers that assist in differentiating them from true pressure-induced skin trauma. First, the lesions tend to be multiple in nature; the ulcers are almost always partial-thickness or stage II lesions; the lesions may or may not be directly over a bony prominence; and finally, the lesions are typically surrounded by other characteristics of perineal dermatitis (eg., diffuse blanchable erythema). When caring for patients who are incontinent of urine and feces, health care providers are faced with the challenge of preventing perineal dermatitis and decubitus ulceration as a result of the decreased tissue tolerance to trauma. True decubitus ulcers result from compression of the soft tissue between the bony prominence and the external surface [44]. When moisture, urine, and feces have caused maceration and overhydration of the epidermis, the skin and tissues are less tolerant of the pressure force. Stage II decubitus ulcers, partial-thickness skin lesions like abrasions, are most commonly attributed to friction and shearing forces [36]. It is likely incontinence plays a critical role in the development of stage II decubitus ulcers.

Prevention of Urinary and Fecal Incontinence

Prevention of incontinence relates to early diagnosis of reversible treatable causes of incontinence. Transient urinary incontinence may be caused by several treatable conditions such as delirium, infection, atrophic vaginitis, restrictions in mobility, fecal impaction, polyuria, and drug side effects [2]. Delirium or acute confusional states may include incontinence as an associated finding that dissipates with treatment of the underlying cause of confusion [2]. Immobility that often accompanies acute illness in the elderly can contribute to urinary incontinence, as can unfamiliar environments (hospitalization, recent transfer to nursing home, or changing rooms within the same facility). Unfamiliar environments exact changes in the schedule of the elderly, impose new routines, and inflict barriers and obstacles such as bed rails or shared toileting facilities to overcome [36]. Prevention of incontinence related to restricted mobility involves use of environmental manipulation. For example, providing urinals or bedpans within easy reach, use of a bedside commode, or scheduled toileting programs may resolve the incontinence [2].

The role of fecal impaction in producing urinary incontinence is not entirely clear. Probably the bolus of stool in the rectum provides mechanical obstruction of the urinary outlet with a resulting overflow-type of incontinence and reflex bladder contractions induced by rectal distension [36]. Fecal impaction is also a transient cause of fecal incontinence, as liquid stool seeps around the fecal bolus. Disimpaction resolves the incontinence [2, 37].

Infection refers to symptomatic urinary tract infection with possible dysuria and urgency. The dysuria and urgency may simply defeat the person's ability to toilet in time to prevent incontinent episodes. The same holds true for polyuria states. The patient may simply be unable to reach the toilet in time to prevent incontinence. Atrophic vaginitis or urethritis may present with some symptoms similar to infection: dysuria, dyspareunia, burning on urination, urgency, and sometimes with urinary incontinence. The treatment is directed towards the restoration of the vaginal and urethral tissues to a state of health. Generally, conjugated estrogen either orally or topically will remedy the situation [2].

Finally, a wide variety of medications can precipitate urinary incontinence in elderly patients. A thorough medication history is essential, and it may be necessary to stop the culprit drug, switch to an alternative or modify the dosage schedule in order to treat the incontinence [2, 37].

Reversible fecal incontinence is commonly caused by fecal impaction, diarrhea states, and enteral feedings. Fecal impaction causes incontinence by providing an obstacle to stool passage with resultant overflow incontinence of watery diarrhea [38] being the most common cause of fecal incontinence, predominating among the elderly and those in extended care facilities [38]. Usually, the patient exhibits continuous leakage of fluid stool [38]. Diagnosis can usually be made by digital rectal examination. Removal of the fecal mass and maintenance of a bowel program contribute to future fecal continence.

Diarrhea states cause fecal incontinence by overwhelming the fecal continence mechanism. Diarrhea states can be caused by a number of factors. Of importance are gastroenteritis and fungal superinfections. Immunocompromised patients are at particular risk for virally or bacterially induced diarrhea. A stool culture should be performed in any patient with diarrhea of unknown origin. Treatment is based on the results of culture and sensitivity tests. Fungal superinfections occur in patients who have undergone aggressive antimicrobial therapy which can destroy the normal flora of the gut and result in diarrhea with incontinence. Use of products with the lactobacillus organism, such as yogurt or buttermilk, may prevent fungal superinfection with resulting diarrhea [38].

Diarrhea states can also be caused by enteral feedings. Enteral feedings are commonly associated with diarrhea and incontinence. Usually the diarrhea and incontinence are attributed to the formula in the feeding; however, the diarrhea is more likely caused by underlying malnutrition [38]. The underlying malnutrition results in edema of the intestinal wall and resultant malabsorption [38]. Interventions to prevent diarrhea from enteral feedings include use of an isotonic formula, institution and advancement of feedings gradually (starting at 50 cc/h), and use of formulas with fiber or bulking agents [38]. Prevention of incontinence is always the ideal; however, there are types of urinary incontinence which are not amenable to prevention and must be dealt with on a more permanent basis.

Management of Incontinence

Management of incontinence is dependent on assessment and diagnosis of the problem. Assessment parameters to be addressed include: history, physical examination, environmental assessment, voiding/defecation diary, laboratory studies, and other diagnostic studies [40]. The history is critical to assess accurately the problem. History taking should elicit information on patterns of urinary/fecal elimination and past/current management program, patterns of incontinence, characteristics of the urinary stream/fecal mass, sensation of bladder/rectal filling, and a focused review of systems and medical-surgical history [2, 40]. The physical examination is designed to gather specific information related to bladder/rectal functioning and thus is limited in scope. A limited neurologic examination should provide data on the mental status and motivation of the patient/care giver, specific motor skills, and back and lower extremities. The genitalia and perineal skin are assessed for signs of estrogenization, pelvic descent, perineal skin lesions and perineal sensation, and bulbocavernosus response in females, and penis/scrotal contents, rectal and prostate, and bulbocavernosus response in males [2, 37, 40].

The environmental assessment should include inspection of the patient's home or nursing home facility to evaluate for the presence of environmental barriers to continence. The voiding/defecation diary is the real tool for management of continence in patients without congnitive impairment. The diary provides baseline data on the problem and so provides a mechanism for determining therapy effectiveness for the future [37]. The diary may provide valuable information for diagnostic purposes. In cognitively impaired patients, the care giver may complete the diary, and management strategies again can be identified from the baseline data.

Laboratory tests help to rule out infections and other pathology responsible for the incontinence. Some specialized studies are helpful in further evaluation of the condition. Urodynamic studies for urinary incontinence provide valuable data related to the pathology. Even in nursing home populations, simple bedside urodynamics can be a useful clinical tool to elicit more specific data on urinary function [37]. Management strategies for incontinence are grouped into three main areas for this discussion: behavioral management, containment strategies, and skin protection guidelines.

Behavioral Management

Patients at risk for decubitus ulcer development are not candidates for all methods of behavioral management. The most successful behavioral management strategies for the frail cognitively impaired patient typically at risk of decubitus ulcer development include prompted voiding and scheduled toileting programs. Both strategies are care giver dependent and require a motivated care giver to be successful. Scheduled intake of fluid is an important underlying factor for both strategies.

Scheduled toileting or habit training is toileting on a planned basis. The goal is to keep the person dry by assisting them to void at regular intervals. There can be attempts to match the interval to the individual patient's natural voiding schedule. There is no systematic effort to motivate patients to delay voiding or to resist the urge to void. Scheduled toileting may be based on the clock (toileting the patient every 2 h) or based on activities (toileting the patient after meals and before transferring to bed). Several studies have demonstrated improvement in continence status in some patients [41, 42].

Prompted voiding has been shown to be effective in dependent and cognitively impaired nursing home incontinent patients [43, 44]. Prompted voiding involves use of a toileting schedule (every 2 h) similar to habit training or scheduled toileting. Prompted voiding supplements the routine with teaching the incontinent patient to discriminate their continence status and to request toileting assistance [2, 43]. The three major elements in prompted voiding include monitoring the incontinent patient routinely, prompting the patient to use the toilet, and praising the patient for maintenance of continence [43]. Prompted voiding results in a 40%–50% reduction in frequency of daytime incontinence and 25%–33% of urinary incontinent patients in nursing homes respond to the therapy [44]. Both of these behavioral management strategies have the added benefit of moving the patient at routine intervals which should relieve pressure over bony prominences and reduce the risk of decubitus ulcer development by allowing reperfusion of the tissues.

Containment Strategies

Underpads and briefs may be used to protect the skin of patients who are incontinent of urine or stool [36]. These products are designed to absorb moisture, wick the wetness away from the skin, and maintain a quick-drying interface with the skin [36]. Studies with both infants and adults demonstrate that products designed to present a quick-drying surface to the skin and to absorb moisture do keep the skin drier and are associated with a lower incidence of dermatitis [30, 36]. It is important to note that the critical feature is the ability to absorb moisture and present a quick-drying surface, and not whether or not the product is disposable or reusable. Regardless of the product chosen, containment strategies imply the need for a check and change schedule for the incontinent patient so wet linens and pads may be removed in a timely manner. Underpads are not as tight or constricting as briefs and may be alternately used [45]. The effects of water on the skin could be reversed and tempered by simply allowing the skin to dry out between wet periods [28]. Use of briefs when the patient is up in a chair, ambulating, or visiting another department, and use of underpads when the patient is in bed is one suggestion for combining the strengths of both products [44].

External collection devices may be more effective with male patients [45]. External catheters or condom catheters (Texas catheters) are devices applied to the shaft of the penis to direct the urine away from the body to a collection device. Newer models of external catheters are self-adhesive and easy to apply. For patients with a retracted penis, a special pouching system, similar to an ostomy pouch, is available – the retracted penis pouch [45]. A key concern with use of external collection devices is routine removal of the product, and inspection and hygiene of the skin.

There are special containment devices for fecal incontinence as well. Fecal incontinence collectors consist of a self-adhesive skin barrier attached to a drainable pouch. Application of the device is somewhat dependent on the skill of the clinician and the patient should be put on a routine for changing the pouch prior to leakage to facilitate success. The skin barrier provides a physical obstacle on the skin to the stool and helps prevent dermatitis and associated skin problems. In fact, skin barrier wafers without an attached pouch can be useful in protecting the skin from feces or urine [44].

Skin Protection

The use of a structured skin care regimen on a small sample of incontinent gero-psychiatric inpatients has not been validated for the efficacy of the treatment in preventing perineal dermatitis. Suggested guidelines for the prevention and prediction of decubitus ulcers in adults [43] recommend use of moisturizers for dry skin and lubricants for reduction in friction injuries. Moisture barriers may protect the skin from the effects of moisture. The success of the particular product is linked to how it is formulated and the hyrophobic properties of the product [44]. Generally, pastes are thicker and more repellent of moisture than ointments. A quick evaluation is the ease with which the product can be removed with water during routine cleansing. If the product comes off the skin with just routine cleansing, it probably is not an effective barrier to moisture. Use of mineral oil for cleansing some of the heavier barrier products, such as zinc oxide paste, will ease the removal from the skin.

Measures to reduce friction are also important in this patient group. Exposing the skin to moisture, urine, and feces makes the skin more vulnerable to friction-induced injury. Use of overhead trapeze bars for those patients who are able to assist with movement and turning sheets used as lifters will facilitate patient repositioning with less friction trauma to the skin. Use of agents, such as cornstarch, to decrease friction, application of transparent film dressings or other protective dressings to the affected area are recommended to decrease skin injury due to friction [43]. Additionally, avoiding the semi-Fowler's position in bed will help decrease patient sliding. The semi-upright position causes friction injury to the epidermis and shearing force to underlying soft tissue as the patient slides down the bed. Use of a foot board and positioning a pillow under the lower legs are measures to help maintain the upright body position in bed.

References

1. McCormick K (1991) From clinical trial to health policy: research on urinary incontinence in the adult, part 1. J Profess Nurs 7:147
2. Urinary Incontinence Guideline Panel (1992) Urinary incontinence in adults: clinical practice guidelines. AHCPR publ no 92-0038. Agency for Health Care Policy and Research, Public Health Service, US Department of Health and Human Services, Rockville
3. Ouslander J, Kane R, Abrass I (1982) Urinary incontinence in a nursing home. JAMA 248:1194–1198
4. Sier H, Ouslander J, Orzeck S (1987) Urinary incontinence among geriatric patients in acute-care hospital. JAMA 257:1767–1771
5. Lavien DH (1992) Sympathetic approach to fecal incontinence in the elderly. Participate 1:3
6. Hu TW (1990) Impact of urinary incontinence on health-care costs. J Am Geriatr Soc 38:292–295
7. Sparks SM (1992) Nurse validation of pressure ulcer risk factors for a nursing diagnosis. Decubitus 5(1):26–35
8. Gosnell DJ (1989) Pressure sore risk assessment: a critique. II. Analysis of risk factors. Decubitus 2:40–43
9. Norton D (1989) Calculating the risk: reflections on the Norton scale. Decubitus 2(3):24–31
10. Braden B, Bergstrom N (1989) Clinical utility of the Braden Scale for predicting pressure sore risk. Decubitus 2:44–51
11. Gosnell DJ (1989) Pressure sore risk assessment: a critique. I. The Gosnell scale. Decubitus 2:32–39
12. Spector WD (1989) Correlates of pressure sores in nursing homes: evidence from the National Medical Expenditure Survey. J Invest Dermatol 102[Suppl]:42S–45S
13. Allman RM, Laprade CA, Noel LB, Walker JM, Moorer CA, Dear MR, Smith CR (1986) Pressure sores among hospitalized patients. Ann Intern Med 105:337–342
14. Pase MN (1994) Pressure relief devices, risk factors, and development of pressure ulcers in elderly patients with limited mobility. Adv Wound Care 7:38–43
15. Ek AC, Boman G (1982) A descriptive study of pressure sores: the prevalence of pressure sores and characteristics of patients. J Adv Nurs 7:51–57
16. Towey AP, Erland SM (1988) Validity and reliability of an assessment tool for pressure ulcer risk. Decubitus 1:40–48
17. Spector WD, Kapp MC, Tucker RJ, Steruberg J (1988) Factors associated with presence of decubitus ulcers at admission to nursing homes. Gerontologist 28:830–834
18. Oot-Girimini BA (1993) Pressure ulcer prevalence, incidence and associated risk factors in the community. Decubitus 6:24–32
19. Brandeis GH, Ooi WL, Hossain M, Morris JN, Lipsitz LA (1994) A longitudinal study of risk factors associated with the formation of pressure ulcers in nursing homes. J Am Geriatr Soc 42:388–393
20. Berlowitz DR, Wilking SV (1989) Risk factors for pressure sores: a comparison of cross-sectional and cohort-derived data. J Am Geriatr Soc 37:1043–1050

21. Bergstrom N, Braden B (1992) A prospective study of pressure sore risk among institutionalized elderly. J Am Geriatr Soc 40:747-758
22. Allman RM, Goode PS, Patrick MM, Burst N, Bartolucci AA (1995) Pressure ulcer risk factors among hospitalized patients with activity limitation. JAMA 273:865-870
23. Maklebust J, Magnan MA (1994) Risk factors associated with having a pressure ulcer: a secondary data analysis. Adv Wound Care 7:25-42
24. Smith DM (1995) Pressure ulcers in the nursing home. Ann Intern Med 123:433-442
25. Berg RW, Buckingham KW, Stewart RL (1986) Etiologic factors in diaper dermatitis: the role of urine. Pediatr Dermatol 3:102-106
26. Cooke JV(1921) The etiology and treatment of ammonia dermatitis of the gluteal region of infants. Am J Dis Child 22:481-492
27. Leyden JJ, Katz S, Stewart R, Kligman AM (1977) Urinary ammonia and ammonia-producing microorganisms in infants with and without diaper dermatitis. Arch Dermatol 113:1678-1680
28. Willis I (1973) The effects of prolonged water exposure on human skin. J Invest Dermatol 60:166-171
29. Berg RW, Milligan MC, Sarbaugh FC (1994) Association of skin wetness and pH with diaper dermatitis. Pediatr Dermatol 11:18-20
30. Zimmerer RE, Lawson KD, Calvert CJ (1986) The effects of wearing diapers on skin. Pediatr Dermatol 3:95-101
31. Buckingham KW, Berg RW (1986) Etiologic factors in diaper dermatitis: the role of feces. Pediatr Dermatol 3:107-112
32. Lyder CH, Clemes-Lowrance C, Davis A, Sullivan L, Zucker A (1992) Structured skin care regimen to prevent perineal dermatitis in the elderly. Nurs 19(1):12-16
33. Brown DS, Sears M (1993) Perineal dermatitis: a conceptual framework. Ostomy/Wound Management 39:20-25
34. Brown DS (1993) Perineal dermatitis: can we measure it? Ostomy/Wound Management 39:28-31
35. Schnelle JF, Adamson G, Cruise PA, AL-Samarrai N, Sarvanjh F, Uman G, Ouslander JG (1996) Skin disorders and moisture in incontinent nursing home residents: intervention implications (in review)
36. Kemp MG (1994) Protecting the skin from moisture and associated irritants. J Gerontol Nurs 20:8-14
37. Kane RL, Ouslander JG, Abrass IB (eds) Essentials of clinical geriatrics, 2nd edn., chap. 6: incontinence. McGraw-Hill Information Services, Newyork, pp 139-190
38. Basch A, Jensen L (1992) Management of fecal incontinence. In: Doughty D (ed) Urinary and fecal incontinence: nursing management. Mosby Year Book, St Louis, pp 235-268
39. Jensen LL (1990) Fecal incontinence. In: Jeter KF, Faller N, Norton C (eds) Nursing for continence. Saunders, Philadelphia, pp 223-240
40. Gray M (1992) Assessment of patients with urinary incontinence. In: Doughty D (ed) Urinary and fecal incontinence: nursing management. Mosby Year Book, St Louis, pp 47-94
41. Schnelle JF, Newman DR, Fogarty T (1990) Management of patient continence in long-term care nursing facilities. Gerontologist 30:373-376
42. Panel for the prediction and prevention of pressure ulcers in adults (1992) Pressure ulcers in adults: prediction and prevention. Clinical practice guideline, no 3. AHCPR publ no 92-0047. Agency for Health care policy and Research, Public Health Service, US Department of Health and Human Services, Rockville
43. Schnelle JF (1990) Treatment of urinary incontinence in nursing home patients by prompted voiding. J Am Geriatr Soc 38:356-360
44. Ouslander JG, Schnelle JF, Uman G, Fingold S, Nigam JG, Tuico E, Bates-Jensen B (1995) Predictors of successful prompted voiding among incontinent nursing home residents. JAMA 273:1366-1370
45. Jeter KF (1990) The use of incontinence products. In: Jeter KF, Faller N, Norton C (eds) Nursing for continence. Saunders, Philadelphia, pp 209-220

Additional Concepts

18 Legal Aspects of Medical Malpractice: Cases Involving Decubitus Ulcers

G.L. Young Jr. and S.A. Larson

Lawsuits are divided into two broad categories, civil and criminal. A civil action is brought to enforce, redress, or protect private rights [1]. Criminal lawsuits, on the other hand, address public rights and public safety.

Criminal cases are further divided into two categories, felonies and misdemeanors. A felony is a crime graver or more serious than a misdemeanor. Many statutes define a felony as any offense punishable by death or imprisonment for a term exceeding 1 year [2]. A misdemeanor is an offense lower than a felony and generally is punishable by fine, penalty, forfeiture, or imprisonment other than in a penitentiary [3].

Medical malpractice lawsuits are generally civil actions based in tort principles. A tort is a private or civil wrong or injury. It involves a violation of a duty imposed by general law or otherwise upon all persons occupying a specific relation to each other. A tort always involves a violation of some duty owing to the plaintiff, and generally that duty must arise by operation of law and not by mere agreement of the parties [4].

Elements of a Medical Malpractice Claim

Medical malpractice claims encompass all liability-producing conduct arising from the rendition of professional medical services [5, 6].

In most states of the United States, the law of medical malpractice is based in tort principles. The elements of a medical malpractice claim require that the patient-plaintiff establish the elements of duty, breach, causation, and damages [5, 6].

The first element requires that the patient-plaintiff establish that the physician-defendant owed a duty or obligation to the patient. The duty of a physician to a patient requires the physician to act in accordance with specific norms or standards established by the medical profession, commonly referred to as "standards of care" [5, 6].

The second element requires that the patient-plaintiff establish that the physician-defendant breached the duty of care owed to the patient. To establish a breach of duty, the plaintiff must show that the physician acted or failed to act in accordance with the standards of care owed to the patient as set forth by the medical community. The standards of the medical community require the physician to exercise such reasonable care, skill, and diligence as other similarly situated health care providers in the same general line of practice ordinarily have and exercise in a like case [7].

Third, the patient-plaintiff must establish that the physician's breach of duty owed to the patient is causally related to the patient's alleged injury [8]. Legal causation is broadly defined and differs from medical causation in that legally plaintiff must only show a reasonable, close causal connection between the physician's conduct and the patient's injuries. The legal cause is not necessarily the most immediate cause.

The fourth and final element of the plaintiff's medical malpractice claim is damages. The plaintiff must establish actual loss or damage has been incurred as a result if the physician's breach of the standard of care [5]. Damages may include physical, financial, or emotional injury. The courts are becoming exceedingly liberal in what constitutes emotional injury.

Damages can be both compensatory and punitive. Compensatory damages are intended to make the patient-plaintiff whole for his injury. Compensatory damages are awarded to recompense the patient for pecuniary loss incurred as a result of the malpractice [9]. Compensatory damages are generally covered by malpractice insurance.

Punitive damages, on the other hand, are intended to punish the health care provider for egregious behavior. In order to recover punitive damages, the plaintiff must establish that the health care provider's conduct was intentional or was done with reckless indifference to the rights of others [10]. Obviously, there can be no insurance coverage for punitive damages. Public policy cannot allow coverage for acts which are intentional or performed with indifference to the rights of others. Allowing coverage for punitive damages would be tantamount to condoning such conduct. Punitive damages are rarely awarded, but are a legitimate concern for physicians.

The plaintiff must establish all four of the above elements (duty, breach, causation, and damages) to present a medical malpractice claim against a physician. The plaintiff must establish each of the elements by a "preponderance of the evidence". A preponderance of the evidence means proof that allows the fact finder to find the existence of a fact at issue is more probable than not [11].

Medical Malpractice Issues Concerning Decubitus Ulcers

Medical malpractice claims alleging negligent treatment by health care providers leading to decubitus ulcers are filed frequently and these lawsuits are on the rise. These claims involve many recurring issues.

In medical malpractice claims involving decubitus ulcers, the patient-plaintiff alleges that no health care provider was monitoring skin integrity or evaluating the risks for developing decubitus ulcers. Once the ulcers develop, the patient-plaintiff alleges that the health care providers failed to properly care for the ulcers.

Documentation becomes extremely important to the plaintiff's position in these cases. The health care provider must document the findings of an examination. This includes the need to document negative findings. Specifically, the health care provider needs to document any areas of skin breakdown noted on examination. It is also important to document that areas without skin breakdown were evaluated and skin was intact. If the negative findings are not documented, the plaintiff will infer at trial that these areas were not assessed on examination.

Treatment plans must also be documented. Initial treatment plans must be noted, as well as an evaluation of the effectiveness of those treatment plans. Specifically, documentation will prove helpful in the medical malpractice claim if it demonstrates that the treatment plan was evaluated at regular intervals for effectiveness and the physician chose to either continue with the current regimen or to change that regimen.

Many institutions maintain practice manuals with policies on the prevention and treatment of decubitus ulcers. If such a policy exists, the plaintiff will review the medical records during the course of litigation to determine if the policy is properly implemented. While documentation does not determine whether patient care was within the standards of care, the institution's adherence to its own policy will affect the jury's opinion of the diligence of medical care in that institution. Accordingly, if a policy exists concerning the prevention or treatment of decubitus ulcers, that policy must be enforced.

Case Illustration 1

A stroke patient was admitted to a nursing home. During his stay at the nursing home he developed decubitus ulcers and ultimately required a below-the-knee amputation. The attending physician and the nursing home were sued. The physician was eventually dismissed and the nursing home settled for $80, 000 in 1994.

The factual background involves a patient post cerebrovascular accident with a history of diabetes and diabetic neuropathy. The patient was paralyzed on admission, unable to speak, and had difficulty swallowing.

On admission, the nursing staff assessed the patient and noted the plaintiff was at increased risk for developing decubitus ulcers secondary to immobilization, decreased circulation, and concerns about his nutritional status. The admitting nurse started a nursing care plan which included assessment of skin integrity to prevent the development of decubitus ulcers.

The nursing home maintained a practice manual with a policy for the prevention of decubitus ulcers and a separate policy for the treatment of decubitus ulcers once they occurred. Each of these policies required extensive documentation by the nursing staff with regular updates. Further, a skin care evaluation sheet was to be placed in the patient's chart so that every 8 h the nursing staff could document that the skin was evaluated. The nursing care plan which documented skin integrity and evaluation of treatment plans was filled out sporadically. The skin care evaluation sheet was never placed in the patient's chart.

The nursing policy also required that the patient be turned every 2 h to avoid further breakdown. The nurses were required by the policy to document the turning every 2 h. This documentation was not done.

In preparing the defense of this case, the attorneys ran into a common problem with nursing home cases. The nurses who cared for this patient no longer worked at that nursing home at the time the lawsuit was filed. Once the former nursing home employees were located, they either could not remember caring for this patient or did not want to get involved in the litigation process. The turnover rate of employees in nursing homes creates difficulty in keeping track of the whereabouts of the nursing staff. Also, when the former nurses were contacted, they had no recollection of the plaintiff. More specifically, the nurses had no recollection of turning the plaintiff or assessing his skin integrity.

The defense, therefore, was forced to rely on the nursing supervisors to testify that the practice of the nurses in that institution was to turn patients at risk for decubitus ulcers at least every 2 h and to regularly assess skin integrity, thus complying with their own policy.

The nursing home appeared negligent simply because they had failed to comply with their own documentation policies. Further, a jury is unlikely to believe the testimony of the nursing supervisor that the policies were complied with generally when the only clear evidence is that the nursing staff did not comply with the documentation portion of the policy.

During the litigation process, it became necessary to understand that the documentation was a weakness in the case and that a jury could likely find that the nursing home was negligent by breaching its own policies. That weakness is handled by a strong causation defense.

To refute the causation element of the plaintiff's case, the defense must show that even if the plaintiff had been turned every 2 h, he would have developed decubitus ulcers anyway. In other words, decubitus ulcers could not be prevented in this patient. The plaintiff had multiple risk factors for developing decubitus ulcers, including decreased circulation due to diabetes and stroke, immobility, and poor nutrition.

Expert testimony was also used to establish that the plaintiff's decubitus ulcers would have developed regardless of the turning schedule. The expert wrote that a 2-h turning schedule is arbitrary and has no relation to the needs of individual patients. The expert opined that each patient's skin integrity is different. Some patients would need to be turned every 10 min and others could be turned every 10 h to prevent decubitus ulcers.

The medical profession has established this arbitrary norm of turning immobile patients every 2 h. That norm is currently the standard of care and is implemented in the policies of most institutions. This rule hurts the medical profession in the context of medical malpractice litigation. By establishing such a norm, the message is conveyed to plaintiffs and juries alike that all decubitus ulcers will be prevented with a 2-h turning schedule.

Documentation in nursing homes is often duplicative. Certainly that was the situation in the case illustrated here. If the nurses complied with the extensive documentation required by the policy, there would be no time to implement patient care. The lesson here is that policies should be purposeful to make documentation efficient and to promote effective patient care procedures.

Case Illustration 2

An 88-year-old, terminally ill man's family sued the nursing home where he stayed before his death. The family alleged that inadequate care contributed to his death. The jury awarded $2.7 million [12].

The family alleged that the nursing home violated his rights to proper hygiene, nutrition, and medical care. The nursing home failed to provide a proper bed and mattress to prevent decubitus ulcers and allowed him to lie in his own body waste.

The defense argued that this man arrived at the nursing home in poor health with advanced Alzheimer's disease and cancer.

The jury was outraged when shown a picture of the plaintiff's condition and awarded $719, 000 in compensatory damages and $2 million in punitive damages.

Trends

American juries are awarding higher and higher damage awards in cases involving the elderly. Sympathy in our society for the elderly is growing.

Increasing government regulation of nursing homes also adds to increasing jury awards in cases involving older patients. The "typical" nursing home patient is elderly and at risk for developing decubitus ulcers for a variety of reasons.

The United States government now maintains over 100 regulations that a nursing home must comply with in order to qualify for Medicare/Medicaid funding [12]. Medicare and Medicaid are government-funded insurance agencies for the elderly and impoverished. Nursing homes rely heavily on those funds and so must comply with the government regulations in order to participate.

The government regulations in turn make the plaintiff's case easier to prove because plaintiffs can now get a hold of these statistics to establish the overall negligence of a nursing home.

Conclusions

Medical malpractice lawsuits involving the development of decubitus ulcers are on the rise in the United States. Plaintiffs in medical malpractice actions must prove that the physician owed a duty to that plaintiff, that the physician breached that duty, that the breach caused injury to the plaintiff, and that the plaintiff suffered damages.

These requirements of plaintiffs are easily met in medical malpractice cases involving the elderly, including decubitus ulcer cases. Jurors are instructed not to let sympathy enter their deliberations. However, it becomes increasingly difficult for people to set aside their emotions as sympathy for the elderly grows in our society. Often, these sympathies lead to extremely high verdicts against physicians and other health care providers.

The main defense against decubitus ulcer lawsuits is documentation. Positive as well as negative findings must be documented in patients' charts. Skin care must be assessed and reassessed on a regular basis.

Finally, health care providers must set attainable standards and goals for themselves. The amount of documentation required by an institution must be carefully assessed to avoid unnecessary duplication and to prevent time lost from patient care. Each institution must comply with its own policies and procedures.

References

1. Gilliken V. Gilliken (1990) 248 NC 710, 104 SE 2d 861, 863. In: Black's law dictionary, 6th edn. West Publishing Co., St. Paul, MN
2. Black's law dictionary, 6th edn (1990) West Publishing Co., St. Paul, MN (1990) (See also Model Penal Code Sect. 1.04 (2) and Sect. 6.01; 18 U.S.C.A. Sect. 1 and Sect. 3559)
3. Black's law dictionary, 6th edn. West Publishing Co., St. Paul, MN (1990) (See also 18 U.S.C.A. Sect. 1, Sect. 19, and Sect. 3401)
4. Coleman v. Yearly Meeting of Friends Church (1990) 27 Cal. App. 2d 579, 81 P.2d 469, 470. In: Black's law dictionary, 6th edn. West Publishing Co., St. Paul, MN
5. Hamil v. Bashline (1978) 481 Pa 256, 392 A. 2d 1280
6. Schroeder v. Perkel (1981) 87 NJ 53, 432 A. 2d 834
7. Parker v. Collins (1992) 605 So. 2d 824 (Ala 1992); See Shelton v. United States 804 F. Suppl. 1147 (E.D. Mo. 1992)
8. Parris v. Uni Med, Inc. (1993) 861 SW2d 694 (Mo. Ct. App. 1993)
9. Pa. Standard Civil Jury Instructions (1978) Sect. 601
10. Smith v. Brown (1980) 283 Pa. Super. 116, 423 A.2d 743; See Claiborne and Hughes Convalescent Center v. State Dept of Health 881 S.W. 2d 671 (Tenn. App. 1994); See also Montgomery Health Care Facility, Inc. v. Ballard 565 So. 221 (Ala. 1990)
11. Braud v. Kinchen (1990) La.App., 310 So. 2d 657, 659. In: Black's law dictionary, 6th edn. West Publishing Co., St. Paul, MN
12. Felsenthal E (1995) In: Wall Street Journal, September 5

19 Can Do, Ought To? Decision: Is It Truly Dilemma?

E.C. Bradley

I have chosen a title for this chapter which I expect will evoke strong disagreement. It suggests that many situations presenting for our decision are not ethical dilemmas at all but rather perplexing problems charged with economic, social, and extended therapeutic considerations. Much of this situational complexity can be attributed to the increased longevity of the human species, its own ability to enhance and prolong its biologic existence through its probing to discover and utilize technologic advances, and the economics of supply and variable demand. The conceptual development of this chapter dealing with ethical considerations in the care of patients with decubitus ulcers may erroneously suggest an absolutism in which all decision must conform to the set-forth objective principles in order to achieve any moral righteousness. There is no intent to command the individual conscience. I cannot, and any effort to do so would itself render this undertaking unethical. Yet, I do not endorse subjectivism. Furthermore, there is some more fundamental guidance than autonomy, paternalism, beneficence on which these qualities of human conduct are based. The nature of the human person is that fundamental. That is a simple enough statement. To be sure, complexity arises and shadows our vision of the person when we are prompted to ask: when does life begin; when does it end; is there an essential difference between biologic life and human existence; what and who determines the acceptable equality of life; what are the fundamental rights of a person; when can they and when must they be exercised; and what is the dutiful relationship to others? Perhaps I can rally some allies in believing that there are few moral dilemmas. All would agree there are many difficult decisions in caring for a patient and discerning the better good is becoming more demanding in our world of high-tech, misdirected economic values, and legal pseudo-solutions.

As a physician for over 40 years and having only recently become an ordained priest, I am viewed by many as having some suddenly infused insight into ethical problems within our medical profession. I have opinions and reflections on experiences gained through the journey of my own professional life and as a member of Ethics Committees of several hospitals. If anyone believes I labor with pre-formed judgments and lack a certain open-mindedness, I can only acknowledge they are correct and immediately point out their luxury, which few can enjoy, i.e., of being right and wrong at the same time. Concerning principles for conduct, I am not open-minded. Does anyone form a judgment without pre-apprehension? Needless to say, in the application of principle to the particular, all circumstances must be assessed and decisions made without sacrificing principle, otherwise a situational ethic dominates. Obviously, dialogue is often extremely important to the process, and participants must be careful listeners and caring contributors. Many physicians seek such dialogue with their peers, with nurses and paramedical personnel and appropriately with patient and family members.

Custom Versus Ethic

We know in some fashion there is distinction between custom and ethic. Custom applies to practices, indifferent to appraisal as right or wrong. Examples are table manners and modes of dress. They arise from the sophistication of a society, technologic advance, and are most often subject to change. Ethic, however, refers to a more fundamental aspect of human conduct arising from man's understanding of his own value, that of other beings, and the environment of life. Being honest, telling the truth, and acting justly are but a few examples. Moreover, these fundamental objectives in human judgment, volition, and action are obviously relational and therefore already imply the necessity of considering rights, duty, freedom, and responsibility. The judgments we make and the actions we pursue are subject to the information we seek and acquire together with the feasibility, overall purpose, anticipated and potential consequences, and the risks and freedom to act. Our conduct is, therefore, the object of our scrutiny, hopefully fewer times as hindsight, and more often and with greater refinement as antecedent. Ethics, then, acknowledges a right and a wrong in human conduct and basically asks what I or we ought to do, and what I or we should not do. Ethics is reasoned morality and although relational, the moralness is not relative to individual whim or majority consensus. There is objective truth. The challenge is to discover it and apply it to the circumstances of our existence. Often the statement is heard at the outset of groups discussion in matters of ethics: "There is no right or wrong answer." The intention, of course, is to encourage attendants to become participants, but already discussion is doomed to the frustration of relativism and/or the capture by legal code. Either creates dilemma. There is a right and there is a wrong in human conduct. If we acknowledge that truth and also that we, individually as well as collectively, can formulate a distinction between right and wrong, we need to discover why we make such distinction and how consistent we are in the judgments we make.

Circumstances contribute to and modify our decisions but we must be wary of the subtleness with which circumstance can lure us into compromising the very foundation of our moral conduct.

"Good" Defined

It would be foolish to believe anyone of us seeks other than the "good." In the Nicomachean Ethics, Aristotle [1] explains that, whenever a being seeks, it seeks only good, a good that satisfies an appetite, a good which fulfills its function, a good which perfects, completes, which is proper to the being whether or not the good is delectable and/or useful. Furthermore, this onto-logic good is not arbitrary, depending on my or someone's choosing it to be so. This good is coterminus with "being" and we are to be careful not to mistakenly identify the good primarily with that which appeals or is concluded to be useful. It is not rational to ignore the perfective good and attend the pleasurable and/or the useful since the latter will be such to some individuals and not to others, and will change in its apparency with time and circumstance.

Begging that simplicity not be construed as insult, it must be evident to everyone that there is a difference between acts of the human and human acts. This distinction is essential to our discussion of any aspect of ethics. Only human acts involve deliberation and volition, assent and consent. The human species is able to choose with its ability to abstract. We are able to compare experiences of the past with those of the present, examine the differences in each presentation, abstract the commonality, the universal, and formulate conclusions and project courses of action. The human species is able to abstract from the accidentals to the essence of an object. The human species is not bound by the enticement of circumstance. Risking brevity so as to avoid unnecessarily prolonged pressure on the fundamental philosophic seat for all ethical discussion, let me conclude this paragraph by merely stating the human species is able to abstract to what is the proper, the befitting, the perfective, the intrinsic good.

Every being is good but all beings are not good for everything. Man is good! Why? What gives man his goodness? Certainly man's choices are arbitrary and man can make erroneous judgments and conduct himself unfittingly and therefore immorally. The moral good is a necessity arising from the nature of man's being.

In ethics, we focus on human acts which are the product of intellectual deliberation, acquiescence, assent and volition, consent. Even in the act of considering this process itself, we are reflecting on the immediate undertaking as we formulate ideas, relate them to other ideas, provide structure for con-clusion and even presentation to other intelligent beings. And the dynamic goes on with acceptance of some ideas, rebuttal of others, clarification, and additions. All this aims at perceiving the "common thread" devoid of the variation induced by the accidentals, the "data of sense," and finally coming to conclude: this is what I ought to do; this is what I must not do.

The human has dominion over his activity, the ability to reflect on his activity and even upon himself. The human must have responsibility therefore for his activity. Since this humanness is the essential of all others of his kind, man stands in a relationship of equality with other humans. The distinctions of age or sex, or race or beliefs, or state of health, or intellectual ability, or career or social rank do not alter this essential equality. This common essence, the communion of nature, provides the foundation of social relationship and re-sponsibility toward the common good as well as the individual good. We each have a role to play and we, each, must be free to direct our minds to truth and our wills to goodness. This integrity of conscience is a right which no other person, or group of persons can violate or make effort to coerce or possess in any way. Reasoned morality dictates this integrity of conscience must not be warred against directly or indirectly by any individual or society. Indirect coercion, perhaps, is exemplified by the illogical concluding mandate of Pennsylvania Law regarding the care of the terminally ill [2].[1]

Human society is constituted by persons of unique dignity, irreplaceable, and not merely by a summation of individual members whose identity merely allows for statistical analysis relative to economic needs, food supply, disease control, or any other undertaking where the person is but a contribution to the analysis and projected policy. The person has rights founded in the very nature of his being. The fright to life is fundamental and from it arises the right to health. No other person(s) gives that right. It is self-possessed as inviolable. Such a right carries with it a duty or obligation to preserve his health. There is a duty to exercise the right through the ordinary or natural means of fulfillment. There is the obligation for others to recognize the person's right and not to interfere with the exercise of that right. To acknowledge the right but intentionally frustrate the person's exercise of it would be morally wrong since there would be a denial of the community of nature and segregate one or more individuals to unequal status. There is also, again arising from the common essence, a responsibility on the part of the person to the society, its health, its well-being, its existence, its vital functions. Such union can easily be understood as a moral bond and since the whole cannot be greater than the sum of its parts, the society of man exists as a moral union of persons with rights and duties toward themselves, others, and the common good.

Personal Rights

Earlier it was stated that the person has the right to health, to promote his well-being. Moreover, it is a duty that he do so. The question should be asked: how absolute is that duty? Is it an obligation for the person to pursue the impossible; to seek the cure at all costs; to direct all efforts at one aspect of his unwellness which aspect is an incidental concomitant, albeit an important one; to jeopardize the financial stability of his family; to undertake some venture which would likely render a long-lasting burden for others? Clearly, there are many instances when a person may elect to avoid the disproportionate effort and select more appropriate means and even avoid treatment altogether when the outcome is reasonably judged to be unalterable. These are judgments concerning obligation and arise from personal right and duty to oneself and to society. The person has a duty to preserve his well-being and has the right to avoid measures he judges inappropriate, unnatural, or extraordinary. The

---

[1]"If an attending physician or other health care provider cannot in good conscience comply with a declaration . . . the attending physician or health care provider shall make every reasonable effort to assist in the transfer of the declarant to another physician or health care provider *who will comply with the declaration*" 1992 Apr 16, P.L. 108, No.24 S 5408.

definition of such qualifications must not be left to ignorance but presumes understanding of these possible measures and this may, indeed, necessitate the informed advice by many others of varying disciplines and relationships. Care, however, must be exercised so as to not coerce.

This coming-together to assist the decision maker is a demonstration of the social nature of man but this immediate need does not constitute a society. Society has a permanence and is a moral union with rights similar to and because of its members. It must take steps to achieve its goal through a diversity of socially responsible functions. As there are bound to be differences of opinion as well as changing horizons in the pursuit of the common good, it is inevitably necessary to establish an authority who directs the measures pursuant of the common good. It is important to note that society exists for its members and not the reverse. Yet, the needs of the common social good can place limitations on the exercise of a person's right. There is no need to distinguish acquired or privileged rights from natural rights for we are addressing the person's right to life and well-being, and society's obligation to not only respect those rights but to actively protect and enhance the exercise of them.

Since the person has an obligation to exercise his natural right to life and well-being through ordinary means, the conscious and deliberate failure to do so would be to avoid the good. This is not "what a person ought to do." The ordinary means are those which are readily available and usable, and offer a reasonable hope for success. The person also has a right to extraordinary means but the exercise of that right is conditional and does not carry the weight of intrinsic obligation. I say intrinsic to distinguish possible circumstances which may suggest obligation to the elector. For instance, the deliberating person may judge, appropriately, his position of singular responsibility to a needy group. On the other hand, pursuit of extraordinary means may be morally unjustifiable when such election involves enormous expense to responsible agents, be that family or society.

Role of Society

Society is obligated to protect the freedom of conscience of persons in their choosing to exercise their fundamental rights. Society, in its governance, is naturally obligated to make every reasonable effort to assure equal opportunity for each person to fulfill the intrinsic obligations accruing from fundamental rights. Society also has its own fundamental right to life and well-being and the obligation to use the ordinary means to preserve and enhance its realization of those rights. Its life and well-being are inseparably bound to the rights of persons and the common good. Through its authority, a corollary to its existence, society also has the obligation to encourage, facilitate, man's quest for the greater good, for advancing the proven extraordinary to the ordinary status. History testifies to the ever-present ordinary in the extraordinary and discovery of it merely awaits the ingenuity of the rational species and the distribution of that discovery to his justice in the market place. Society, then, has both an immediate obligation as well as a remote one toward the common good. The remote is dependent on the immediate in that, if the immediate is not well executed, the remote will not come to fulfillment because society has become less vital. The immediate obligation must be exercised carefully and caringly in order to preserve life and well-being. The ordinary way of doing that is through the recognition of rights and the properties of rights. Limitation in the exercise of a right is the restriction to certain boundaries and these are mainly determined by the extent of obligations. Since society has the immediate obligation to preserve the common good, since the person has the obligation to preserve his life through ordinary means, since society exists for its members, that society has a right to ration the use of extraordinary means. Indeed, the exercise of that right becomes obligatory when common good is threatened. The appropriateness, the moral rectitude, in effecting such limitation on the exercise of a person's right, heralds justice and the identification for swift condemnation, any political, social, or economic preferences or exclusions. Are humans capable of such behavior? History and psychology might say, "No!" Yet, as we speak not of behavior, but of conduct and its morality, we also maintain the hope that the human will continue to search for what ought to be done and avoid what should not be done. Although subject to errors and to judgments clouded by ignorance and to choices shrouded in self-centeredness and insecurity, the nature of the person will allow him to reflect on his dignity and make the necessary and appropriate corrections for his journey.

Before commencing with the second portion of this chapter, the practical application of the first relative to the patient with decubitus ulcer(s), more properly termed pressure ulcer, let me briefly note some important relationships. As a physician, I am in a covenant relationship with my patient. The possessive pronoun is a purposeful expression not of dominance but rather of trust and respect. This quality in relationship must exist and must grow as the process of recognized need and effort to restore health unfolds. This quality is mutually necessary. As a physician, I am also in a relationship with other members of my profession, the patient's family, and society. That relationship is basically one of responsibility, varying in specifics, but it is not one of covenant.

Prevention and Management

Decubitus ulcers are existent in an enormous number of patients. Estimates vary from 1.5 to 3.0 million [3]. Probably this figure would be significantly increased if account could be made of those living in private circumstances. The costs of conservative therapies and more aggressive treatment approach $5 billion annually [3]. Although immobilization and nutritional status are major contributors in the development of decubitus ulcers, the aging process probably contributes to the incidence with the changes in vascular supply to skin, loss of elastic fibers, and other natural alterations. The pathogenesis and treatment are covered elsewhere in this text and attention will be primarily given to the moral issues in caring for the patient who has or who is likely to have a decubitus ulcer.

Because there are known predisposing factors to such ulceration, the first moral "ought" is to identify the patient at risk and to perform, or have performed, the prophylactic measures. The ethical obligation would direct a careful assessment of the patient as to their general health, their nutritional status, mental responsiveness, mobility, bowel and bladder function, as well as the specifics of treatment programs in certain circumstances, e.g., fracture management and spinal injuries. To avoid, if possible, the development of a decubitus ulcer is a greater good than to experience the benefit of treating one. The Norton scale [4] and the strategies outlined in the recent United States Department of Health and Human Services publication [5] provide useful information. Apart from the efficacy of directing and educating those personnel who will provide the treatment measures, there is the moral obligation to do so, that the patient best be served. To inform the patient and/or responsible family member(s) or surrogate is in keeping with the right to know and the covenant relationship which exists between physician and patient. The prevention of ulceration in, as well as the treatment of the patient who has developed this etiologically multifactorial complication often involves the use of means which are of limited availability, extremely expensive, and of variable success. I refer to air-fluidized beds, inflated mattresses, and other devices used to reduce the pressure over bony prominences. Again, the decision to use such means should be based not only on scientifically recognized benefits and limitations but also on the likelihood of their promoting the overall well-being of the specific patient. How long should they be used for efficacy? Does this patient have a very limited life expectancy? Systemically, is the patient stable? Is the patient's prognosis good? Hopefully, the reader will note the emphasis is on the patient, not on the ulcer. Obviously, the patient is more than the object of the doctor's scientific pursuit and truly in partnership with the physician in the quest for well-being. As the person of primary concern, the patient has the right to know the nature of proposed interventions and as a person with the right to self-appraisal and self-determination, the patient is free to accept or reject other than the conventional therapy. What was said of special instruments can be said of films, foams, and other wound-care products. Likewise, surgical interventions to provide tissue cushions over bony prominences must be included in this garden-of-means subject to moral reasoning on the part of patient and physician. Neither participant may demand, coerce, or deceive the other in the decision process. Must conventional therapy be used and accepted? Considering the serious complications of decubitus ulcers if left unattended and the contrasting simplicity of conventional therapies, such as relief from pressure through regular repositioning and ambulation, removal of necrotic tissue, and proper cleansing and aeration, one could reasonably conclude that conventional therapy must be accepted and implemented. Yet it also must be obvious that the ethics of an action can only be predicated of its possibility. No one can be obliged to the impossible. Scarcity of personnel, demands of acute problems with other patients, the physical state of the patient with the decubitus ulcer may render needed scheduled body repositioning virtually impossible. The extent of surgical debridement needed to promote wound healing may not be within the tolerable limits for a specific patient.

Finally, the disproportionate efforts of therapies directed at an ulcer when the patient has little or no time to enjoy the healing is a misdirected expenditure of time, personnel, and money. The simplicity of conventional therapies is itself a quality necessitating judgment. Simply put, can it or any portion of it be carried out? If the next question is whether it ought to be done, attention must be focused on the patient as a whole, not in isolation but as a contributing and responsible member of society.

Resource Allocation

It would be a welcomed circumstance if all proven treatment modalities were available for use in appropriately selected patients. This is not the case and probably never will be. There is a natural rationing, if I may call it that. Yet if rationing is fundamentally because of the economic limitations of the patient, such prohibition of professionally judged needed therapy is immoral. That economic limitation may be with the patient's own inability to pay, the insurance agency's policies, or society's refusal to address the need. There is ample reason to cite society for immorality in governance and appropriation when its expenditures are directed toward special interest groups and undertakings of questionable value in promoting the common good. It is not a question of idealism versus realism. It is the fact that we ought to be moral and should not be immoral. As long as we, individually and as a society, sincerely try to be, we will conduct ourselves ethically. Difficulties present for decision making and the practical implementation of those decisions is often impeded and to varying degrees, but let us not confuse the ultimate effort at decision with dilemma. If the intention and deliberation of means-to-be-used are consonant with the end, namely, the good of the patient, then certainly the choice to be made will not be between equally unfavourable alternatives. If one were to retort: "But how does anyone decide what that good is?", there is perhaps an unsettling answer: "You must look to yourself, devoid of accident and circumstantial distinction and see the other's uniqueness to be that of your own." The additional response to such a question is: "It's not *anyone* who must decide. It is *you*."

References

1. Aristotle (1925) Nicomachean ethics, book I, Chap 1, 1094a; translated by WD Ross. Oxford. The Clarendon Press
2. Commonwealth of Pennsylvania, Advanced directive for health care Act April 16,1992, Chap. 54, Sect. 5409a
3. Cowart V (1987) Pressure ulcers preventable, say many clinicians. JAMA 257:589–593
4. Norton D (1989) Calculating the risk: reflections on the Norton scale decubitus 2:24–31
5. US Department of Health and Human Services (1992) Pressure ulcers in adults: prediction and prevention. Clinical practice guideline no 3. Rockville

20 Decubitus Ulcers in Animals

S.F. Swaim, R.R. Hanson Jr., and J.R. Coates

Decubitus ulcers are a major health care problem in the United States. They are also a problem for veterinarians in both small pet animals (dogs) [1–6] and large animals (horses). As with humans, prevention is a major part of dealing with decubitus ulcers; however, once they develop, treatment becomes necessary just as with humans.

Naturally Occurring Decubitus Ulcers in Small Animals

Certain breeds of dogs are predisposed to decubitus ulcers because of a neurologic condition associated with the breed. The dachshund and Pekingese, for example, have chondrodystrophic degeneration of the intervertebral discs [7]. Intervertebral disc herniation in these breeds can result in paraplegia and occasionally tetraplegia. During neurologic recovery, these dogs are subject to decubitus ulcer formation. Another breed-associated neurologic condition that can result in decubitus ulcers secondary to temporary tetraplegia that may follow surgical intervention is the cervical vertebral instability/malformation syndrome seen in Doberman pinschers, Great Danes, and other large or giant breed dogs. These are two common examples of breed-associated neurologic conditions that can result in decubitus ulcers. As with humans, any neurologic condition that results in paraplegia or tetraplegia can predispose to decubitus ulcers.

Decubitus ulcers may also result from damage to peripheral nerves. Trauma to a forelimb with damage to the ulnar nerve that causes motor nerve deficit in the forelimb flexor muscles is an example. The abnormal weight distribution on the paw resulting from this deficit may lead to an ulcer at the proximolateral aspect of the metacarpal paw pad [8, 9].

Decubitus ulcers are also associated with orthopedic abnormalities in dogs [4–6]. Of course, the orthopedic–neurologic pathology caused by spinal trauma may have decubitus ulceration as a secondary factor to the paraplegia or tetraplegia associated with the condition. Animals immobilized from multiple long bone and/or pelvic fractures are also subject to decubitus ulcers. Related to orthopedic conditions causing dermal decubitus ulcers are the decubitus ulcers that develop over bony prominences as the result of an improperly applied or padded coaptation cast or splint [1, 5, 10, 11]. These lesions usually result from light pressure over a prolonged period [1]. Again, comparatively, orthopedic conditions common to humans and small pet animals can predispose to dermal pressure lesions.

As in humans, debilitated animals and those convalescing from severe injuries or illnesses that are unable or unwilling to change body positions are subject to decubitus ulcer development. Predisposing factors to decubitus ulcers include: (a) lessening of padding between skin and bone that results from disease, atrophy, or loss of adipose tissue; (b) loss of tissue elasticity; (c) malnutrition (hypoproteinemia, anemia, vitamin deficiencies); (d) skin maceration; (e) soft tissue contusion; (f) skin chafing; (g) skin friction and stretching; (h) skin irritation from urine and feces; (i) skin burns and scalds; and (j) improper nursing care [3–6].

Greyhound dogs have a very angular conformation, short hair, and thin skin. Thus, they are quite subject to development of decubitus ulcers especially when they become debilitated [4, 12, 13].

Another condition that can result in a dermal decubitus ulcer is elbow hygroma. The hygroma is a fluid-filled cavity surrounded by a dense wall of fibrous tissue (Fig. 1). Hygromas are seen in young large or giant breeds of dogs (e.g., German shepherds, Great Danes, bull mastiffs, and Irish wolfhounds) secondary to repeated pressure or trauma over the olecranon [14, 15]. The condition is often seen in large or giant breeds of dog that tend to lie in sternal recumbency on unpadded surfaces, thus placing pressure on skin over

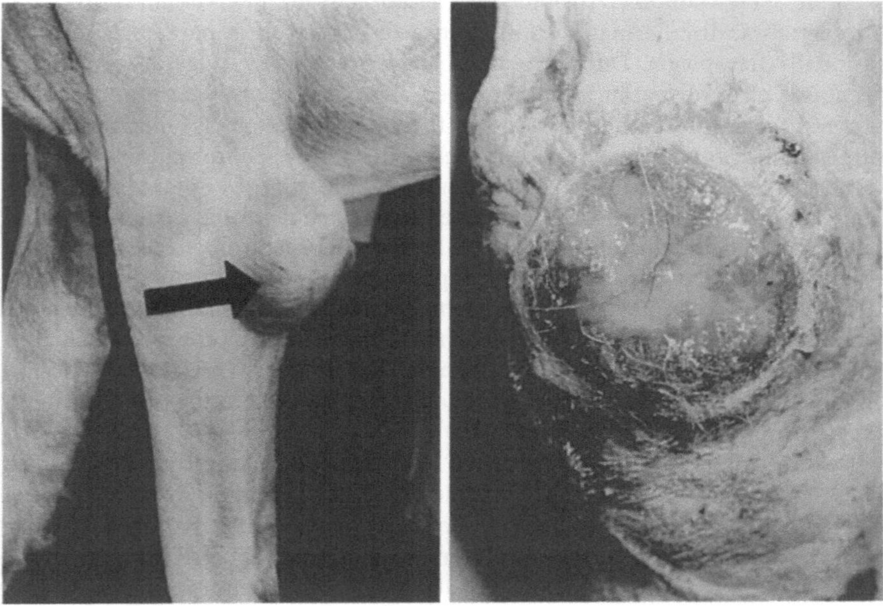

Fig. 1. Elbow hygroma (*arrow*) over the olecranon of a bull mastiff dog

Fig. 2. Chronic elbow ulcer following wound dehiscence after surgical excision of an elbow hygroma on a Irish wolfhound (From [14] with permission)

the olecranons. Large dogs in hot weather may be more prone to elbow pressure lesions as they seek to lie in the shade on hard cool surfaces, i.e., concrete patios. After surgical excision of an elbow hygroma, wound dehiscence may result in a chronic nonhealing ulcer as the animal continues to lie in sternal recumbency and place pressure over the surgical site [14] (Fig. 2). Hygromas may become infected and form abscesses that rupture, with the result being a chronic open wound or ulcer over the olecranon.

Hip dysplasia may also predispose to elbow hygroma and elbow lesions in large dogs. The pain associated with the condition may render the dog less able to protect the elbow from traumatization when attempting to lie down [5]. In other words, as the dog attempts to lie down in sternal recumbency, the pain in the coxo-femoral joint becomes so great that the dog drops on the olecranons rather than easing onto them. This traumatizes the skin and may be the beginning of elbow hygroma and possible ulceration problems.

Location and Pathogenesis of Dermal Pressure Lesions

As in humans, decubitus ulcers in dogs develop over bony prominences [5] (Fig. 3). Most of the decubitus ulcer sites are on the lateral aspect of the dog because recumbent dogs usually are in lateral recumbency. Owing to their greater weight, decubitus ulcers are more of a problem in large dogs, especially over the greater trochanter (Fig. 4), whereas smaller paraplegic dogs that tend to sit up on their perineal region for long periods tend to develop decubitus ulcers over the ischial tuberosities [3] (Fig. 5).

In dogs, as in humans, the primary pathologic change of decubitus ulcers is tissue ischemia with its resultant necrosis as soft tissues are compressed between a bony prominence and the surface on which the animal is resting. With improperly applied casts or bandages, the cast or splint material causes the compression.

Pressure on the soft tissues associated with a developing decubitus ulcer causes focal intravascular changes which result in vascular occlusion and tissue

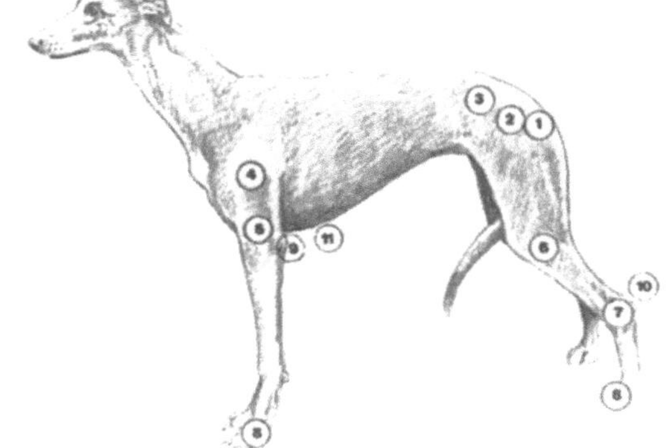

Fig. 3. Areas over bony prominences that are prone to decubitus ulcers. *1,* Ischiatic tuberosity; *2,* greater trochanter; *3,* tuber coxae; *4,* acromion of scapula; *5,* lateral epicondyle of humerus; *6,* lateral condyle of tibia; *7,* lateral malleolus; *8,* sides of fifth digit; *9,* olecranon; *10,* calcaneal tuber; *11,* sternum. (From [5] with permission)

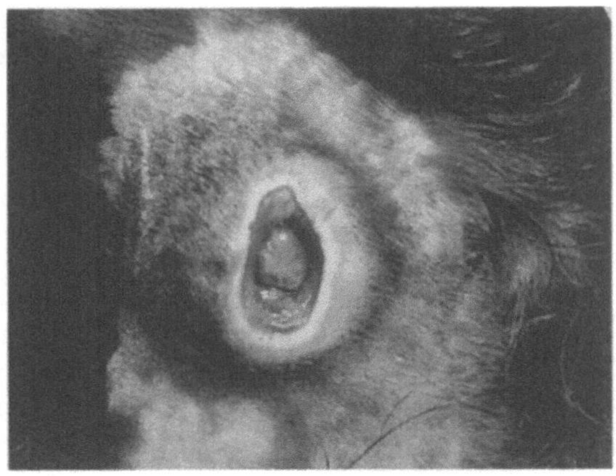

Fig. 4. Decubitus ulcer over the greater trochanter of an Irish setter. (From [45] with permission)

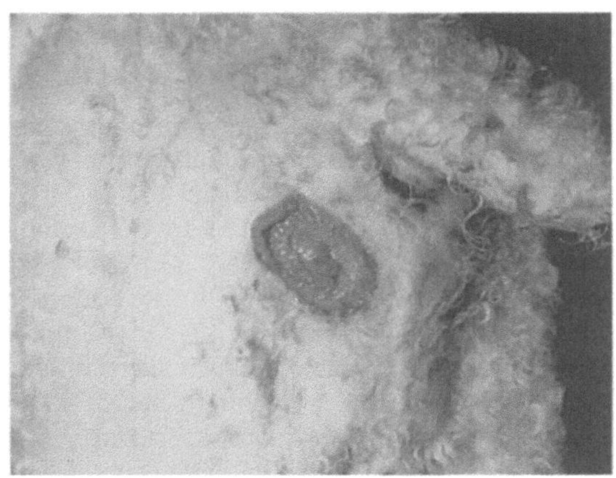

Fig. 5. Decubitus ulcer over the ischial tuberosity of a toy poodle. (From [45] with permission)

ischemia. The degree and severity of ulceration varies with the extent of vascular occlusion [16]. Biochemical changes take place within the ischemic skin and contribute to necrosis. It has been theorized that damage to the compressed skin also occurs during reperfusion with reoxygenation of ischemic tissue after pressure is released. The endothelium of vessels is damaged by oxygen free radicals that form [17].

Thromboxane B_2, a measurable stable metabolite of thromboxane A_2, has been identified in tissues of naturally occurring decubitus ulcers and impending decubitus ulcers in greyhound dogs [12]. In addition, in greyhound dogs, this pathobiochemical has also been identified in early dermal pressure lesions induced over bony prominences by application of coaptation casts with only stockinette lining and no padding [13, 18]. Thromboxane A_2 contributes to the already present dermal ischemia and causes vasoconstriction and intravascular platelet aggregation which leads to vascular thrombosis and thus restricted vascular flow to the tissues as progressive dermal ischemia develops

[18]. Research indicates this as a factor in pathogenesis since the systemic administration of a thromboxane antagonist (a thromboxane synthetase inhibitor) in a greyhound dog model for dermal pressure lesions resulted in lower thromboxane tissue levels, fewer physical dermal abnormalities, and fewer severe histopathologic changes in the pressure-exposed skin of treated dogs than of untreated dogs [18, 19].

Preventive Measures

As with humans, the goal in animals is prevention of decubitus ulcers, and numerous measures are available for this. Some methods are the same as in humans, but others are modifications of techniques used with people. Still other techniques are unique to veterinary medicine due to the nature of the patient.

Padding. Padded bedding is a primary means of preventing decubitus ulcers. Blankets, coated or closed-cell foam pads, air mattresses, water mattresses, sheepskin pads, or artificial fleece pads have been described for providing a padded surface [1–7]. Sheepskin pads and foam rubber mattresses help provide some air circulation under the animal and help wick moisture (i.e., urine) away from the skin. Placing these on grates or racks also helps separate the animal from urine and feces [1, 3, 7]. Foam rubber with a convoluted, "egg-crate" design has been found to provide a good bedding surface. In evaluation of dogs with severe paraparesis or paraplegia resulting from thoracolumbar spinal trauma, it was found that the Schiff-Sherrington posture was followed by pelvic limb spasticity. This neurologic status resulted in some dogs maintaining a posture distributing weight on the ischial tuberosities, thus predisposing the area to decubitus ulcer development. Vinyl-covered convoluted foam rubber pads (Comfy Dog Bed; J. & M. Stuart Co., Inc., St. Louis, Missouri) were quite effective in helping prevent decubitus ulcers in this area [20]. An artificial fleece (Unreal Lamb Skin, Alpha Protech, North Salt Lake, Utah) over these vinyl-covered foam rubber pads has also been found effective in helping prevent decubitus ulcers in dogs. The fleece provides an additional dry soft surface to the bedding. A factor that veterinarians have to deal with that their counterparts in human medicine do not encounter is the tendency of some dogs to bite, chew, or scratch mattresses and foam pads.

Proper padding of coaptation casts is important in preventing pressure lesions over bony prominences. Evaluation of the dermal effects of different configurations of cast padding in coaptation casts on dogs indicated that absence of cast padding can result in dermal pressure injury over sharp prominences. In some areas, localized cast padding may settle around larger prominences and increase pressure to potentiate dermal pressure injury. Although pressure over bony prominences may be elevated immediately after applying full-length cast padding and a coaptation cast, some compacting of the padding occurs and this provides the best form of cast padding to prevent dermal pressure injury [11].

Inspection. The veterinarian and veterinary technician have a challenge that their counterparts in human medicine do not have in that their patients are hirsute. Thus, the hair coat will conceal skin that is undergoing the early changes associated with an impending decubitus ulcer. It is important for animal care personnel to part the hair over bony prominences and observe the underlying skin, looking for hyperemia, moisture, and easily epilated hair [1, 3–6].

If an animal tends to lick or chew at a bandage or cast, it may just be the nature of that animal to do so. However, the animal may be indicating an underlying dermal pressure lesion because of an ill-fitting cast or bandage. It is wise to remove the cast or bandage and check for pressure lesions. Likewise, if a cast or bandage has an offensive odor or an internally derived stain over a bony prominence, it should be removed and the tissues checked for pressure wounds.

Positioning. As with humans, changing the body position of an animal unable to or unwilling to change its own position should be done frequently to help prevent decubitus ulcers [1–6]. Ideally, position should be changed every 2 h [1, 3]; however, a range of 1–5 h has been described [6]. Positions should alternate between left lateral, sternal (prone), and right lateral [1, 3]. When a dog is placed in sternal recumbency, positioning the pelvic limbs caudally in extension helps prevent joint contraction problems [1]. Some dogs that are able to change their position will prefer and will get into their preferred position (sometimes with difficulty). This is when decubitus ulcers begin to develop. In dogs that do not cooperate with periodic attempts to change their position, barriers (cardboard boxes, pads, etc.) are used to restrict their movement [3].

Occasionally slings are used to support tetraplegic and tetraparetic dogs in a standing position for 2–4 h daily [7]. The dog's limbs are placed through holes in the sling material which is suspended from a frame (Fig. 6). This is probably the most effective way of keeping pressure off the skin overlying the tuber coxae, trochanter major, and acromion of the scapula on large dogs. For paraplegic or paraparetic dogs, wheeled carts that support the pelvic area are often used as part of the rehabilitation of the dog. These carts provide mobility for the dog and help keep pressure off bony prominences on the hindquarters.

Skin Hygiene. Keeping the skin clean and dry and free of urine and feces is an important factor in preventing decubitus ulcers in dogs [1–6]. Clipping the hair of the perineal area, especially on dogs with long hair, facilitates cleaning in the presence of fecal incontinence [3]. A closed collection system can help prevent urine scalding and skin maceration in patients with urinary incontinence. However, this requires proper maintenance [3]. Whirlpool or warm-water baths two to three times daily help keep the skin clean and promote circulation [6].

Nutrition. Animals, like humans, require proper nutrition as part of the preventive routine for decubitus ulcers [3–6]. A high-protein, high-carbohydrate diet with vitamin supplements has been advocated [4, 6].

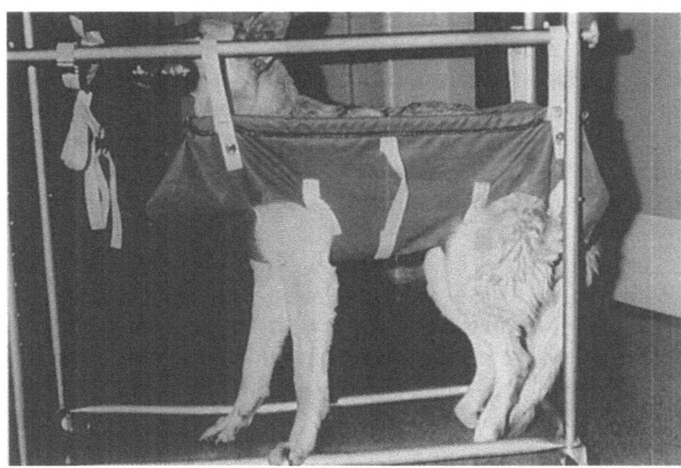

Fig. 6. A sling being used to help prevent decubitus ulcers in a large dog. (courtesy Dr. D.C. Sorjonen)

Innovative Bandaging. Because of the nature of the patient being dealt with and the fact that they cannot be reasoned with, it is often necessary to apply innovative bandages and splints. These keep pressure off skin over a bony prominence or prevent the animal from assuming a posture that would place pressure on skin over a bony prominence.

A "donut" bandage can be placed over a bony prominence on the lateral aspect of a limb (i.e., lateral malleolus) to keep pressure off of the skin. Such a bandage is made from a rolled and tightly taped hand towel that is cut to the appropriate length and the ends are taped together to form a "donut." This is taped to the limb with the "donut hole" over the lesion [5] (Fig. 7) . Although this type of bandage is not advocated in treating decubitus ulcers in people,

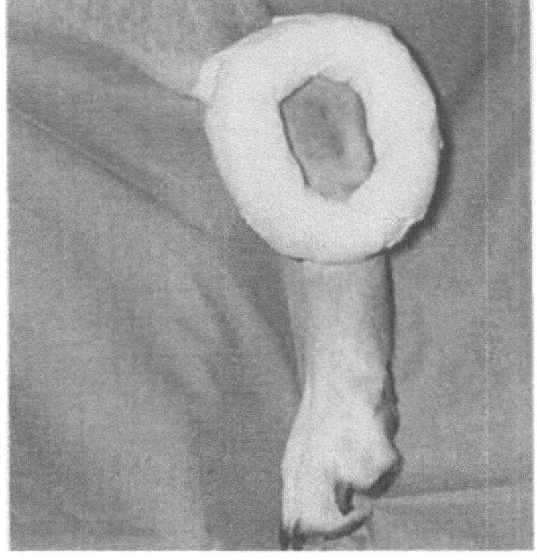

Fig. 7. A "donut" bandage made from a taped and rolled hand towel. The bandage is taped over the lateral malleolus area. (From [5] with permission)

they have been used in keeping pressure off decubitus ulcers and decubitus ulcer repair sites on the lower limbs of dogs. Donut bandages are difficult to hold in place around decubitus ulcers over bony prominences higher on the limbs, e.g., over the acromion of the scapula or greater trochanter. As they slip out of position, they can place pressure over the wound. If they do stay in place on these heavier and higher areas, there is the potential for them to impair healing by the pressure they place on vasculature in the tissue near the periphery of the ulcer.

Another pressure relief bandage that has been used to keep pressure off the olecranon area is a pipe insulation bandage. Two or three pieces of foam rubber pipe insulation of the proper length and diameter are split lengthwise and a hole large enough to accommodate the olecranon is cut in the center of each piece of split rubber (Fig. 8a). The pieces are stacked and taped together.

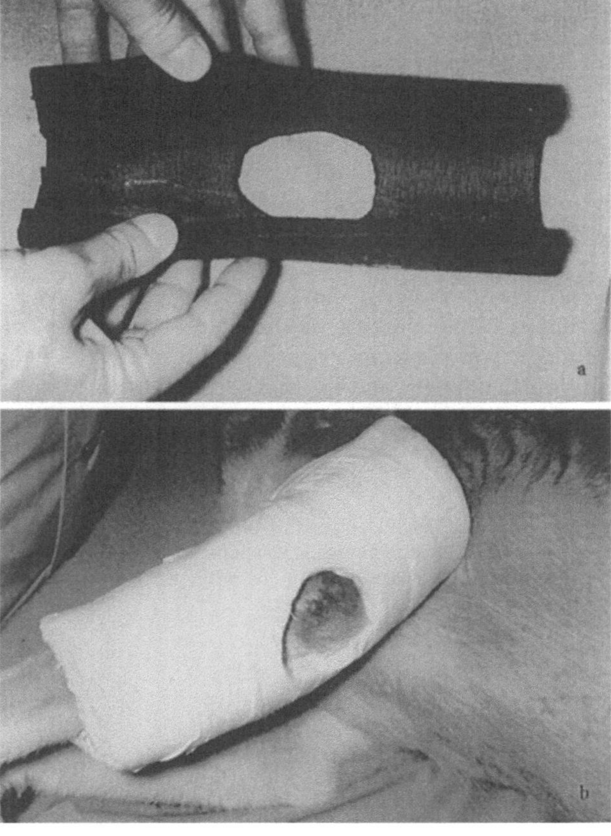

Fig. 8a,b. Pipe insulation split lengthwise with a hole cut in its center to fit over an impending decubitus ulcer, ulcer, or repair site (**a**). Two pieces of pipe insulation stacked and taped together and affixed with the hole over the olecranon area after the cranial surface of the elbow has been well padded (**b**). (From [5] with permission)

With the radial-humeral joint in extension, the cranial surface of the joint is padded well with cast padding material. The foam rubber pad is placed on the caudal aspect of the limb with the hole over the olecranon. The padding and foam rubber pad are taped in place (Fig. 8b). The bulky padding on the flexion surface of the joint helps prevent joint flexion and thus keeps the dog out of sternal recumbency. This, with the foam rubber padding on the olecranon area, keeps the dog from putting pressure on the olecranon area. On obese dogs with a short humeral area a spica-type bandage is sometimes needed to keep the bandage from slipping distally [5].

Another method of keeping pressure off the olecranon area by keeping the dog from bending its elbow to get in sternal recumbency is to place an aluminum rod splint in the front of the elbow bandage. The splint bridges the radial-humeral joint (Fig. 9).

On small paraplegic dogs that tend to sit on their perineal area, decubitus ulcers over the ischial tuberosity can be prevented by placing side splints along each side of the dog so they extend beyond the perineal area. One piece of aluminum splint material can be bent in a "U" shape and placed on the dog such that the base of the U extends beyond the perineal area (Fig. 10). Such a splint must be removed daily to accommodate defecation. One straight splint on either side extending beyond the perineal area is a bit more awkward, but precludes their removal for defecation since the perineal area is left unobstructed. The extensions of the splints beyond the perineal area prevent the dog from getting the ischial area in contact with the surface on which it is resting [5, 21].

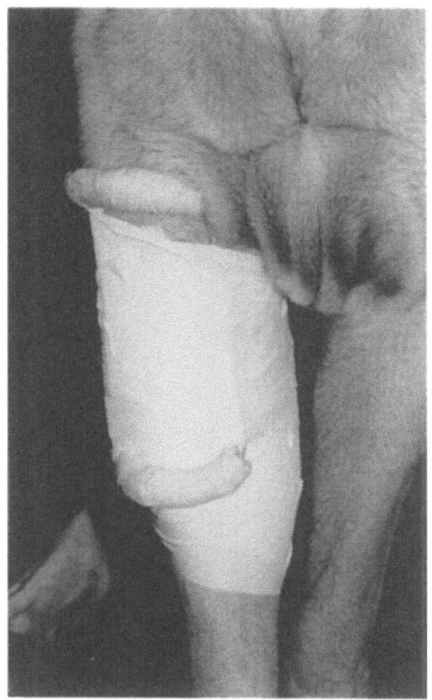

Fig. 9. A splint made from aluminum splint rod incorporated in the cranial surface of an elbow bandage. This prevents elbow flexion to keep pressure off of the olecranon area. (From [45] with permission)

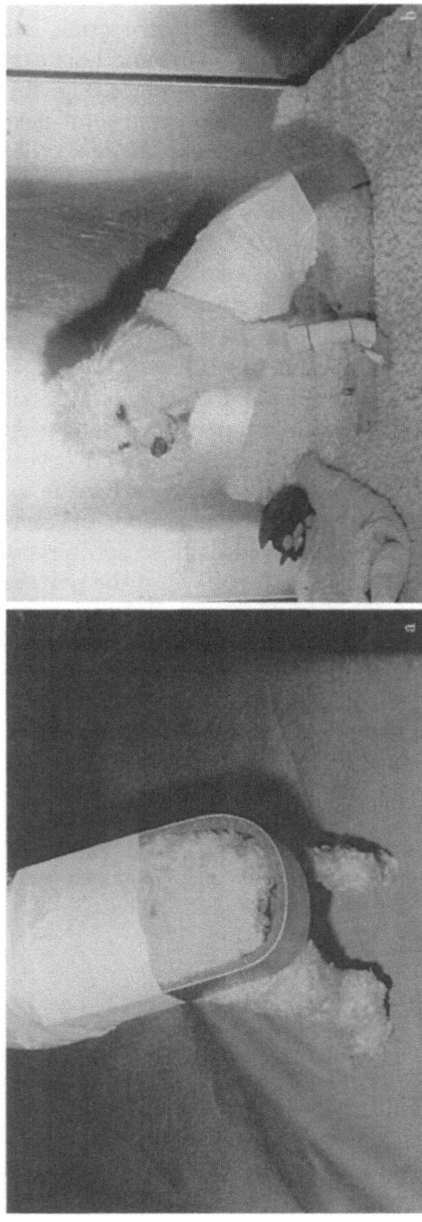

Fig. 10a,b. A piece of aluminum splint bent in the shape of a "U" and affixed to a body bandage (a). The base of the U keeps pressure off an ischial tuberosity decubitus ulcer (b)

Classification and Treatment

As with humans, decubitus ulcers in animals are graded from I to IV as to their severity (Table 1).

A major part of treating decubitus ulcers is relieving the pressure over the ulcer. The adage that "anything can be placed on a decubitus ulcer but the patient" holds true for animals as well as people. Therefore, many of the factors presented as preventive measures also apply in the therapy of decubitus ulcers. Wound debridement, stimulation of healthy granulation tissue and wound contraction, and surgical wound closure are the wound management principles used in treating decubitus ulcers. The following is the general treatment regimen used by one author (SFS) in managing decubitus ulcers [5].

General Wound Management

Grade I ulcers may be treated by periodic wound cleansing and removal of sloughing surface tissue. The wound is allowed to heal by second intention.

Grade II ulcers are surgically and/or bandage debrided (wet-to-dry bandage) to cleanse the wound and free it of necrotic tissue. After a healthy bed of granulation tissue has formed, the wound is either allowed to heal by second intention or it is closed by secondary closure. When secondary closure is used, efforts are made to keep suture lines away from bony prominences.

Grade III ulcers with undermining of surrounding skin are debrided of nonviable tissue and treated as open wounds until a healthy bed of granulation tissue is present. Either wet-to-dry or dry-to-dry bandages are used. When pockets are present in the undermined skin a 5-mm diameter Penrose drain is placed at the most dependent area. Secondary closure is performed once a healthy bed of granulation tissue has formed.

With grade IV ulcers, infected tissue, to include any infected bone, is removed. Sinus tracts and pockets are excised or opened and debrided. From this point, management is like a grade III ulcer with regard to bandaging, drain placement, and secondary closure.

Table 1. Classification of decubital ulcers (after Swain and Henderson 1990)

Ulcer type	Characteristics
Grade I	1. Dark reddened area that does not blanch on pressure. 2. Epidermis and upper dermis may slough.
Grade II	1. Full-thickness skin loss down to the subcutaneous tissue.
Grade III	1. Ulcer extends through the subcutaneous tissue down to the deeper fascia. 2. Wound edges may be undermined.
Grade IV	1. Ulcer extends through the deep fascia down to the bone. 2. Osteomyelitis or septic arthritis may be present.

Fig. 11a,b. Debridement of wound edges of a decubitus ulcer over the lateral humeral epicondyle area. **a** Skin for creating transposition flap for surgical repair (*F*). **b** Transposition flap covering the ulcer (*F*). (From [45] with permission)

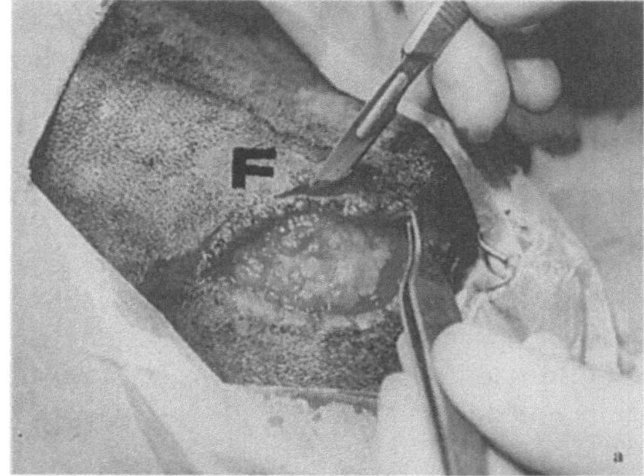

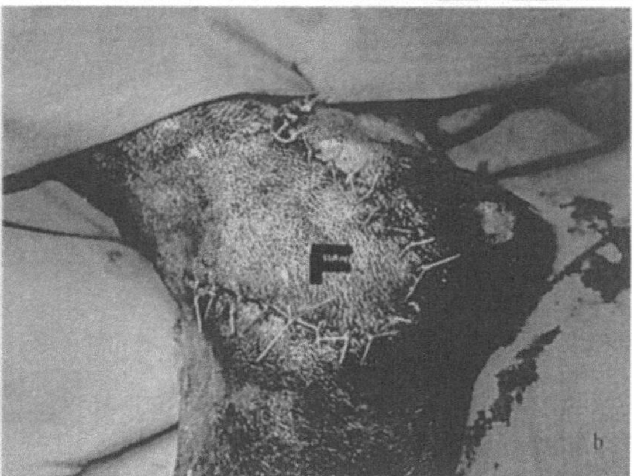

Owing to the size and/or location of some ulcers, a local skin flap may be necessary for closure (Fig. 11). An axial pattern skin flap based on the thoracodorsal vessels has been used to correct an elbow pressure ulcer in an Irish wolfhound [14] (Fig. 12). A similar potential flap that could add bulk over the olecranon area would be a myocutaneous flap containing the latissimus dorsi muscle transposed off the side of the dog [22]. Muscle flaps from the cranial sartorius and rectus femoris muscles have been used successfully to treat decubitus ulcers over the greater trochanter in dogs [23].

Topical Medications

There are many topical medications that may be used in treatment of decubitus ulcers. Those mentioned in this chapter are primarily those used at the Auburn University College of Veterinary Medicine. Following surgical and/or bandage debridement of a wound, the goal is to control infection and stimulate the development of a healthy bed of granulation tissue in the ulcer. Topical anti-

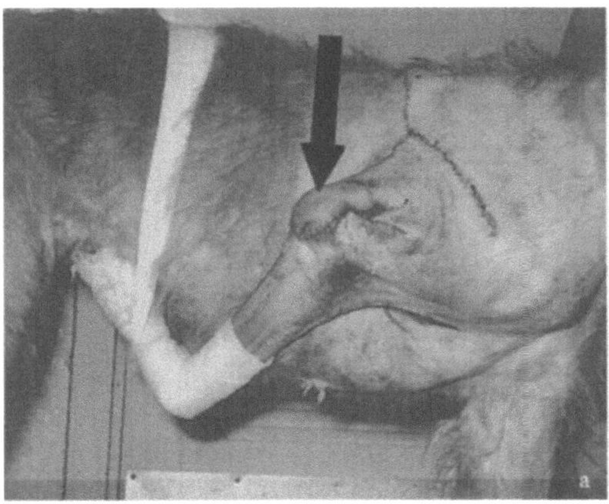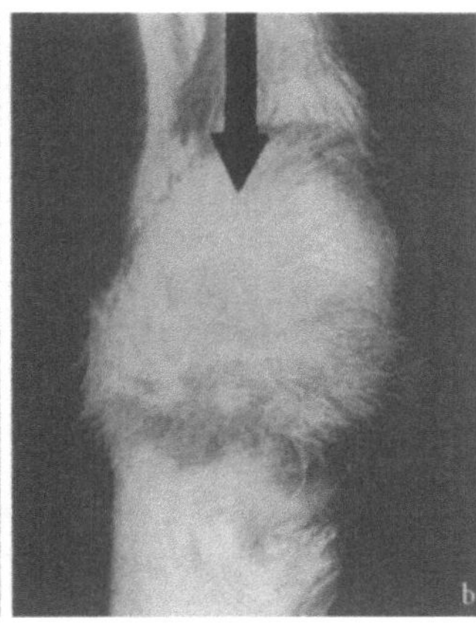

Fig. 12. a Axial pattern flap based on the thoracodorsal vessels (*arrow*) used to correct a chronic elbow ulcer. **b** Final appearance of elbow after completion of flap correction (*arrow*). (From [14] with permission)

biotics do not necessarily enhance granulation tissue development. They help control infection. However, once a healthy bed of granulation tissue is developed, topical antibiotics may help control surface bacteria, but the granulation tissue serves as a barrier to control against deeper infection. If deeper tissue infection is a factor, systemic antibiotics are indicated with the selection being based on culture and sensitivity tests.

There are topical medications that are used to help stimulate the formation of granulation tissue in wounds. One veterinary compound is Granulex (Pfizer Animal Health, West Chester, Pennsylvania), which contains trypsin as an enzymatic debriding agent and the angiogenic stimulant balsam of Peru. An acemannan-containing hydrogel topical dressing, Carravet (Carrington Laboratories, Inc., Irving, Texas), has also been used to stimulate granulation tissue formation. Acemannan is a macrophage stimulant, enhancing the production of the cytokines interleukin-1 and tumor necrosis factor [24]. These two cytokines in turn stimulate angiogenesis in wounds [25].

Hydrophilic agents are also used to enhance wound healing. These medications pull body fluids through the wound tissues to bathe them from the inside. A dry starch copolymer flake dressing, Avalon, Copolymer Flakes (Summit Hill Laboratories, Navesink, New Jersey), and a hydrophilic dextran polymer, Debrisan (Johnson and Johnson Products, Inc., New Brunswick, New Jersey) have been used for this purpose [26].

Contact (primary) bandage materials used in decubitus ulcer therapy are adherent gauze sponges when using wet-to-dry or dry-to-dry bandages. Once debrided, the wounds are covered with a nonadherent bandage such as a Telfa pad (The Kendall Co., Boston, Massachusetts), Release Nonadherent Dressing (Johnson and Johnson Products, Inc., Arlington, Texas), or Hydrasorb sponge (Kenvet, Animal Care Group, Ashland, Ohio). These are used in combination with the above medications.

Naturally Occurring Decubitus Ulcers in Large Animals

Horses that are recumbent for long periods of time, particularly those with postanesthetic myopathies, neurologic disease, limb fractures, or laminitis, are most prone to develop decubitus ulcers (Fig. 13). As in other species, in horses, decubitus lesions usually occur as a result of prolonged pressure in a relatively small area of the body that leads to tissue ischemia followed by necrosis [27, 28]. The condition is particularly serious when it occurs near a joint because infection of the synovial spaces can result [29]. Pre-existing conditions which accelerate the onset of decubitus ulcers in horses include some of the same factors associated with decubitus ulcers in dogs, such as loss of subcutaneous padding as a result of disease, malnutrition, skin friction, urinary and fecal incontinence, inadequate nursing care, or poor skin hygiene [28].

Although no detailed pathologic or pathobiochemical studies have been reported for pressure lesion pathogenesis in large animals, it is reasonable to assume that these changes would be similar to those occurring in tissues of other species. Lesions are initially characterized by an erythematous reddish-purple discoloration. There is progression to oozing, necrosis, and ulceration. The resultant ulcers tend to be deep, undermined at the edges, secondarily infected, and very slow to heal [30].

Casting of limbs in large animals, along with considerable movement by the animal, may cause friction sores underneath the casting material. Although the sores are not classified as decubitus ulcers, they nonetheless create full-thickness skin lesions that can have mortal results if not cared for properly (Fig. 14). To reduce the chances of friction sores, the fiberglass casting material must conform to the limb as perfectly as possible. Excessive padding compresses inside the cast, resulting in increased movement of the limb with resultant friction sores.

Reluctance to bear weight on a cast when a horse had originally borne weight on it is one of the initial signs of an ill-fitting cast. Swelling of a limb

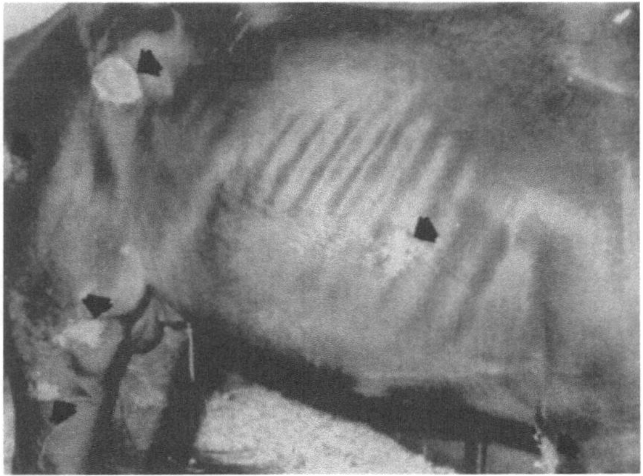

Fig. 13. Decubitus ulceration (*arrows*) present in a horse recumbent for an extensive period due to chronic laminitis. (From [45] with permission)

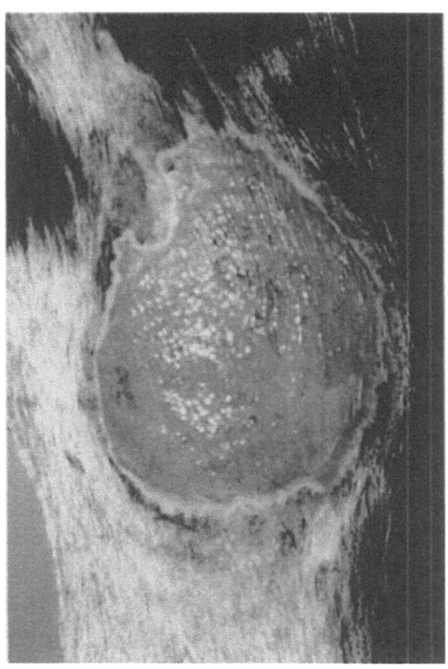

Fig. 14. Movement sore of medial aspect of the carpus that developed under a cast for repair of a limb fracture

above a cast, moisture of the cast, or any foul odor emanating from above or within the cast area warrants cast removal, limb evaluation, and new cast application. Skin necrosis or wound dehiscence can progress to the point where the damage from the cast is worse than the original lesion that led to cast application [31, 32].

Postanesthetic myopathies occur in horses in which there is hypoperfusion during anesthetic recumbency because of inappropriate positioning and inadequate padding. It is particularly a problem in heavy-muscled breeds. When the myopathy and neuropathy are local, it resolves many times with symptomatic treatment. However, the generalized myositis associated with hypotension may be so severe that the horse is unable to stand and ultimately requires euthanasia. Such horses are in extreme pain and require aggressive supportive therapy [33].

Preventive Measures

During anesthesia, careful attention to patient positioning, padding, and limb support is critical for the prevention of postoperative neuropathy and myositis [34]. Facial, radial, and peroneal nerve paresis may be produced by even short periods of lateral recumbency on hard surfaces. If the horse is in lateral recumbency, the undersurface, especially the shoulder and hip, should be padded. Inner tubes, air mattresses, dunnage bags, or foam padding (15-20 cm thick) have all been used. The limbs that are dependent should be pulled forward to protect major nerves. Halters should be removed to prevent facial nerve paralysis. The nondependent limbs should be supported to prevent undue compression of and impaired blood flow to the large chest and thigh muscle masses. No unpadded ropes or tape should be used for positioning. In dorsal recumbency, the horse's back and neck should be padded and the legs should be loosely extended to prevent compression and impairment of blood flow caused by limb flexion. Postoperative myositis has been linked to hypotension; therefore, the anesthetist should monitor blood pressure closely to prevent hypotension [34].

In the recumbent horse, preventive measures should be taken in any horse which remains recumbent for more than 3 h. These measures include bandaging the lower extremities to prevent self-inflicted trauma and having clean dry bedding free from excreta [35, 36]. The horse's lateral recumbency should be changed every 6 h. It is preferable to maintain the horse in a sternal position to minimize pulmonary congestion and prolonged weight-bearing on skin surfaces over bony prominences. A body sling is useful to assist the horse to stand. This decreases muscle damage and the likelihood of decubitus ulcer development. Slings may also improve a horse's attitude in addition to increasing limb use and circulation [35] (Fig. 15). Slings should be used on an individual basis since some horses do not tolerate them well. One author (RRH) has found that stall bedding made with a 40-cm thickness of peat moss above a clay-based floor works well in minimizing the incidence of decubitus ulcers. The peat moss reduces shearing forces and skin friction, and acts as a drying agent by allowing excessive moisture to wick away from the skin. It is imperative that the top level of the peat moss be changed frequently to prevent the build up of urine and feces. Plastic-covered pillows can also be used to minimize decubitus ulcers (Fig. 16). If approximately 40 pillows are placed on one side of a 3.6 × 3.6-m stall above a straw base, the horses will learn to lie on the side of the stall with the pillows. Although more expensive than peat moss, it is a cleaner method and equally as effective.

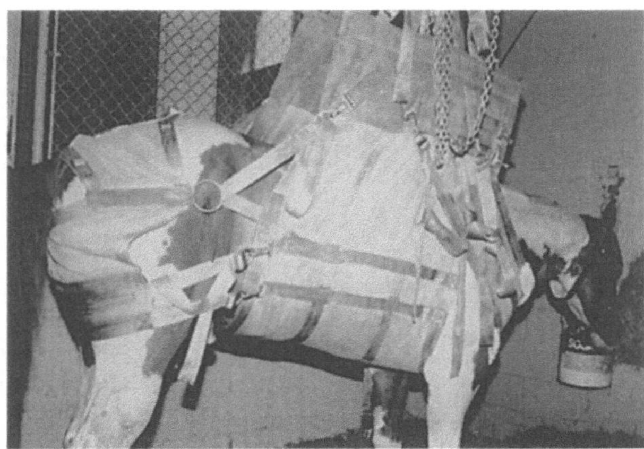

Fig. 15. A body sling assisting a horse to stand. (From [45] with permission)

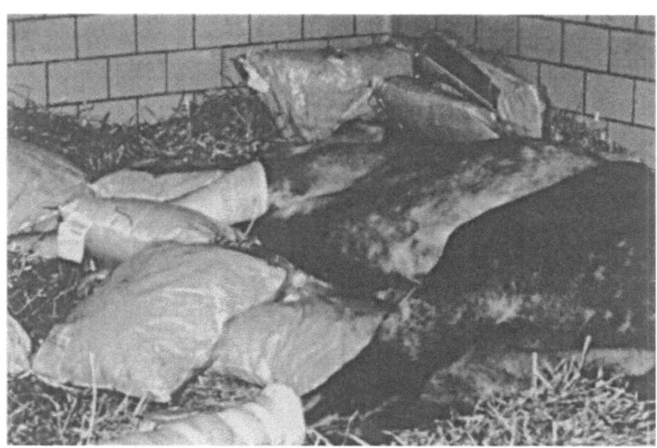

Fig. 16. Plastic-lined pillows above a straw base used under a recumbent horse to minimize decubitus ulcer development. (From [45] with permission)

Treatment

Severe myositis develops rapidly in horses totally recumbent for more than 24 h that have not received proper care. To minimize the problems associated with recumbency and self-induced trauma, the previously mentioned precautions should be employed as soon as possible. This minimizes further pressure to major muscles and other susceptible areas. Slinging the horse should be attempted if feasible [35]. Any skin sores or abrasions should be cleaned and lavaged twice daily with saline and antiseptic solutions to avoid secondary infections [31, 35, 36]. Topical antibiotic ointments, aluminum and magnesium hydroxide solutions (Maalox, William H. Roarer, Inc., Ft. Washington, Pennsylvania), emollient creams (Silvadene cream, Marion Laboratories, Inc., Kansas City, Missouri) otic cleaning solutions (Oti-Clens, Pfizer Animal Health, West Chester, Pennsylvania), and granulated sugar have all been advocated to aid in healing of decubitus ulcers [29, 36].

If spontaneous urination is not observed, the bladder should be manually expressed per rectum or it should be catheterized aseptically. If prolonged recumbency is anticipated, and indwelling urinary catheter may be advisable. Urine scald should be prevented by application of petrolatum or other water-repellent ointments to areas likely to become wet with urine [35]. However, prolonged use of oil-based ointments may lead to maceration of tissues.

Adequate nutrition is necessary to promote healing of decubitus ulcers. A protein deficiency can result in general debilitation and increased susceptibility to tissue breakdown. Severe anemia can cause a low oxygenation of tissue and lead to the death of tissues subjected to pressure. Anorexia and decreased food intake result in nutritional and caloric deficiencies that delay the healing process [35, 36]. Affected horses should be fed a high-roughage, high-protein, and vitamin-supplemented diet [29, 35, 36].

Fig. 17. A split-thickness mesh graft has been applied to the palmar aspect of the third metacarpus following cast removal and repair of a limb fracture

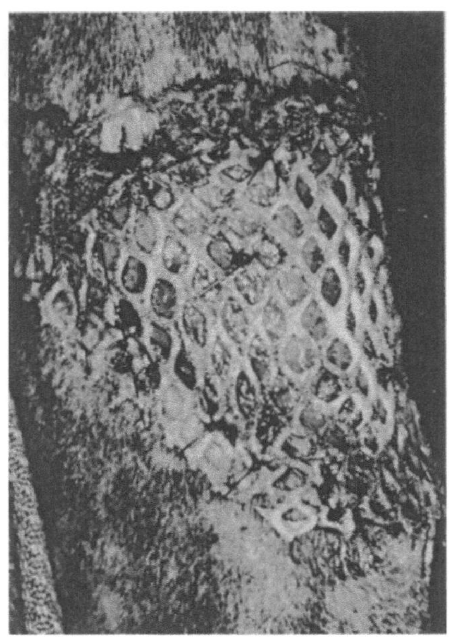

The most important aspect of therapy, however, is to identify and correct the cause of the prolonged recumbency so the patient can stand. Surgical treatment of decubitus ulcers is not as frequently performed in horses as it is in humans and small animals [29]. Surgical debridement of infected granulation tissue, undermined and traumatized skin, and infected muscle and bone, along with primary closure of the remaining skin defect has been used successfully. The use of skin flaps and grafts, and myocutaneous flaps has not been specifically described for correcting equine decubitus ulcers. If such procedures were used, it would only be after correction of the condition causing the recumbency that resulted in the ulcer [29]. Skin grafts have been used to correct limb lesions resulting from improper casting (Fig. 17).

Induced Dermal Pressure Lesions in Animals

Since decubitus ulcers are a major health care problem in the United States, research on the prevention and treatment of these wounds is certainly in order. Thus, animal models have been used for such research.

Over the years, various animal models have been described for the study of decubitus ulcers. Pressure applied to the ischial area of rabbits with and without spinal cord transection was used in early studies of decubitus ulcers. Using this model, it was concluded that there was an inverse relationship between pressure and its duration required to produce a pressure lesion. The most severe pathologic changes occur in deep muscle with only minimal changes in the skin, and pressure necrosis was similar in paralyzed and normal rabbits [37].

Decubitus ulcer studies have been performed using dogs. In one study, pressure was applied over the greater trochanter and lateral aspect of the tuber ischii by a pneumatic piston apparatus. Both high pressure for a short time and low pressure for a prolonged time resulted in muscle necrosis [38].

Using the pneumatic piston pressure device, pressure has been applied to hamstring muscles of normal and paraplegic rats. Low constant pressure for a short period caused the most damage. Application of equal amounts of alternating pressure was less damaging to tissue. No microscopic differences were noted between normal and denervated tissue after applying either constant or alternating pressure [39].

Pigs have also been used in decubitus ulcer studies. Eight days following spinal cord transection, mechanical pressure was applied to the posterior iliac spine in pigs. In addition, friction was applied to areas of pressure. It was found that friction increases the susceptibility to skin ulceration at a constant pressure of less than 500 mmHg, and friction with repetitive pressure of only 45 mmHg resulted in skin ulcers. As with the earlier work in dogs, it was found that there was an inverse relationship between the magnitude and duration of pressure in producing decubitus ulcers [40].

In a 1981 report, a computer-controlled electromechanical pressure applicator was used on normal and paraplegic pigs to produce decubitus ulcers over the greater trochanter. It was found that muscle was more susceptible to pressure damage than skin. High pressure in a short time (500 mmHg–4 h) caused muscle damage, whereas skin destruction required high pressure over long duration (800 mmHg–8 h). It was hypothesized that the pressure duration threshold for production of decubitus ulcers is lowered markedly following changes in soft tissue coverage due to paraplegia, infection, and repeated trauma [41].

In a more recent study using spinal-transected pigs, an automatic computer-controlled system was used to apply pressure over the greater trochanter for periods of 4–16 h. Since 6 weeks were allowed between spinal cord transection and pressure application, considerable muscle atrophy was present. Results indicated that spinal-transected animals developed pressure lesions at lower pressures than in normal animals. It was stated that the difference was due to the marked soft tissue atrophy [42].

The pig has also been used as an animal model to study the physiologic characteristics of cutaneous wounds induced by a device that applied both pressure and temperature over a 5-h period. Twelve 5.6-cm diameter sites along the backs of pigs were subjected to pressure and temperature, and were evaluated using various parameters to include histopathologic evaluation [43]. This model was used to further evaluate the quantitative relationship between the severity of induced decubitus ulcers and the causal factors of variable pressures, temperatures, and time. These studies were performed to define critical thresholds for changes in cutaneous function related to these causal factors, with clinical implication for establishing safety standards for such things as warming devices [44].

With its natural proprensity to develop decubitus ulcers, the greyhound dog could be considered as a model for decubitus ulcers, utilizing the naturally occurring wounds that occur in this breed. In addition to this, a model has been established for experimentally inducing early dermal pressure wounds on greyhounds. A short-limb walking cast on one pelvic limb of greyhound dogs has been found to produce lesions over bony prominences that have physical characteristics, pathobiochemical (thromboxane B_2) changes, and histopathologic characteristics that are consistent with early decubitus ulcers [13]. This model has been used to evaluate the efficacy of a systemically administered thromboxane synthetase inhibitor in helping prevent or reduce the severity of dermal pressure lesions. All three of the above-mentioned dermal pressure parameters were less severe in treated dogs than in the placebo-treated control greyhounds [19]. The greyhound induced dermal pressure technique could also be used for dermal reperfusion injury studies, whereby no medications are administered during the presence of dermal pressure. Dermal pathologic changes could be assessed following pressure relief (cast removal). Factors that are not present in the greyhound induced dermal pressure model that are often present in the naturally occurring decubitus ulcer patient are hypoproteinemia and malnutrition [13].

References

1. Betts CW (1986) General nursing and client education. In: Betts CW, Crane SW (eds) Manual of small animal surgical therapeutics. Churchill Livingston, New York, pp 391–407
2. Kunkle GA (1994) Necrotizing skin diseases. In: Birchard SJ, Sherding RG (eds) Manual of small animal practice. Saunders, Philadelphia, pp 330–335
3. Pavletic MM (1993) Atlas of small animal reconstructive surgery. Lippincott, Philadelphia, pp 114–120
4. Swaim SF, Angarano DW (1990) Chronic problem wounds of dog limbs. Clin Dermatol 8:175–186
5. Swaim SF, Henderson RA (1990) Small animal wound management. Lea and Febiger, Philadelphia, pp 52–86
6. Swaim SF, Votau K (1975) Prevention and treatment of decubital ulcers in the dog. Vet Med Sm Anim Clin 65:1069–1074
7. Knecht CD (1987) Principles of neurosurgery. In: Oliver JE, Hoerlein, Mayhew IG (eds) Veterinary neurology. Saunders, Philadelphia, pp 408–415
8. Gourley IM (1978) Neurovascular island flap for treatment of trophic metacarpal pad ulcer in the dog. J Am Anim Hosp Assoc 14:119–125
9. Read RA (1986) Probable trophic pad ulceration following traumatic denervation: report of two cases in dogs. Vet Surg 15:40–44
10. Holmberg DL (1990) Tissue handling. In: Whittick WG (ed) Canine orthopedics. Lea and Febiger, Philadelphia, pp 146–157
11. Swaim SF, Vaughn DM, Spalding PJ, Riddell KP, McGuire JA (1992) Evaluation of the dermal effect of cast padding in coaptation casts. Am J Vet Res 53:1266–1272
12. Vaughn DM, Swaim SF, Milton JL (1989) Evaluation of thromboxane in pressure wounds. Prostaglandins Leukot Essent Fatty Acids 37:45–50
13. Swaim SF, Bradley DM, Vaughn DM, Powers RD, Hoffman CE (1993) The greyhound dog as a model for studying pressure ulcers. Decubitus 6(2):32–40
14. Pope ER, Swaim SF (1986) Chronic elbow ulceration repair utilizing an axial pattern flap based on the thoracodorsal artery. J Am Anim Hosp Assoc 22:89–93

15. Muller GH, Kirk RW, Scott DW (1989) Small animal dermatology. Saunders, Philadelphia, pp 762–795
16. Barton AA (1973) Pressure sores reviewed by electron microscope and thermographically. Geriatrics 28:143–147
17. Parish LC, Witkowski JA (1987) The decubitus ulcer: reflections of a decade of concern. Int J Dermatol 26:639–640
18. Swaim SF, Vaughn DM, Riddell KP, Powers RD (1992) Use of a thromboxane synthetase inhibitor in the presence of dermal pressure. Am J Hosp Pallia Care 9:21–23
19. Swaim SF, Bradley DM, Vaughn DM, Powers RD, Hoffman CE, Beard ML (1994) Evaluation of a thromboxane synthetase inhibitor in the prevention of dermal pressure lesions. Wounds 6:74–82
20. Coates JR, Sorjonen DC, Simpson ST, Cox NR, Wright JC, Hudson JA et al. (1995) Clinicopathologic effects of a 21-aminosteriod compound (U74389G) and high dose methylprednisolone on spinal cord function after simulated spinal cord trauma. Vet Surg 24:128
21. Swaim SF (1995) Bandaging techniques. In: Bistner SJ, Ford RB (eds) Handbook of veterinary procedures and emergency treatment. Saunders, Philadelphia, pp 550–561
22. Pavletic MM (1993) Pedicle grafts. In: Slatter DH (ed) Textbook of small animal surgery. Saunders, Philadelphia, pp 295–325
23. Chambers JN, Purinton PT, Moore JL, Allen SW (1990) Treatment of trochanteric ulcers with cranial sartorius and rectus femoris muscle flaps. Vet Surg 19:424–428
24. Tizard IR, Carpenter RH, McAnalley BH, Kemp MC (1989) The biological activities of mannans and related carbohydrates. Mol Biother 1:290–296
25. Wahl LM, Wahl SM (1992) Biological processes involved in wound healing: inflammation. In: Cohen IK, Diegelmann RD, Linblad WJ (eds) Wound healing: biochemical and clinical aspects. Saunders, Philadelphia, pp 40–62
26. Swaim SF (1990) Bandages and topical agents. Vet Clin North Am 20:47–65
27. Swaim SF (1980) Surgery of traumatized skin: management and reconstruction in the dog and cat. Saunders, Philadelphia, pp 60–62
28. Shappell KE, Little CB (1992) Special surgical procedures for equine skin, In: Auer JA (ed) Equine surgery. Saunders, Philadelphia, pp 272–284
29. Greenough PR, Johnson L (1988) The integumentary system: skin, hoof, claw and appendages. In: Oehme FW (ed) Textbook of large animal surgery. Williams and Wilkins, Baltimore, pp 166–167
30. Scott DW (1988) Large animal dermatology. Saunders, Philadelphia, pp 66–67
31. Stashak TS (1987) Adams' lameness in horses. Lea and Febiger, Philadelphia, pp 852–855
32. Stashak TS (1991) Equine wound management. Lea and Febiger, Philadelphia, pp 264–272
33. Robertson SA, Green SL, Carter SW, Bolen EM, Brown MP, Shields RP (1992) Postanesthetic recumbency associated with hyperkalemic periodic paralysis in a quarter horse. J Am Vet Med Assoc 201:1209–1212
34. Heath RB (1981) Complications associated with generalized anesthesia of the horse. Vet Clin North Am 3:45
35. Wilson JH (1987) Eastern equine encephalomyelitis. In: Robinson NE (ed) Current therapy in equine medicine. Saunders, Philadelphia, pp 345–347
36. Johnston J, Whitlock RH (1987) Botulism. In: Robinson NE (ed) Current therapy in equine medicine. Saunders, Philadelphia, pp 367–370
37. Groth KE (1942) Klinische Beobachtungen und experimentelle Studien über die Entstehung von Dekubitus. Acta Chir Scand 87[Suppl]:76 (English Summary pp 198–200)
38. Kosiak M (1959) Etiology and pathology of ischemic ulcers. Arch Phys Med Rehabil 40:62–69
39. Kosiak M (1961) Etiology of decubitus ulcers. Arch Phys Med Rehabil 42:19–29
40. Dinsdale SM (1974) Decubitus ulcers: role of pressure and friction in causation. Arch Phys Med Rehabil 55:147–152
41. Daniel RK, Priest DL, Wheatley DC (1981) Etiologic factors in pressure sores: an experimental model. Arch Phys Med Rehabil 62:492–498

42. Daniel RK, Wheatley DC, Priest DL (1985) Pressure sores and paraplegia: an experimental model. Ann Plast Surg 15:41–49
43. Leland K, Kokate J, Kveen GL, Oakes SG, Wilke MS, Sparrow EM, Iaizzo PA (1994) A porcine model for temperature-augmented pressure ulcers. Proc Annu Symp Adv Wound Care 129
44. Kveen GL, Wilke MS, Sparrow EM, Iaizzo PA (1994) The effects of pressure intensity, temperature, and duration on wound causation and severity. Proc Annu Symp Adv Wound Care 129
45. Swaim SF, Hanson RR, Coates JR (1996) Pressure wounds in animals. Compend Cont Educ 18:203–219

Subject Index

Springer and the environment

At Springer we firmly believe that an international science publisher has a special obligation to the environment, and our corporate policies consistently reflect this conviction.

We also expect our business partners – paper mills, printers, packaging manufacturers, etc. – to commit themselves to using materials and production processes that do not harm the environment. The paper in this book is made from low- or no-chlorine pulp and is acid free, in conformance with international standards for paper permanency.

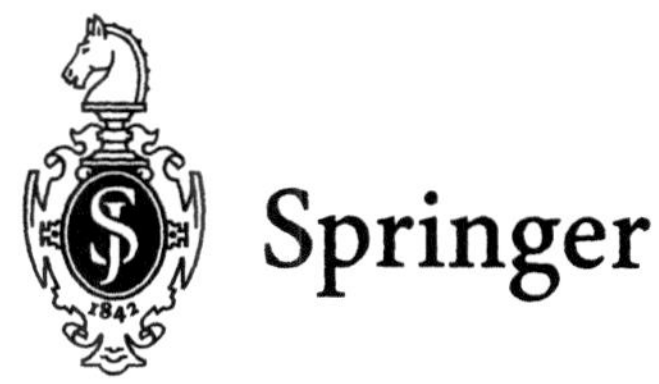

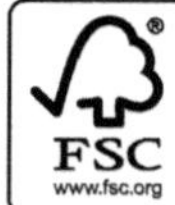

MIX
Papier aus verantwortungsvollen Quellen
Paper from responsible sources
FSC® C105338

If you have any concerns about our products,
you can contact us on
ProductSafety@springernature.com

In case Publisher is established outside the EU,
the EU authorized representative is:
Springer Nature Customer Service Center GmbH
Europaplatz 3, 69115 Heidelberg, Germany

Printed by Libri Plureos GmbH
in Hamburg, Germany